CONSTRUCTING PARIS

THE WELLCOME INSTITUTE SERIES IN THE HISTORY OF MEDICINE

Forthcoming Titles

Cultures of Psychiatry
edited by Marijke Gijswijt-Hofstra and Roy Porter

Drugs On Trial:
Experimental Pharmacology and Therapeutic Innovation
in the Eighteenth Century
Andreas-Holger Maehle

Academic enquiries regarding the series should be addressed
to the editors W. F. Bynum, V. Nutton and Roy Porter at
the Wellcome Institute for the History of Medicine,
183 Euston Road, London NW1 2BE, UK

CONSTRUCTING PARIS MEDICINE

Edited by
Caroline Hannaway and Ann La Berge

First published in 1998
by Editions Rodopi B. V., Amsterdam – Atlanta, GA 1998.

© 1998 Hannaway and La Berge

Typesetting by Alex Mayor, the Wellcome Trust.
Printed and bound in The Netherlands by Editions Rodopi B. V.,
Amsterdam – Atlanta, GA 1998.

All rights reserved. No part of this book may be reprinted or reproduced or utilized in any form or by any electronic, mechanical, or other means, now known or hereafter invented, including photocopying and recording, or in any information storage or retrieval system, without permission in writing from the Wellcome Institute for the History of Medicine.

British Library Cataloguing in Publication Data
A catalogue record for this book is available from the British Library
ISBN 90-420-0681-1 (Paper)
ISBN 90-420-0691-9 (Bound)

Caroline Hannaway and Ann La Berge
Constructing Paris Medicine – Amsterdam – Atlanta, GA:
Rodopi.– ill.
(Clio Medica 50 / ISSN 0045-7183;
The Wellcome Institute Series in the History of Medicine)

Front cover (and back cover inset):

A collection of digitally edited images from a folding plate in Henri Meding's *Paris Medical 1852-53*, after p. 352. Courtesy of the The Wellcome Institute Library, London.
Design by A. Mayor

© Editions Rodopi B. V., Amsterdam – Atlanta, GA 1998

Printed in The Netherlands

To Owen Hannaway and Marshall Fishwick
for their support and encouragement

Contents

	Notes on Contributors	viii
	Preface	xii
1.	Paris Medicine: Perspectives Past and Present *Ann La Berge and Caroline Hannaway*	1
2.	Before the Clinic: French Medical Teaching in the Eighteenth Century *L. W. B. Brockliss*	71
3.	Was Anatomical and Tissue Pathology a Product of the Paris Clinical School or Not? *Othmar Keel*	117
4.	Pious Pathology: J.-L. Alibert's Iconography of Disease *L. S. Jacyna*	185
5.	Corvisart and Broussais: Human Individuality and Medical Dominance *W. R. Albury*	221
6.	Laennec and Broussais: The "Sympathetic" Duel *Jacalyn Duffin*	251
7.	Dichotomy or Integration? Medical Microscopy and the Paris Clinical Tradition *Ann La Berge*	275
8.	Faithful to its Old Traditions? Paris Clinical Medicine from the Second Empire to the Third Republic (1848–1872) *Joy Harvey*	313
9.	Paradigm Lost or Paradise Declining? American Physicians and the "Dead End" of the Paris Clinical School *John Harley Warner*	337
	Bibliography	385
	Index	397

Notes on Contributors

W. R. Albury completed his Ph.D. in the History of Science and a Postdoctoral Fellowship in the History of Medicine at the Johns Hopkins University, before moving to the University of New South Wales in Sydney, Australia. He is now Professor of History and Philosophy of Science in the School of Science and Technology Studies and Associate Dean of the Faculty of Arts and Social Sciences at UNSW. His historical research interests include French biology and medicine from the late eighteenth to the late nineteenth century, aetiological theories in twentieth-century American psychiatry, and depictions of the interior of the body from Renaissance illustrations to early X-ray images. He has also published on the sociology of scientific knowledge.

His address is: School of Science and Technology Studies, UNSW, Sydney, NSW 2052, Australia; e-mail: WR.Albury@unsw.edu.au.

L. W. B. Brockliss is a Fellow and Tutor in Modern History at Magdalen College, Oxford. For 20 years he has worked on the history of education, science, and medicine in early modern France and has published widely in the field. His book *French Higher Education in the Seventeenth and Eighteenth Centuries: A Cultural History* (Oxford University Press) appeared in 1987. From 1985 to 1992 he was editor of the annual publication *History of Universities*. In 1997, he has published, with Colin Jones, a social and cultural history of French medicine from the sixteenth century to the French Revolution, titled *The Medical World of Early Modern France* (Oxford University Press).

His address is: Magdalen College, Oxford OX1 4AU, U.K.

Jacalyn Duffin is a haematologist and historian who teaches history, medicine, and philosophy at Queen's University in Kingston, Ontario. Her research interests are in nineteenth- and twentieth-century medicine, medical iconography, medical saints, and medical education. She is the author of *Langstaff: A Nineteenth-Century Medical Life* (University of Toronto Press, 1993) and *To See With a Better View: A Life of R. T. H. Laennec* (Princeton University Press, 1998).

Her address is: History of Medicine, 78 Barrie Street, Queen's University, Kingston, Ontario, K7L 3N6, Canada; e-mail: duffinj@post.queensu.ca.

Caroline Hannaway is a Historical Consultant to the National Institutes of Health, Bethesda, Maryland. She edited the *Bulletin of the History of Medicine* for eleven years and was Director of the Francis C. Wood Institute for the History of Medicine of the College of Physicians of Philadelphia. Her research interest in French medicine is longstanding and she has published a number of articles on eighteenth- and early nineteenth-century French medical institutions, health issues, and epidemics. Her current research project is analysing with Victoria Harden the National Institutes of Health response to AIDS and she has co-edited with Victoria Harden and John Parascandola, *AIDS and the Public Debate: Historical and Contemporary Issues* (IOS Press, 1995).

Her address is: 316 Suffolk Road, Baltimore, MD 21218-2521 U.S.A.; e-mail: channaway@aol.com.

Joy Harvey is Associate in the Department of the History of Science at Harvard University. She is the author of *Almost a Man of Genius: Clémence Royer, Feminism, and Nineteenth-Century Science* (Rutgers University Press, 1997). She has been an Associate Editor on the Darwin Correspondence Project, Cambridge University Library and has taught history of science and science, and women in science and medicine. She is currently editing a dictionary of women scientists with Marilyn Ogilvie for Routledge, Kegan Paul; translating a history of immunology written by Anne Marie Moulin; and completing a biography of Dr. Mary Putnam Jacobi.

Her address is: 29 Kidder Avenue, Somerville, MA 02144, U.S.A.; e-mail: jharvey368@aol.com.

Stephen Jacyna is Senior Research Fellow at the Wellcome Institute for the History of Medicine. He is the author of *Nineteenth-Century Origins of Neuroscientific Concepts* (with Edwin Clarke) and *Philosophic Whigs: Medicine, Science, and Citizenship in Edinburgh, 1789-1848*. His monograph *Lost Words: Narratives of Language and the Brain* is due to appear next year.

Notes on Contributors

His address: Wellcome Institute for the History of Medicine, 183 Euston Rd, London, NW1 2BE; email s.jacyna@wellcome.ac.uk

Othmar Keel is Professor of the History of Medicine at the Université de Montréal. His books and articles are largely concerned with the history of European medicine (18th–19th century) and the history of public health in Québec. Recent publications include *Polysémie de la santé: Institutions et pratiques sociales en France et au Québec (1750–1980)* (Paris: Ecole des Hautes Etudes en Sciences Sociales/Centre National de la Recherche Scientifique, 1994), joint editor with Jean-Pierre Goubert; *Santé et société au Québec: XIXe-XXe siècle* (Montréal: Boréal, 1997), joint editor with Peter Keating; and *Vers un système de santé publique au Québec* (Montréal: Presses de l'Université de Montréal, 1997), with Georges Desrosiers and Benôit Gaumer. His forthcoming book *Etudes sur l'histoire de la médecine clinique et de la pathologie, XVIIIe–XIXe siècle* will be published by the Presses de l'Université de Montréal. Since 1987, he has been Co-Editor of the journal *Bulletin Canadien d'Histoire de la Médecine/Canadian Bulletin of Medical History*.

His address is: Département d'Histoire, Université de Montréal, C.P. 6128, Succursale Centre-Ville, Montréal, Québec, H3C 3J7, Canada: e-mail: Keel@cam.org.

Ann La Berge is Associate Professor of Science and Technology Studies at Virginia Polytechnic Institute and State University. She is the author of *Mission and Method: The Early Nineteenth-Century French Public Health Movement* (Cambridge University Press, 1992) and the co-editor (with Mordechai Feingold) of *French Medical Culture in the Nineteenth Century* (Rodopi, 1994). She is working on a study of technology and the clinical tradition in nineteenth-century France, focusing on medical statistics and medical microscopy.

Her address is: Program in Science and Technology Studies, Center for Interdisciplinary Studies, Lane Hall, Virginia Tech, Blacksburg, VA 24061, U.S.A.; e-mail: alaberge@vt.edu.

John Harley Warner is Professor of the History of Medicine and Science and of American Studies at Yale University, New Haven. In addition to articles on the history of professional culture, clinical medicine, and the ideals of science in medicine, his publications include *Against the Spirit of System: The French Impulse in Nineteenth-Century American Medicine* (Princeton University Press, 1998), and *The Therapeutic Perspective: Medical Practice, Knowledge, and Identity*

Notes on Contributors

in America, 1820–1885 (Harvard University Press, 1986; paperback edition with new preface, Princeton University Press, 1997). He is now studying the clinical practice of narrative, focusing on the epistemological, aesthetic, and moral choices involved in the transformation of the patient record in the United States.

His address is: Section of the History of Medicine, Yale University School of Medicine, L132 SHM, P.O. Box 208015, New Haven, CT 06520-8015, U.S.A.; e-mail: WarnerJH@MASPO3.MAS.yale.edu.

Preface

Constructing Paris Medicine is the result of a collaborative endeavour. A group of scholars interested in examining what the advent of the Paris Clinical School has meant for medicine and how historians have interpreted the developments associated with it began to discuss the topic in an informal way in the early 1990s. A conference was organized by Caroline Hannaway and Ann La Berge at the College of Physicians of Philadelphia in February 1992 to provide the opportunity for a more formal discussion of how well the views of the two best-known historians of Paris Medicine in the twentieth century, Erwin H. Ackerknecht and Michel Foucault, have stood the test of time and in what ways new scholarship might provide insights on one of the most important transitions in the history of medical thought. The result was a valuable set of essays interpreting the historiography of Paris Medicine and re-examining many of the standard tropes and figures associated with this school. We are pleased to present these to a larger audience in this volume.

Not only has this project resulted in new thinking about Paris Medicine as the essays included amply demonstrate, but several of the authors have gone on to develop individual monographs on various aspects of the subject. What had seemed a settled area of scholarship is once more in the arena for debate. The historians involved in the project come from several countries around the world, including Britain, Canada, the United States, and Australia. The editors and organizers had also planned for a contribution from France. But the sad death of Roselyne Rey, who was to write on "Respiration, Asphyxia and Experimental Physiology in the Early Nineteenth Century" with reference to Bichat, Magendie, and Le Gallois for the volume, meant the loss of her particular insights.

Many people and organizations have assisted in the development of this project and the making of the volume. We thank the National Endowment for the Humanities for its support and the College of Physicians of Philadelphia for sponsoring the conference.

Preface

Individual thanks are due to Russell C. Maulitz for helpful advice, Janet Tighe and Carla Jacobs for conference and project-related activities, Moira Rogers for research support for Ann La Berge, Jennifer Gunn for bibliographic research, and John Parascandola for friendly assistance. Thomas Broman, Guenter Risse, Roy Porter, and Colin Jones provided useful comments and W. F. Bynum not only offered advice but made publication a reality.

1

Paris Medicine:
Perspectives Past and Present

Ann La Berge and Caroline Hannaway

1. The French Revolution and Institutional Change: 1794

Nineteen ninety-four was the bicentennial of the Revolutionary restructuring of French medical education. The year 1794 has been taken to be the demarcation between the old and the new medicine. It has provided a point of rupture for those who have wanted to argue for the distinctiveness of the Paris Clinical School from the medicine that came before. As such, 1794 provides a useful and historically justified starting point for an examination of what was Paris Medicine in the early nineteenth century.

With the reform of medical education in 1794 the existing faculties of medicine in Paris and the provinces were abolished[1] and replaced by three *Ecoles de Santé*: Paris, Montpellier, and Strasbourg. In keeping with Revolutionary ideals, medical education was now to be free, without restriction, and open to all. Medical education was also to be fundamentally reconstituted. The more theoretical training that had supposedly dominated Old Régime faculties was to be replaced by clinical training in hospitals. Furthermore, the longstanding distinctions in education and professional status between surgeons and physicians were abolished; henceforth all practitioners would receive the same education and the same degree. The professional level of surgery was raised to that of medicine in recognition of the high status that French surgeons in large towns had come to enjoy in the eighteenth century. The hands-on training of surgery influenced all medical education. Thus, in 1794, a series of reforms was initiated that transformed the face of medicine and medical education.

The medical profession itself remained unregulated until 1803 when a law established two grades of medical practitioners: one, physicians with a doctoral degree from one of the three recognized medical schools; and two, the *officiers de santé*, practitioners with some practical experience and a degree from one of the secondary schools of medicine that were slowly established throughout the nation to train these personnel.[2]

With this Revolutionary legacy and the resulting rise of Paris clinical medicine to international prominence, the Paris School has ever since been identified as the starting point of modern scientific medicine. The history of Paris Medicine has been written by many, first by contemporary commentators and critics, including foreigners who studied in Paris and reported on their experiences, and later by various interpretators beginning in the mid-nineteenth century. Important twentieth-century accounts of Paris Medicine include Paul Delaunay's 1949 study, *D'une Révolution à l'autre*, Erwin Ackerknecht's 1958 conference presentation, *La Médecine à Paris entre 1800 et 1850*, Michel Foucault's 1963 *La Naissance de la clinique*, and Erwin Ackerknecht's 1967 *tour d'horizon*, *Medicine at the Paris Hospital, 1794-1848*. The last continues to be the standard text on the subject.[3]

2. The Need for Reinterpretation

By the early 1990s it became apparent to several historians of French medicine that, in the light of additional research and new interpretive strategies that had emerged since the 1960s, Paris Medicine merited re-examination. There was a growing realization that Ackerknecht had demarcated his subject idiosyncratically, and some historians wanted to explore the impact of Foucaultian analysis on the history of Paris Medicine. The "received view" of what constituted Paris Medicine seemed to have become a kind of "myth". Curiously, this was also the starting point for Ackerknecht in 1953 when he began to examine the centrality of Broussais for Paris Medicine. He commented: "Yet perusal of some recent textbooks of medical history seems to indicate that the details of the genesis of the Paris School have fallen largely into oblivion and that a subtle process of mythologizing this part of our medical history is underway."[4] Like Ackerknecht, those involved in this volume decided to take a fresh look at a classic story in the history of science and medicine. Indeed it is a classic story in French history in general, since it has been told within the context of a certain view of the French Revolution, the political and social event upon which the medical revolution and ensuing developments were dependent for valorization.

The goal of the group involved in this endeavor is to reinterpret Paris Medicine by incorporating some of Foucault's insights and by challenging certain aspects of Ackerknecht's delineation of clinical medicine, even while acknowledging Ackerknecht's pioneering and central importance in the field. The aim is to place in context those who first discussed the Paris School, as well as those, including Ackerknecht and Foucault, who have continued the examination of its significance for medical history, and for French history at large.

This essay looks at the construction of the entity that we are calling Paris Medicine. It will examine what emerged as the dominant "myth" of the Paris School as it was first developed in the early nineteenth century; then look at later analyses in the nineteenth and twentieth centuries by members of the French medical community and historians. The word "myth" is used in the same sense as that of Robert Gildea in his recent work, *The Past in French History*, to mean "in the sense not of fiction, but of a past constructed collectively by a community in such a way as to serve the political claims of that community".[5] The essay will discuss how and why the "myth" was continued and suggest that for twentieth-century chroniclers it was employed not so much to serve political and professional claims as to satisfy certain personal agendas. By re-evaluating the story of Paris Medicine, the group will create its version of the "myth", which, it hopes, will speak to the needs and agendas of scholars in the 1990s.

3. The "Received View", or the "Myth" of Paris Medicine

Paris Medicine is a shorthand way of referring to the Paris Clinical School of the nineteenth century and the developments in medicine associated with it. To cite two venerable but commonly consulted standard histories, Richard Shryock in his *Development of Modern Medicine: An Interpretation of the Social and Scientific Factors Involved* says:

> The emergence of medicine from the confusion of the eighteenth century into the relatively clear and critical atmosphere of modern science was the achievement of no single time or place. Yet so far as one can put his historical finger on the process, it can best be pointed out in Paris during the half century between 1800 and 1850.[6]

Erwin H. Ackerknecht more picturesquely indicates in his *Short History of Medicine* (1955) that the first great step forward in scientific medicine was achieved when medicine, like "the legendary

Paris Medicine: Perspectives Past and Present

Baron von Munchhausen who pulled himself out of a swamp by tugging on his own pigtails", rescued itself from the morass of eighteenth-century theories and systems and concentrated on "clinical observation, checked and complemented by extensive and intensive studies on the autopsy table". Ackerknecht goes on to say "France, particularly Paris, was the starting point for this new type of medicine and it was in the hospitals of Paris that it reached its climax".[7] The rise of scientific medicine and the development of the Paris Clinical School have been linked in essential ways in the chronology of medicine's evolution.

The characteristics of Paris Medicine that gave it this prideful place include: (1) the rise of pathological anatomy, or the systematic correlation of clinical observations of the external manifestations of disease with the lesions found in the organs at the time of autopsy; (2) the transformation brought about in clinical observation by its being made not just on dozens of cases but on thousands; (3) the change in clinical activity from primarily listening to the patient's story to making an active physical examination of patients through large-scale application of new and revised methods of diagnosis, i.e. percussion, auscultation and, most notably, the appearance of that symbol of modern medicine, the stethoscope; (4) the hospital as the locus of medical activity and research, to the extent that the designation "hospital medicine" was applied by Ackerknecht to the period as a whole; and (5) the use of medical statistics in the analysis of case histories and the evaluation of therapy. Agreement on all of these elements as important contributions is apparent in history of medicine textbooks throughout the twentieth century. For example, the most recent survey of nineteenth-century medicine, W. F. Bynum's *Science and the Practice of Medicine in the Nineteenth Century* (1994), sees 1794 as the year of change for French medicine, reiterates the importance of hospital-based medicine in Paris for medical education and research, and indicates the importance of the development of clinical observation and pathological anatomy, the new methods of diagnosis, and the numerical method.[8]

The pantheon of physicians of the Paris Clinical School is also well established and of long standing. The names of Philippe Pinel (1745–1826), Jean Nicolas Corvisart (1755–1821), Xavier Bichat (1771–1802), René Théophile Laennec (1781–1826), François Broussais (1772–1838), Jean Cruveilhier (1791–1874), Pierre Rayer (1793–1867), Gabriel Andral (1787–1876), Jean-Baptiste Bouillaud (1796–1881), and Pierre Louis (1787–1872) are all linked with key developments in clinical medicine and pathological anatomy. The spotlight may shine more brightly on one man or another depending on who is writing about them or an author's nationality, but all these figures are notable in particular ways. A frequently mentioned consequence of the rise of the Paris Clinical School, contributing in no small measure to its significance, is that its fame was such that students from all over Europe, from across the Channel, and from across the Atlantic flocked to benefit from its opportunities, its facilities, and its teachers. On their return home, these medical voyagers worked to spread the new gospel in their native lands. A favourite estimate of Paris Medicine as a magnet is that of Carl Wünderlich in 1841, "Thither came almost all the youth of the medical world. Nowhere are conditions more splendid, more multifarious than in Paris."[9] But, alas, such splendour did not endure indefinitely. The decline of the School's influence in the mid-nineteenth century is attributed to laboratory medicine's gaining precedence over clinical experience and the rise of Germany as the new Mecca of medicine.

One of the factors that adds to the lustre of French achievements is that, at first blush, Paris was not the most likely place for clinical medicine to be transformed. Henry E. Sigerist expresses a theme that is reiterated by others when he says in his *Great Doctors* (1933), "In Paris the old medical faculty persisted like a fossil, its one thought being to stand upon the ancient ways, to maintain its traditional rights." In contrast to Leyden, Göttingen, and Vienna, Sigerist goes on to say, "at the Paris faculty, as of old, 'learned doctors' were discussing ancient texts, and were breeding a type of physician which belonged to days long past".[10]

Political transformation is seen as laying the groundwork for medical change. The French Revolution abolished the established system of medical education and regulations governing practice, and made possible new institutions, new programmes, and new professional structures. It also solidified Paris's position as the centre of medical as well as political, economic, and social life in France. Some of the benefits for French medicine were the unification of medicine and surgery;[11] the opening of the profession to new talent; greater control over the operations of hospital facilities for medical personnel; and greater access to these institutions for physicians and medical students. Last, but by no means least, the heart of the change in medical thinking at that time, which has had major and continuing ramifications, was a different outlook on diseased persons and diseases. Clinicians no longer simply saw sick individuals, they saw diseases.

It is worth noting that in many depictions these changes in French medicine came swiftly and with dislocation. Henry Sigerist claims that:

> France, whose medical institutions had hitherto been obsolete, acquired betwixt night and morning the most admirable institutions for teaching and research. This was not a mere change of framework, the entire mental attitude of the doctors was modified. They no longer looked backward, but forward. They were eager to scan all the new trends, and they took up their duties with zeal.[12]

In fact, he concludes that "By the opening of the nineteenth century, French clinical medicine was far in advance of that of other lands, and guided the progress of medical science for several decades."[13] Knud Faber, in his *Nosography, The Evolution of Clinical Medicine in Modern Times*, records that "The violence with which clinical medicine was completely revolutionized in the course of a few decades by these important and striking discoveries (about disease) will always remain one of the wonders of medical history."[14] And Jean-Charles Sournia in his 1992 *Histoire de la médecine* echoes Faber by claiming that "In the course of its history, medicine has never known a break as brutal as that of the beginning of the nineteenth century. In several decades, disease became something different, it was no longer a subject of discussion, but of material observation."[15]

While the version distilled from general histories of medicine presented thus far may provide a simple answer to the question of what was Paris Medicine, a review of past historiography and recent research shows that historical reality is more complex.

4. Constructing Paris Medicine (1794–1836)

The Paris School acquired definition as an entity in the early nineteenth century. References to the School of Paris (Ecole de Paris) abound in the French medical literature of the time and later. By this was meant not an educational institution but the ideas, persons, and circumstances comprising the development of clinical medicine and pathological anatomy in France.

The new medicine began when Antoine Fourcroy wrote the report that led to the Revolutionary reform of medical education in 1794. He set out ideals to which the School should aspire: it was to provide the best medical teaching in Europe so that the French would surpass other nations in medical science as they had already done in other areas.[16] Fourcroy's report embodied the notion developed by later chroniclers of Paris Medicine: a recognition that France had been lagging behind, but now should not only catch up, but move ahead of others. By 1803, when Fourcroy was again writing on medical reform, some of his goals had already been fulfilled. He reported that, since the reform of 1794, medicine had never been taught as well as it now was in the three revamped French medical schools.[17] A sampling of early nineteenth-century accounts reveals the acceptance of Fourcroy's vision.

Pierre Rayer, who later became a specialist in diseases of the kidneys and Dean of the Paris Faculty of Medicine, when writing his M.D. thesis in 1818, describes himself as a "student of that celebrated school which has seen pathological anatomy produce fruits on its own ground beyond all expectations".[18] Some early nineteenth-century accounts add an adjective to the designation calling it the anatomical school of Paris. The emphasis on exact observation thought to be characteristic of the school is recognized in other descriptions. For example, Elisha Bartlett, the ardent American proponent of medical things Parisian, refers to the "Modern School of Medical Observation".[19] Exactly when the designation Paris Clinical School appeared is unclear, although it probably dates to the first half of the nineteenth century. Certainly Charles Daremberg refers to the great school of the medical clinic in his *Histoire des sciences médicales* of 1870.[20] But labelling Paris Medicine a school did not disguise from nineteenth-century contemporaries the fact that matters were not clear-cut. Much medical writing was devoted to polemics, particularly about conceptions of disease and therapy, and rival groups spent great energy in supporting the supremacy of the ideas and works of their chosen masters. There is without doubt in these early references a sense of new direction but the path to take was not firmly signposted.

In 1818 Rayer noted that the Paris School had not created pathological anatomy, but that this approach had become its principal defining characteristic, and pointed out that: "thanks to the attention of the Paris School of Medicine, France has no longer anything to envy of her neighbours, in this regard as in many others".[21] Rayer recognized that Paris Medicine was initially a borrower and follower in pathological anatomy and clinical medicine.[22] For him, in the development of clinical medicine, the sequence was first Leyden, then Edinburgh, Vienna, and Pavia. There was no priority dispute. Contemporary commentators thus noted that initially Paris lagged behind other European medical centres.

Writing in 1836, Jean-Baptiste Bouillaud, a specialist in diseases of the heart and brain, offered a similar genealogy as he described the origins of Paris Medicine:

> New clinical establishments were being organized little by little in the various countries of northern Europe, as well as in Italy. Padua, Rome, Pavia, Genoa, Florence, Milan, Naples, Turin, Bologna, etc. became seats of clinical teaching... . While so many countries had been enjoying for many years the immense benefit of clinical teaching, France, which later would have over them such superiority in this genre, was completely deprived.[23]

If this was the case where did Paris Medicine's claim to fame come from, if it was initially a borrower and a follower? Bouillaud answers the question:

> Whatever the case may be, it was really only after the new organization of the medical schools [in 1794], that France shone among all the other nations, and took that surge [forward] which made her surpass all her rivals with regard to clinical teaching.[24]

Guillaume Dupuytren, for twenty years the chief surgeon at the Paris Hôtel-Dieu, provided his version of the origins of Paris Medicine. The occasion was a speech given at a public meeting of the Paris Faculty of Medicine on 22 November 1821:

> The needs of the war that France began with Europe brought about the creation of the *écoles de santé*. We will remember for a long time the care that was taken in the choice of the masters and students who were supposed to compose these famous schools. From all parts of France they called the most distinguished men and the students who were the most appropriate to benefit from the lessons of such masters. The successes of Desbois [de Rochefort], of Desault, and of Corvisart [in courses before the Revolution], have made us realize the advantages of clinical teaching too much for it to be forgotten in this Institute of medical sciences.[25]

Later in his speech, Dupuytren continued:

> It was with such methods that Corvisart raised the reputation of the *clinique interne* of the Charité [Hospital] to the level of, if not above, all known clinics; and it was there that, during nearly fifteen years, were formed nearly all of those that France considers today her best trained physicians; finally, it was there that a great number

of foreign physicians came to perfect their skills.[26]

And Bouillaud, adding to Dupuytren's version, noted: "You know what a dazzling light Corvisart's star spread over the whole first period of clinical medicine in France; a period forever memorable, and which will constitute one of the most remarkable eras in the general history of this kind of teaching."[27]

Although Bouillaud, Dupuytren, and most later commentators recognized the contributions of pre-Revolutionary clinical teachers, they believed that the clean sweep of the Revolution made Paris Medicine unique – and indeed possible. With the Revolution Paris Medicine caught up with other nations and then surpassed them.

Rayer in 1818, Bouillaud in 1836: the accounts are similar and noncontroversial. There was agreement that if clinical teaching and pathological anatomy were two defining characteristics of Paris Medicine, they were not a Parisian creation. Parisian physicians had borrowed from foreign models to create their own version of the clinic and the pathological anatomical approach.

In the birth of the Paris Clinic, the work of the early clinical teachers bore much fruit. By 1836 Bouillaud was able to proclaim: "Paris is today, without contradiction, the classic city for clinical teaching; in this regard, as in so many others, the capital of France is truly the queen of the world."[28] No modesty there. Bouillaud not only elevated Paris Medicine to the best of all medicines, he designated Paris as the best of all cities.

While there was consensus about the origins of the School, Paris Medicine had different meanings for different people. Foreign students and observers of the Paris School took away what they found useful for their own situation back home.[29] For example, Charles Cowan, the British translator of Pierre Louis's *Pathological Researches on Phthisis* (1836) emphasized exact observation: "From this moment [the publication of this work of Louis] may be dated the presence of that strong impression of the necessity of exact observations, by which the *School of Paris has been since so distinguished* [italics added] and which is now gradually pervading the medical institutions of the continent and of our own country..."[30] Cowan saw Paris as a model to be emulated.

What was characteristic and special about Paris Medicine for F. Campbell Stewart, an American physician writing in 1843, was the large number of patients to observe in institutional settings. But in this Paris was not unique; other European cities had large hospital populations. What set Paris apart was access to the patients and the ability to gain practical experience easily and cheaply:

> Where such a number of sick persons are congregated together as are constantly to be met within the wards of the Paris hospitals, great facilities must necessarily be afforded for the study of disease in all its multiplied forms and varieties; and as no difficulty exists in gaining a free and easy access to most of them, it may be asserted that in no part of the world can the same practical experience be acquired by the attentive student as in the French capital.
>
> The professional reader, who is not already aware of the nature and extent of these institutions, will be surprised to find that there exists anywhere such a vast and inexhaustible field of observation for gaining practical knowledge and experience of disease.[31]

Access was easy because of the many private/public courses taught outside the Faculty in hospitals and elsewhere.[32] These courses constituted a complementary and, indeed, almost parallel medical education for students, especially for foreign students, many of whom already had their medical degrees. Stewart stated this clearly:

> It is very much the custom in Paris, as I have already stated, for young men to deliver lectures on such branches of the profession as they have been paying particular attention to; many of them are public, but in some cases the lecturers demand small fees for attendance on their courses. *The most useful of these are practical lectures given by the internes at the hospitals with which they are connected* [italics added]; many others, however, merit the attention of students who may be visiting Paris, and I will subjoin a list of such as may be attended with much advantage. The prices for such as are not gratuitous, vary from 10 to 50 francs a month, which is their usual duration.[33]

While many contemporaries commented on what Paris Medicine meant to them, the account of Paris Medicine that has served as the foundation of its later reputation was that of Jean-Baptiste Bouillaud, a student and leading disciple of Broussais and a central figure in the Paris School. Bouillaud's discussion, in his *Essai sur la philosophie médicale* (1836), already referred to above, became the source on which nineteenth- and twentieth-century analyses were based.

The principal discourse which influenced Bouillaud and other nineteenth-century chroniclers of Paris Medicine was French Enlightenment positivism. Progress was the driving force of history, science, and medicine; reason was the prime mover of progress. It is familiar ground. But in examining how physicians actually wrote their accounts, then the engine of history appears to be individual genius, assisted by progress, which was both evolutionary and inevitable.[34] These writers followed in the tradition of Enlightenment historians, for whom history of science was about great individuals,[35] in their emphasis on the power of the individual physician. In fact, their accounts of Paris Medicine are principally stories of individual accomplishments with the aid of important institutional underpinnings.

Another element common in this approach to the history of science and medicine, indeed of French history in general, was the emphasis on linear progress punctuated by revolutions. These revolutions are made by men, not socioeconomic forces. Bouillaud, for example, outlined five laws of scientific and medical progress: (1) individual genius is the driving force of history; (2) progress proceeds intermittently, at an even pace, with normal periods being punctuated with revolutionary periods; (3) an important component of progress is the production and propagation, or popularization, of knowledge; (4) resistance and opposition, characterized by conflict, is a necessary part of progress; and (5) science is constrained by political realities.[36] Bouillaud's analysis of Paris Medicine followed these five laws, and, in general, other accounts were similar in their historiographical orientation.

Bouillaud's study was important for both Ackerknecht and Foucault. Ackerknecht seems to have relied quite heavily on Bouillaud's account as he offers a strikingly similar interpretation of the major events in the story of Paris Medicine to that of Bouillaud. For Bouillaud, Paris Medicine was not monolithic, but complex and multifaceted. He commented, and Ackerknecht uses this very quote: "In an epoch in which the confused noise of a thousand opposing voices reigns in the medical world, you can only make yourself heard by speaking loudly."[37] And surely Bouillaud exaggerated for rhetorical effect to present his point of view – that of a disciple of Broussais and an eclectic – as a voice of positivistic clarity in a mass of confusion.

An important theme espoused by Bouillaud is that disputation and resistance were necessary for progress in medicine. Why? They clarify the issues. According to Bouillaud: "Medical disputes ... are the inevitable accidents of scientific progress: they are like storms which purify the atmosphere; we must be resigned to them."[38]

Bouillaud recognized dynamic tension, as exemplified in the

"medical duel" of Broussais and Laennec, as one of the important characteristics of Paris Medicine. According to him, in a sense, differing opinions gave Paris Medicine its richness and dynamism. For Bouillaud, Paris Medicine displayed conflict and tension between vitalists and mechanists and between spiritualists and materialists.[39] The tension between these viewpoints was one of the strengths of the entity.

Paris Medicine functioned within the context of political tension. In Bouillaud's account, the fundamental tension between royal, or central power – and the government control of French medicine – and the liberal aspirations of many Parisian physicians was exemplified by the government's overhaul of the Faculty of Medicine in 1822 and the replacement of liberal by royalist faculty. While physicians were asserting the freedom of doctors, the central government was increasing its hold over medicine. Bouillaud emphasized the intensely political nature of Paris Medicine. French medicine functioned at the pleasure of the government.[40]

Bouillaud imposed a tripartite division on the Paris School: (1) the partisans of the present, or the pro-Broussaisists; (2) the partisans of the past, or the anti-Broussaisists; and (3) the eclectics.[41] Bouillaud was not uncritical of his mentor Broussais nor was he negative toward Broussais's opponents. Bouillaud, in fact, grouped himself with the eclectics. This was in keeping with his vision of Paris Medicine, for in eclecticism Bouillaud and others, such as Andral and Rayer, sought to construct a whole out of the disparateness within Paris Medicine. Eclecticism was an integrative movement that sought a synthesis following the "Broussais wars".[42]

Individuals figured prominently in Bouillaud's account. Pinel and Bichat were the "two men who ... founded a school of medicine and physiology, which had all Europe for its disciple".[43] By this comment Bouillaud recognized the centrality of Paris Medicine and argued for a diffusionist model. Although France was indebted to others in the areas of pathological anatomy and clinical medicine, Pinel and Bichat had created their own model of medicine and physiology that was both indigenous and distinctive, which they then exported. Bouillaud thus presents a dynamic picture of the flow and interchange of ideas, methods, and practices at the Paris School.

Knowledge and practice moved from centre to periphery, but the centre changed. By the 1830s Paris was the centre from which ideas and practices were disseminated to an ever wider periphery, including North America and North Africa. Bouillaud cites the example of Laennec, showing how 300 students, young doctors from all over Europe, came to learn and practise stethoscopic observations under him, then carried their knowledge and skills with them when they returned home.[44]

Bouillaud waxed eloquent about the brilliance of Paris Medicine: "If the medical epoch that we just covered [that of Pinel and Bichat] is brilliant, that which followed and of which it is left to me to give an account, is no less. This new era is perhaps the most glorious that has yet existed for medicine."[45] Bouillaud was not a humble man and the most brilliant era was his own! Self-promotion figures prominently in Bouillaud's account. Bouillaud recognized physiology, by which he meant both the experimental physiology of François Magendie, who occupied a central place in his account, and also the physiological medicine of his mentor, Broussais, as one of the crowning achievements of Paris Medicine. Bouillaud indeed lumped them together, referring to "this programme of the modern physiological school" and linked them in physiological reform and revolution.[46]

Bouillaud's Paris Medicine was "scientific medicine". He self-assuredly proclaimed:

> Whatever it may be, thanks to all the improvements in methods of observation already known and to the acquisition of new methods, the various branches of pathology have been cultivated in our day with a precision, an exactitude, up to now unknown. It is thus that medicine has definitively constituted itself on the same bases as the other physical sciences, and that it will have the right from now on to figure among the exact sciences, after having been for so long considered as a conjectural art.[47]

Bouillaud believed, as did other physicians of the Paris School, that medicine could be modelled after the physical sciences and could achieve the same kind of certainty that they possessed. But again, this attitude conflicted with a strong vitalist/humanistic tradition, coming from Montpellier, and exemplified by Bichat and, later, Laennec and Récamier. According to this, the physical sciences could never serve as a model for medicine or the natural sciences, because living systems had too much variability to allow the formulation of certain laws. This line of argument had been expounded by Buffon, and Bichat had excluded the application of the physical and chemical sciences to medicine. Bichat thus exemplified one tradition within Paris Medicine; Bouillaud represented another. By the 1830s Paris Medicine had achieved a working synthesis. With the end of the July Revolution and the accession to the throne of Louis Philippe, France entered a period of political stability. Within the medical community, by 1840, the great Broussais–Laennec quarrel had ended; both Broussais and Laennec had died, and Broussais was being replaced by younger men, such as the conciliatory eclectic Gabriel Andral.[48] Bouillaud recounts that there existed by then an alliance between the former Broussaisists and their opponents:

> This happy fraternity between medicine and physiology, the fraternity no less happy, between this double branch of one and a single science and the physical sciences, that is what really characterizes our epoch and what will be for her one of the most beautiful titles of glory.[49]

In his focus on individual physicians, Bouillaud devoted much attention to Broussais and Laennec, as did most of the nineteenth-century chroniclers. Broussais figured most prominently because, with the publication of his book *Examen de la doctrine médicale généralement adoptée*, he was responsible for the "medical revolution" of 1816, the term used by Bouillaud.[50] In a section devoted to Laennec, Bouillaud states, "Laennec is without contradiction, one of the men whose name honours medical France the most."[51] If Laennec had had enemies in his lifetime, Bouillaud paid fealty to him in 1836. Indeed Bouillaud ranked Laennec second only to Broussais in his pantheon of medical heroes.[52] Of Laennec he said, "But we will not insist too much on these errors of a man who, after M. Broussais, is uncontestably the greatest medical illustration of his epoch."[53]

By referring to Hippocratic medicine, Bouillaud used history to legitimize his construction of Paris Medicine.[54] He was not alone. Physicians of varying persuasions cited Hippocrates to justify particular viewpoints. A typical earlier example was Pinel, who saw Hippocrates as the originator of observational medicine. Thus Hippocrates was associated both with Enlightenment reform and with the development of clinical medicine.[55] Bouillaud wanted to establish a lineage between Greece and France, to portray Paris Medicine as, in a sense, a reincarnation of Hippocratic medicine.[56]

In the end, Bouillaud's message was self-congratulatory: Paris Medicine was the best. Medicine had finally become enlightened, that is, scientific. After surveying the history of medicine from Hippocrates to 1836, Bouillaud concluded: "Such is the way in which medicine was condemned to direct itself up to the epoch in which the culture of anatomy and physiology – both normal and abnormal (pathological) – changed its face completely. In this epoch [of Paris Medicine] begins a great and magnificent era for medicine."[57]

A different perspective on the Paris School of the early nineteenth century is offered by Louis Peisse. If Bouillaud offers the clinician's viewpoint, Peisse provides that of a medical journalist and penetrating critic. Peisse was one of the editors of the *Gazette médicale de Paris* and, although not a physician, was so knowledgeable about medicine that he was made an *associé libre* of the Academy of Medicine.[58] His work *Sketches of the Character and History of Eminent Living Surgeons and Physicians of Paris* was first published in French in 1827–28, with an English translation in 1831.[59] It consisted of admittedly satirical biographical sketches of many of the leading physicians and surgeons of the time. Later, in the 1850s, Peisse published a two-volume work on Paris Medicine, *La Médecine et les médecins: philosophie, doctrines, institutions*, which incorporated his earlier work and included many of the articles he had written as a regular columnist for the *Gazette médicale de Paris* in the intervening years.[60] The discussion of Paris Medicine by Peisse presented here focuses on the earlier work.

Peisse shared many of Bouillaud's views on Paris Medicine, but his emphasis was different. Even more than Bouillaud, Peisse commented extensively on the political nature of Paris Medicine: the rivalries, the parties, and the passions. He had no notion of a value-neutral science. On the medical polemics of the 1820s – the Laennec–Broussais "duel", he commented:

> Medical polemics are the most violent of all polemics. The field of dispute is vast, for medicine is not yet established, whatever may be said at the present day, but on principles which are contested, varying from age to age and from day to day and rarely susceptible of being verified by direct and conclusive experiments.[61]

And in the medical profession it was the "law of opposition and rivalry" which prevailed.[62]

The nature of science was eternal debate, the overturning of facts and systems. Science was characterized by its dynamism. Hence, Peisse dismissed the eclectic programme of synthesis and integration espoused by Bouillaud and Andral, calling it "sheer nonsense".[63]

Peisse equated scientific debates with party quarrels. For him the "spirit of system" was really the "spirit of party". He argued that medical disputes were about power. Paris Medicine exemplified medical politics, not disinterested science. It was not a question of the most accurate system or doctrine prevailing, but of who had the most power. As support for his argument he noted physicians' use of statistics to support any position whatsoever.

Power figures prominently in Peisse's critique. How did Broussais effect a revolution? The answer was power: "for no sudden change is effected, either in the moral or physical world, but by power; and power links itself especially with passion".[64] Peisse's account of Paris Medicine was replete with military analogies and metaphors. Speaking of Broussais's efforts to overturn medical thinking, Peisse commented: "It was important, above all things, that the attack should be made roughly, resolutely, and with unerring directness."[65] His use of the term "duel" to describe the Laennec–Broussais rivalry is apt.[66] Peisse saw Broussais's self-presentation as crucial: "He presented himself from the first as alone with his opinions, declaring of no avail the past and the present."[67] He was the Descartes of Paris Medicine: "It cannot be denied that he [Broussais] has done for medicine what Descartes did for all the other sciences."[68]

Parisian physicians acquired power in part, according to Peisse, by creating a name, a place, and an image, by associating themselves with a system, a procedure, or a discovery. Thus Broussais named his approach "physiological medicine". According to Peisse, Broussais's physiological medicine derived power from its "seductive simplicity".[69] Broussais's "intellectual despotism", that is, the power of his system, was fertile. It spawned hundreds of followers, and they became the "converted".[70] He created his own "school", with his own disciples who spread the good news. If and when he was attacked, Broussais "defends his opinion with violence, and endeavours to subdue by force when he cannot by reason. He wishes to convince in spite of all obstacles".[71]

Peisse also introduced the notion of the physician/scientist as a public man judged by his actions rather than his theories or writings. This public/political nature of science and medicine was one of the central characteristics of Paris – indeed French – medicine and science in the nineteenth century. The example chosen by Peisse is that of Nicolas Desgenettes, a leading army physician and surgeon during the Napoleonic Wars, who later held the chair of hygiene at the Paris Faculty. Peisse commented, "M. Desgenettes has done more in action than in writing, and we must consider him less as an author than as a public man. His name and his glory are attached to the history of our armies."[72] Desgenettes' reputation came from what he did rather than what he said or wrote. His famous self-inoculation with the black vomit of plague was a kind of "science theatre", an act of medical heroism. Peisse used Desgenettes as an example of how one could make oneself into medical hero, without having to wait for the verdict of history.[73]

Another central theme in Peisse is the theatrical nature of Paris Medicine. It was not all seriousness of purpose; it was drama, entertainment, performance, whether in the lectures of the luminaries such as Broussais and Andral, the "great tournaments", that occurred at the Academy of Medicine, or the grand rounds that took place daily in the hospitals of Paris. The theatre of Paris Medicine was played out in medical journals as well, especially when Paris was in the throes of a major medical debate: "The medical journals were divided in the debate and became the theatre of a warm and animated contest."[74]

Peisse exploited the metaphor of Paris and its medical institutions as a theatre in which the physicians were the leading actors: "The Faculty of Medicine, the *hospices de perfectionnement* and *Maternité*, and private practice, are the theatres where the talents and knowledge of M. Dubois have been displayed in all their variety and solidity."[75]

Peisse again used the theatre metaphor in referring to surgeon Philippe-Joseph Pelletan, who distinguished himself as a teacher: "His oratorial superiority was such that we could have wished, for its full display and development, a more extensive theatre and more popular subjects." Pelletan was one of those men who needed an audience to display his talents. In solitude and silence such men were impotent: "They do not enjoy the plenitude of their faculties but when moved by the facilities and momentary excitement of a public assembly, by the enthusiasm of a crowd, and by the sound of their own voice, creating a sort of cerebral fever, which, while it continues, imparts to them unwonted power and activity."[76]

In Peisse's writings there is a pervasive notion of doctors engaged in creating themselves as medical heroes. Peisse thought it unwise to take doctors too seriously. He was reluctant to worship either their science or their medicine. Peisse saw French physicians as consummate public relations men. They participated in a more general French cultural arrogance. As he noted: "Modesty is not a defect of French character. In everything we place ourselves, without ceremony, at the head of all civilized people. In an individual, such vanity is considered caprice, in a nation, virtue."[77]

Peisse satirized Paris Medicine, much as Molière had done two centuries earlier in *Le Médecin malgré lui*. This was medical theatre at its best:

Although physicians no longer walk the streets in black robes, and with magicians' hats, although they do not often speak either in good or in bad Latin, unless it be at the concourse [concours] of *Aggrégés* [sic], there is yet remaining among them matter for comedy. Leeches and warm water, Magnetizers and their somnambulists, the amusing scenes of the *Aggrégation* [sic], the lessons of a professor of 1823, and the course of Récamier! O Gui Patin! Rabelais! and Molière, where are you?[78]

Thus Peisse throws light on the role of individual actors, the political nature of medicine, and Paris Medicine as theatre.

5. Later Nineteenth-Century Constructions of Paris Medicine

Bouillaud set out what became for posterity the principal construction of Paris Medicine. His 1836 work can also be regarded as the end of one era in the history of Paris Medicine. The entity of Paris Medicine, whose creation began with Fourcroy in 1794, was complete. By the 1840s, the beginnings of changes in the history of the School appear. Some contemporaries began to claim that the "great era" of Paris Medicine was over, or at least in serious decline.

As early as 1840, Jules Guérin, the editor of the *Gazette médicale de Paris*, wrote about Paris Medicine:

From this ardour, from this effervescence, from this universal belief, we have passed to a state of indifference, inertia and individualism which would be the death of science if, underlying these appearances of disjuncture of ideas and efforts, there were not some hidden ties, which hold them together and unite them...[79]

This view was reiterated later by Jules Rochard, in his 1875 history of French surgery. Rochard presents a serious indictment of Paris Medicine in the years 1835–1847:

This was the moment when ... the scientific level began to decline in France, and all the writings of the time carry the imprint of this sort of discouragement which follows epochs of agitation and struggle. Medicine, fatigued by the storms raised by the doctrines of Broussais, disgusted with theories and systems, turned toward experimental research and abandoned itself to the cult of individual facts. Each one ploughed his furrow alone, followed his own ideas, his formulas, moved straight ahead without looking to the right or the left, without concerning himself with the work of others: each dreamed of finding his place in the sun, to achieve his own fame, and there resulted a general free-for-all of research without direction...[80]

The view of many that the great era of the Paris Clinical School was over is exemplified by the 1854–1855 debate that took place at the Academy of Medicine over the value of using the microscope in medicine. Some clinicians were opposed to its use. But others in the debate envisaged a new era in which links with the laboratory began to develop. During the debate Armand Velpeau, the chief surgeon at the Charité hospital, coined the description "the Young Paris School" to refer to the up-and-coming generation of physicians and surgeons. Men like Paul Broca, Aristide Verneuil, Eugène Follin, and Charles Robin, who embraced microscopy as well as other laboratory methods and who wanted to integrate clinical and laboratory medicine, were included in this designation. They were the heirs and students of the eclectics.[81]

In the *Moniteur des hôpitaux* Broca recounted what the Paris School meant to him and the other students of the 1840s:

> All of us who compose what they now call the Young Paris School, we were directed by our masters, at our entrance into science, toward the study of pathological anatomy; they said to us, they repeated – they said and repeated above all to those of us who particularly cultivated surgery: If you want to know disease, study lesions first of all, do autopsies, dissect the pathological specimens, inject them, have recourse, if need be, to chemical analysis: in one word, use all the methods of investigation [at your disposal].[82]

The notion of two generations of Paris Medicine, both sharing in a common enterprise, was well expressed by Jules Cloquet in an article by Paul Broca in the *Moniteur des hôpitaux* of 25 November 1854. Broca summarized Cloquet's point of view as follows: "The clinician-micrographers do not constitute a new School, and the Young Paris School, as Velpeau says, is only the legitimate daughter of the Anatomical School to which belong most of our masters."[83] This mid-century viewpoint did not last.

On the occasion of the International Exposition of 1867, the Ministry of Public Instruction commissioned and published several official histories of French medicine. By this time Franco-German rivalry had intensified.[84] A new stridency set in, accompanying the more virulent form of nationalism pervading Europe at the time. Politics and national pride had always shaped Paris Medicine. They became ever more pervasive, as the French struggled to keep up with the Germans not only in science and medicine, but also in population, military might, and economic strength. If parity could not be achieved, the aim was to demonstrate that, at the very least, the

French could use history to their advantage. French historians of science and medicine of the 1870s could show that they had been first in a variety of areas, that, in fact, it was French science and medicine that had laid the groundwork for whatever success the Germans were now enjoying. The previous willingness to grant that French physicians were participating in a common scientific enterprise to which many people and nationalities were making important contributions diminished. France was afflicted with a national inferiority complex, symptomatic of the discourse of degeneration which dominated French political culture from the 1860s on.[85]

In 1867 Claude Bernard, François Magendie's protégé and successor at the Collège de France, wrote the official history of physiology in France.[86] Two separate volumes were published as part of the international exposition mentioned above: one on physiology and one on medicine, indicating a thoroughgoing clinicism, as well as the historical and institutional separation of the two areas. Not surprisingly Bernard expressed reverence for and awarded priority to his mentor Magendie:

> He undertook private courses in experimental physiology founded on vivisection. When he began this teaching it was unique in Europe. It [his course] was frequented by numerous students among whom were many foreigners. It was from this foyer that the young physiologists went out to carry the seeds of the new experimental physiology to the neighbouring schools, where it developed subsequently with such a prodigious rapidity.[87]

Like Bouillaud, Bernard saw experimental physiology as an important component of Paris Medicine, the origin of a new movement, which spread out to Germany, England, and the United States. But Bernard's work has a different emphasis than that of Bouillaud. It conveys the importance of establishing national identity within the context of growing Franco-German rivalry. No matter what other problems beset the nation, this aspect of Paris Medicine was something of which the French could be proud.

Bernard was one of the leading scientific and medical exemplars of the intensifying national rivalry of the 1860s.[88] He was outspoken in his fears that France was falling behind. But if the present was problematic, the past was glorious, and there was hope for the future. Bernard asserted: "The future of experimental physiology belongs to France; it is to Magendie that is owed the glory of having definitively planted the flag of physiological experimentation. That will be one of his titles for the recognition of posterity."[89] Bernard saw himself continuing in a direct line of succession from Magendie. "It is important to point out that France has been the cradle of this renewal [in physiology], to which Lavoisier, Laplace, Bichat, and Magendie have principally assisted."[90] France had many heroes of which to be proud.

Jules Béclard and Alexandre Axenfeld's account of the progress of medicine – the companion piece to Bernard's – is self-congratulatory and also nationalistic. For these authors, medicine included: pathological anatomy, pathological physiology, aetiology, and nosology. A permanent feature of the history of the Paris School, according to Béclard, was the "great debates created in France by the Broussaisist reform".[91] With regard to the rift between Broussais and his opponents over physiological medicine, Béclard says that "history ... can reconcile these enemy brothers [Broussais and Laennec]",[92] and he recognizes the centrality of Broussais's contribution. The perspective of time allowed for the resolution of the Laennec–Broussais quarrel to create a unified picture of Paris Medicine. Béclard was intent on establishing the priority rights of the French in every important medical contribution – from Bouillaud's discovery of endocarditis, to Ribes' work on phlebitis, to French contributions in diseases of the urinary tract, in neurology, and in haematology. Without a doubt, for Béclard, French medicine was the leader.

These nationalistic accounts of the 1860s were followed by works of a different character in the 1870s. Eugène Bouchut, professor at the Faculty of Medicine and physician at the Hôpital des Enfants-Malades, published a two-volume history of medicine and medical doctrines in 1873. In his discussion of Paris Medicine, he venerated Bichat and Laennec, both of whom, he said, deserved the label "immortal".[93] He mentioned the usual list of luminaries of the "French School of the Nineteenth Century", as he called it, including Bayle, Bichat, Broussais, Dupuytren, Laennec, and Cruveilhier.[94] But Bouchut's was not a nationalistic history; it was more detached, less self-congratulatory, and more cosmopolitan. He was not writing what he regarded as a traditional history of medicine, that is, one consisting of philology, linguistics, and chronology, but instead a history of systems of thought.[95] In his account, which ranged broadly from ancient medicine to the nineteenth century, however, the Paris School merited only a minor place.

Writing in the 1870s, American physician Henry Bowditch reflected on the Paris Medicine he knew in the 1830s. Bowditch portrayed the years 1823 to 1837 as dominated by a

Louis–Broussais dialectic. Bowditch saw Louis's work as forming a body of protest against Broussais, whom he felt "had regally governed the medical mind of France, England, America, and in a measure, that of the entire civilized world".[96]

Reviewing Paris Medicine from the vantage point of forty years, Bowditch articulated several themes: the dominance of Broussais and the challenge of Louis as an alternative voice; the post-Broussais triumvirate of the Paris School: Andral, Chomel, and Louis, and the theatrical nature of Paris Medicine; each leading physician had his theatre in which he regularly performed: Andral at the Faculty of Medicine, Chomel at the Charité hospital, and Louis at the Pitié Hospital.[97]

Like his confrère F. Campbell Stewart, Bowditch emphasized the easy access to clinical and scientific instruction as a central feature of Paris Medicine. Most important were the special public and private courses taught outside the formal institutional instruction at the Faculty of Medicine, the Collège de France, and the Muséum d'Histoire Naturelle.[98]

Charles Daremberg, the pre-eminent nineteenth-century French historian of medicine, who taught at the Collège de France, perhaps at first sight surprisingly, wrote only briefly about Paris Medicine. His main interest was his speciality of ancient medicine. But in his *La Médecine: Histoire et doctrines* of 1865, he does single out Bichat, Corvisart, and Laennec for praise and indicates that pathological anatomy and the new diagnostic techniques, such as stethoscopy, constituted the principal contributions of Paris Medicine. Then, in his short chapter on the history and application of pathological anatomy, Daremberg gives pride of place not to a French pathological anatomist, but to Hermann Lebert, an émigré microscopist and clinician from Germany.[99]

Daremberg praised pathological anatomy itself as an area of medical and scientific investigation, as well as the selfless doctors who had pursued this approach: "I want to make [the public] understand ... the importance of pathological anatomy and all the difficulties that it was necessary to overcome to make it one of the most positive and most immediately useful parts of medical science."[100] Pathological anatomy gained strength from the accessory sciences, chemistry, physics, and microscopy. By joining microscopy with pathological anatomy to create pathological physiology, medicine became a positive science. For Daremberg, the microscope was not only a key instrument in the transformation of medicine, but an important symbol of hope for the future.[101]

Daremberg did point out the important didactic role of medical illustration and medical iconography. Neither was new nor unique to Paris Medicine. He cited forerunners, including Baillie and Hunter in England, but argued that it was Dupuytren who gave birth to this genre in its modern form by funding the pathological anatomical illustrations of Cruveilhier and Rayer with his legacy. Lebert, Daremberg maintained, surpassed even these two with the help of his editor J. B. Baillière, who contributed to the rapid progress of pathological iconography by assuring that the work of the artist would equal that of the scholar. Pathological iconography was not the same as art, for Daremberg, however. Art was idea, but pathological iconography was characterized by its realism, its "brutal exactitude". (This at a time when photography was in its infancy.)[102]

Daremberg's view of history as slow, continuous, cumulative, and progressive provided the context for his study.

> We can deplore this inflexible slowness which presides over the development of each part of science; but at the same time we could not but admire how each progressive aspect arrives according to its own schedule and brings with it new [stages]. This is an important lesson for the historian; he learns to respect the past and not to despair over the future, to moderate too much lively ardour and to keep his spirits high.[103]

Thus Paris Medicine illustrates a larger feature of Daremberg's historiography: Paris Medicine gives cause for optimism.

In another of Daremberg's works, his 1300-page, two-volume *Histoire des sciences médicales* (1870),[104] the nineteenth century merits only five pages (1295–1300): the *"Coup d'oeil général sur le XIXe siècle"*. Here Daremberg comments on the Paris School: there was Rupture #1: the Revolution; and Rupture #2: Broussais. The account is reminiscent of Bouillaud. It is the story of French medicine at its zenith with no serious challengers for forty years: 1800–1840. But Daremberg saw no dead end. Microscopy had opened up a new era, and if the future was unpredictable, progress, even if slow, was nevertheless assured.

Other late nineteenth-century evaluations of the Paris School that illuminate developing perspectives include the above-mentioned Jules Rochard's *Histoire de la chirurgie française au XIXe siècle* (1875)[105] and Paul Triaire's *Récamier et ses contemporains* (1899).[106] Both works give detailed accounts of Paris Medicine with variations on the themes laid out by Bouillaud. The discourse is the same: Enlightenment positivism, and an emphasis on individual genius as the driving force of history.

Rochard's history was written within the context of decline following the French defeat in the Franco–Prussian War.

> If we have let the heritage of our fathers fall into the hands of scientific newcomers, it is up to us to deal with it, it is up to us to reconquer it. During the first half of this century our first rank was never contested. France was then the eldest daughter of science; nations which are today our rivals admired us without envying us, and came to acquire in our schools the seed of knowledge that would later blossom in their hands.[107]

Rochard recalled that in the first part of the century, "even our enemies paid homage to us", and he quotes Rudolf Virchow, who in reflecting on the situation from the vantage point of 1872, reminisced: "When German naturalists met in 1822, we had to avow, to be honest, that what one could call German science was still in its infancy. The prevailing science, the elementary science, even the manuals were French ... and this period lasted until after 1830."[108] Rochard poses the question: "Is it true that this splendour has been eclipsed, that we have descended from the rank that the recognition of [other] nations assigned to us?"[109]

The French were wallowing in self-pity at the pre-eminence they had lost. Could it be recaptured by history? This was the question that those who discussed Paris Medicine asked. Although billed as a history of surgery, Rochard's account was as much about medicine as surgery, because, as he notes: "Inseparable in their aims and their essence, they are equally so in their past."[110] The uniting of the two branches during the Revolution made them inseparable in the nineteenth century. Surgery, however, could in some instances be singled out. For example, Rochard maintains that French surgery had held its own *vis-à-vis* other countries better than medicine and science. Nevertheless, he has to admit that "French surgery has no doubt lost the monopoly it exercised during Dupuytren's day".[111]

In Rochard's account the turning point for French medicine was pre-Revolutionary with Desault, but change continued through the reforms of 1794 to Bichat. Rochard gives the story an interesting twist by comparing the contributions of Desault before the Revolution and those of Bichat after with the Hunterian rupture in England. Of Bichat, he comments: "he conceived the idea of reconstituting the entire medical edifice on new foundations, and as he had the prescience of his near end, he set to work with a febrile ardour. Two and one-half years sufficed for him [to produce] his prodigious work." Bichat's *Traité d'anatomie générale* "produced a revolution in science".[112] Not only did Bichat inaugurate pathological anatomy in France, but his ideas were enthusiastically welcomed throughout all of Europe. The Bichatian revolution produced "this anatomo-pathological school which constituted science on new bases and operated in our country a movement analogous to that which Hunter produced in England twenty years earlier".[113]

In a sense Rochard's account might be subtitled "The Rise and Fall of Paris Medicine". He sets the history of the original Paris School within the context of the "rise", or as he calls it, the "élan scientifique", whereas at the time he was writing, Paris Medicine was clearly perceived to be in decline. He singles out the years 1814–1835 as the most brilliant period in French surgery. Curiously, there was an analogy between 1814 and the early 1870s, because the French had suffered military defeats at both these times. Thus Rochard writes of the early period: "it was brilliant above all for our country in that science was a consolation for our misfortunes". He summarizes the great era of Paris Medicine: "The discovery of auscultation, of lithotrity, of iodine and the vegetable alkaloids; the impulsion given to surgical anatomy, to experimental physiology, to pathology, everything ... assured France, in this great movement which took root in 1814, the first place that she occupied up to then [1835] and which she should never have lost".[114]

Rochard identifies two important steps forward in Paris Medicine: (1) the movement in anatomy and pathological anatomy inaugurated by Bichat; and (2) the later incorporation of microscopy into Paris Medicine. For Rochard, as for Bouillaud, dynamic tension was the engine of progress.[115] Rochard emphasizes how Broussais functioned as a catalyst for the development of pathological anatomy, inciting both Laennec and Louis to engage in prodigious research in reaction to his system.[116]

Rochard provides an answer to questions posed earlier: why did Broussais "fall out" of the story of Paris Medicine? How was Laennec redeemed and written back in? "The physiological doctrine, after having excited, from its first appearance, an enthusiasm which we cannot today account for, vanished with the medical generation that it had impassioned, and aroused after it a reaction [that it was] necessary to combat in its turn."[117] In contrast, as Rochard notes, auscultation at first aroused scepticism and indifference, but its reputation only increased with the passage of time: "History has relegated the name of Broussais to the class of false prophets, it has ranked Laennec among the benefactors of humanity. This is how posterity does justice to enthusiasms which are too easy and to precipitous judgments."[118] Rochard discusses more than individual medical heroes. He portrays Paris Medicine as situated within institutions, societies, and hospitals. For him, as for Bouillaud and Peisse, Paris Medicine was intrinsically political.

After the reigns of Dupuytren and Broussais, he believes that Paris Medicine never regained its supremacy. The principal hope on the medical horizon was the French Micrography School, the second great phase in the history of French anatomy. In his brief overview of French medical microscopy, Rochard credits Raspail and Royer-Collard with developing the cell theory long before the Germans Schwann and Schleiden. The impression given is that this was an area that might allow the French to regain their medical supremacy.[119]

The second later nineteenth-century source that merits examination is Paul Triaire's *Récamier et ses contemporains, 1774–1852*, published in 1899. Triaire's goal is to rehabilitate Récamier, who, he contends, was misunderstood in his own time. Like Laennec, Récamier was a vitalist, Catholic and royalist, and had to wait for posterity to redeem him.[120] Triaire writes within a context quite different from that of Rochard. He views the history of French medicine from the perspective of what he calls "the current revolution", that is, the Pasteurian Revolution. This he believes is the only period of French medicine comparable to that of the early nineteenth century.[121] As Triaire puts it, the first third of the nineteenth century was one of the most brilliant periods in the history of medicine. "To find a comparable flowering [of genius] we would have to look to contemporary times; and we know now, by what filiation, by what development of hereditary germs, by which numerous points of contact, the great current School which ends the century, is attached to that no less great which inaugurated it."[122]

Once again, history serves to justify and glorify the existing state of French medicine. For Triaire, French medicine and science had recovered from the defeatism of the 1870s with the sweet revenge of Pasteurism, institutionalized, by the time he was writing, in the Pasteur Institute.[123]

Triaire calls early nineteenth-century French medicine "the most tortured and most glorious of the century". The "prodigious rebirth of French medicine" dated from 1794:

> [The law of 1794] introduced practical studies of anatomy and chemistry into teaching, created the clinic, inaugurated the

laboratory, established dissection rooms, founded hospitals, and it insisted, above all, on this fact, that bedside observation of the sick would become the principal part of teaching.[124]

But for Triaire, as for Bouillaud and others, the history of science and medicine did not just show revolution, but also continuity. Punctuated progress might be the best way to characterize this approach.

> But we ought not forget that this reform ... was a legacy of the eighteenth century, and owed its accomplishment to men, who – like Fourcroy, Thouret, Chaussier – belonged to the old, dissolved institutions. Furthermore, the new School recruited entirely in the old personnel of the Faculty and the two Academies.[125]

Individuals who built the new School included Corvisart, whose reputation was unequalled in Europe, and who bridged the old and new traditions, and Pinel, who founded a "new School by the publication of his famous nosography".[126]

The 1794 reorganization of medical teaching was, according to Triaire, part of the national mission "to show Europe that French scientific genius had not been darkened amidst the ruins amassed by the Revolution".[127] How similar this was to the mission of Triaire's own generation to demonstrate that French scientific genius had not been dampened by the French defeat in the Franco-Prussian War. Just as the French had moved from the "ruins" of 1793–94 to the most glorious period in French medical history, so history had repeated itself at the end of the nineteenth century. With the Pasteurian Revolution the French had avenged themselves.

It is no accident that Paris Medicine is discussed by using the term "construction". This is the way its chroniclers referred to their endeavour. Note Triaire's summing up of the development of the Paris School after 1794:

> Such was the edifice constructed in all its parts. It rested ... on a broad and solid foundation, which could support new construction and brave the centuries. The Architects were incomparable. They respected the past and conserved all that was useful but they also pruned what was sterile: scholasticism, vain argumentation, the Latin language, antiquated forms and apparati. They added to the edifice all the concepts of modernity, which already the Academy of Surgery and the Royal Society of Medicine stood for at the end of the eighteenth century: practical anatomical studies, legal medicine, medical and surgical clinics. They reorganized the teaching of

obstetrics and enlarged the domain of the physical and natural sciences ... This edifice was arranged with a marvellous understanding of current needs and future necessities.[128]

Triaire emphasizes how adaptable the School had been. The result of all this, in his own time, was another great demonstration of French medical and scientific strength in the Pasteurian Revolution. Even the discoveries of Pasteur did not mean the demolition of the Faculty: "not one stone of its walls will be touched", Triaire confidently predicts. The new sciences would be annexed to the old, and the institution, continually rejuvenated, would be able to sustain all its new responsibilities.[129] Thus Triaire portrays the Paris School as a flexible dynamic entity made stronger and better by change.

Triaire's account of Paris Medicine has four turning points: first, Pinel "undertook to reconstitute medicine with the help of analytic procedures and nomenclatures used in mathematics and the natural sciences". With his influential *Nosographie philosophique*, which became "the charter of contemporary medicine", he "botanized" medicine. Pinel's challenge was "Given a disease, find – not its treatment – but its place in the nosological framework".[130] The Broussais revolution ended Pinel's reign so completely that in the later nineteenth century, Triaire notes, nobody knew of Pinel's *Nosographie philosophique*: "it has gone to join so many other preceding systems in the profound forgetfulness of history".[131]

Meanwhile, running parallel to Pinel's system was the founding of pathological anatomy, by which Bichat changed the face of medicine.[132] Triaire contends that Bichat's work "contained the germ of all the modern science we are so proud of".[133] For Triaire, pathological anatomy was practically synonymous with Paris Medicine, exemplified by the work of the luminaries Laennec, Bayle, Dupuytren, Récamier, Cruveilhier, and Andral.[134]

Another transformation was not long in coming with Broussais and his system of "physiological medicine". Triaire compares Broussais with the violent, systematic reformers of the French Revolution. Broussais, he suggests, wanted to demolish the existing structure of medicine, and to construct a new and exclusive system. Comparing Broussais to Paracelsus, Triaire recounts how Broussais took Paris by storm: "His spirit of systematization appears extraordinary today and no one would think it worthy of a serious refutation. But then, the times were ripe for reform..."[135]

Triaire ranks Laennec as "one of the greatest doctors France ever produced".[136] He portrays the rivalry between Laennec and Broussais in a negative light, in which Broussais was rude and aggressive and Laennec above reproach. He describes the creation of Laennec's posthumous reputation, by placing Laennec and Broussais within the context of Restoration politics, in which a majority of the medical community, especially students, was anti-royalist. Laennec's royalist politics and his Catholicism, as well as his vitalism, meant that he had many enemies in his own time. In contrast, Triaire attributes much of Broussais's success to his political ideas, which were in opposition to church and monarchy.[137]

Finally, Magendie inaugurated a new era in Paris Medicine, the era of positivism. Magendie, Triaire contends, exemplifies the modern scientist and the laboratory. For Triaire one era of Paris Medicine always overlaps with another. Magendie's era ran parallel to the reign of pathological anatomy and of the "physiological medicine" of Broussais. With Magendie the "spirit of party" was as alive as it was during the Broussais–Laennec quarrel. Paris Medicine was by nature polemical.[138]

As Triaire aims at restoring the reputation of Récamier, he pays great attention to the vitalist current in Paris Medicine. For a while the negative associations of vitalism, which tended to go hand in hand with royalism and Catholicism, obscured the reputations of luminaries of the Paris School such as Laennec and Récamier.[139] But posterity (in the form of writers such as Triaire) returned these men to their rightful place in the pantheon of medical heroes.

Triaire ends his account of the Paris School with an overview of the dazzling accomplishments of the school up to 1830. The Paris School had been founded to reconstitute science. An elite group of men appeared to take up the challenge, and "Each brought his own building block to the new edifice".[140]

By 1830 the work of this first generation was complete. It had reconstituted medicine, developed surgery, created pathological anatomy, inaugurated tissue pathology, redone therapeutics, and founded gynaecology. Thus, Triaire concludes, sounding much like Bouillaud: "Never – in any historical epoch, in any branch of human knowledge, and in such a short space of time – has such a considerable evolution been as brilliantly concluded."[141] Only in Triaire's time was there an era that rivalled that of the early Paris School.[142]

6. The Twentieth Century

In the mid-twentieth century, Paris Medicine again became the subject of large-scale historical attention. Works on individual figures and particular events primarily characterized the scholarship of the first half of the century.[143] Paul Delaunay's 1948 account of French medicine is set between the great political Revolution of 1789 and that of 1848.[144] His discussion of the 1794 turning point neatly contrasts the "before" and the "after". Although he acknowledges a break, at the same time he notes the continuity of a humanist orientation in medicine, references to classical scholarship, the use of Latin, and the persistence of classical forms. Delaunay has a cyclical view of history, suggesting that there are a limited number of ways to look at health and disease and that as one cycle ends, another emerges to replace it. His account emphasizes evolution. Perhaps for this reason he does not capture the age by naming it Paris Medicine or characterizing it as the Great Age of French Medicine.

For Delaunay, the basic change of 1794 was a move from theoretical to practical studies. What Desbois de Rochefort in medicine and Desault in surgery had done in clinical instruction before the Revolution became the order of the day. At the *clinique interne* Corvisart organized his teaching on the model of that of Stoll in Vienna. France adopted foreign clinical models. Medicine and surgery were unified and all this was done within a new institutional organization of the three *Ecoles de Santé*.

Much of Delaunay's account focuses on the professional and speciality societies where learning and knowledge production took place. Paris Medicine was developed in the midst of "The golden age of learned societies".[145] Delaunay characterizes the period as one of monographs, of specialized learning, but suggests that the real monuments of this age, as well as of others, are the comprehensive works, in this case the medical dictionaries. In these multi-volume works, he believes, the historian can find the style and inspiration of each period better than in articles in the medical press.

Delaunay sees the underlying discourse of the age as system: "systems regulate everything: philosophical, scientific, and medical conceptions, each one submitted, as the geologists say, to a cycle, or moreover to cycles which, after various vicissitudes, return to the point of departure".[146]

Delaunay saw Broussais not as initiating a "revolution" but as preaching a doctrine in opposition to throne and altar, royalists and vitalists, Récamier and Alibert, as well as Laennec and Cruveilhier.

Paris Medicine: Perspectives Past and Present

One cycle followed another. Vitalism was challenged by Broussaisism, which, in turn, was eclipsed by eclecticism and then positivism. Delaunay saw the polemics as one of the principal elements characterizing Paris Medicine. But, unlike Bouillaud (or Ackerknecht), Delaunay does not try to impose unity on diversity. He only uses the term "Paris School" once, although he refers to leading individuals and their particular schools. His history has a revolution at each end, but the dates he uses do not correspond to the industrial and scientific revolutions which Delaunay argues went hand in hand with political revolution.

Delaunay's treatment is broad and comprehensive and includes early nineteenth-century developments in chemistry, physics, physiology, and microscopy. He privileges neither clinical medicine nor pathological anatomy, although both merit significant discussion. He pays careful attention to the Montpellier School as well as the Paris School, and includes foreign developments as readily as French ones. Paris clearly emerges as the place where the action was, but Delaunay's emphasis is on individuals and their particular contributions rather than assessing the overall significance of Paris Medicine. This was, in the final analysis, the "era of heroic battles".[147] Delaunay does not change the historiography of the Paris Clinical School.

The enterprise that was the Paris Clinical School gained prominence in the 1960s by the attention of two scholars of very different stamp. Their names are well known: Michel Foucault and Erwin H. Ackerknecht. The first author of an influential book on Paris Medicine was Michel Foucault, the French philosopher and intellectual historian. Foucault came from a middle class medical family, had a traditional elitist education in Paris, where he studied under the historian and philosopher of science Georges Canguilhem. From his student days, he was obsessed, at least in his early years, with death, disease, and violence, the dark side of human existence. Upon graduation from the *Ecole Normale Supérieure*, he went to Uppsala, Sweden, as a French cultural officer. Besides putting on plays and reviewing films, while there Foucault worked about six hours a day in the library of the University of Uppsala, which has an extensive collection of eighteenth- and nineteenth-century medical books. It was from these that he learned about, and began to identify with, some of the leaders of Paris Medicine, especially Bichat. Foucault already had a background in the history of psychiatry and had done volunteer work for several years at the Ste.-Anne psychiatric hospital in Paris. Foucault's research in Uppsala led to *La Naissance de la clinique: une archéologie du regard médical*, his most historical and, in some ways, least characteristic work.[148]

In 1963 when Foucault published *La Naissance de la clinique* in France,[149] it apparently received little immediate attention. The English translation was not published until ten years later with the title *The Birth of the Clinic: An Archaeology of Medical Perception*.[150] In fact *The Birth of the Clinic* only appeared in English after the English version of one of Foucault's other books, *The Order of Things*, was published in 1970.[151] This latter work marked the beginning of Foucault's rise to the status of intellectual guru for English-speaking academe. In France he had been in the vanguard of intellectual life since 1966. One earlier work of Foucault's must also be mentioned at this point. This is, to translate from the French title, *Madness and Unreason: The History of Madness in the Classical Age*, first published in 1961. It was first published in English in 1965 in a shortened version with the title of *Madness and Civilization: The History of Insanity in the Age of Reason*.[152] It is the work of Foucault's that has perhaps had the greatest long-term impact on the history of medicine.

Foucault saw the three works just noted as a trilogy. When describing his earlier research, his own account of his quest in *The Birth of the Clinic*, written in 1969 when he was a candidate for the Chair of Systems of Thought at the Collège de France, is as follows:

> At the beginning of the nineteenth century [clinical medicine] was in fact linked to established sciences, or those in the process of becoming established, such as biology, physiology, and pathological anatomy. But, on the other hand, it was also linked to a group of institutions such as hospitals, establishments providing care, and teaching clinics, as well as to practices, such as administrative inquiries. I wondered how it was that between these two markers, a knowledge could have arisen, could have changed and developed, offering scientific theory new fields of observation, original problems, and objects that until that point had gone unnoticed; but how, in return, scientific learning had been imported into it, and had taken on prescriptive value, and a quality of ethical norms. The practice of medicine makes up an unstable mixture of rigorous sciences and uncertain tradition, but it is not limited to this; it is constructed like a system of knowledge with its own equilibrium and coherence.[153]

Paris Medicine was important for Foucault, because he found in it –

especially in the anatomical and pathological anatomical tradition of Bichat – a useful historiographical model. Just as Pinel, Bichat, and other physicians had rejected causality in order to focus on locating and describing disease, so Foucault rejected historical causality in his approach to historical topics. Just as Bichat took a tissue section and analyzed it, Foucault attempted to provide a "slice of life" account of Paris Medicine. He focused on ruptures, the new way French physicians developed of looking at disease, the so-called "gaze", and its underlying discourse. Bichat and the other pathological anatomists spoke to Foucault's obsession with the "dark side" of life. Foucault identified with the approach of Corvisart and Broussais that to understand life, it was necessary to study death, and to understand health, it was necessary to study disease. Foucault's biographer James Miller has suggested that all of Foucault's works are a reflection on his own life and problems and the way he worked through them.[154] Paris Medicine, represented by the work of Bichat and the pathological anatomists, spoke to Foucault on a deep, personal level. Broussais was also a model for Foucault: in the violence of his polemic, his recognition that there was no great difference between the normal and the pathological, and that there was a continuum between life and death, health and disease.[155]

The question is not, in the case of Paris Medicine at least, what has Foucault done for the history of medicine? Instead the question to be asked is what did the history of medicine do for Foucault? Some of the Parisian physicians thought in ways that resonated with Foucault's own views, and he used their ideas to structure his own historical/analytical approach. Jean Starobinski, the eminent Swiss historian of the Enlightenment, makes a similar point in a review he did shortly after the publication of the English translation of *La Naissance de la clinique*.[156] But when historians of medicine today talk about incorporating a Foucaultian perspective into their work, they do not necessarily mean turning to *The Birth of the Clinic*. They are more likely interested in Foucault's perception of the role of power, which he began to emphasize somewhat later. The power/knowledge relationship does figure in *The Birth of the Clinic*, but it is not made explicit.[157] It is the discourse underlying his subject.

The Birth of the Clinic is conceived as a study of the structures of medical perception and experience. The period encompassed is 1794 to 1820. For Foucault, *la clinique*, which the English translator rendered as "the clinic", means both clinical medicine and the teaching hospital. Foucault believes that the new way of seeing disease characteristic of the clinic and the new way of saying things about it is linked to the structure of what was visible and invisible. For Foucault new rules govern medical discourse after the birth of the clinic. A predominant role is given to the "gaze" (*le regard* in French, again the translator's choice) in observation both of the patient and of changes revealed internally by dissecting the body, and to adopting the point of view of a knowledge that is based primarily on what can be discovered through autopsy, the "invisible made visible" in Foucault's phrase. As he describes, the status of disease changed when it was freed of metaphysical implications. Sickness and sin were no longer intertwined. This also affected the meaning of death and the conception of the individual. All are linked. Foucault's mode of analysis and his concentration on language mean that he is opposed to the traditional historiography of the history of ideas and to assigning credit to individual medical innovators. Thus he is not interested in investigating the causes of medical change. He is intent on capturing a changed perception of humans and disease.[158]

Medical history was not significantly affected initially by Foucault's work on the clinic. Ackerknecht had read *La Naissance de la clinique* but only refers to it in two footnotes in one chapter of his Paris hospital book as a source for a comment on the paradoxical nature of revolutions. The medical revolution, Ackerknecht says, "which wanted to abolish hospitals, improved them – this revolution, which wanted to abolish official medical teaching, created a new particularly vigorous type of it".[159] Foucault himself does not cite more than two or three items in the secondary literature in the sources for his book, although his work fully demonstrates his command of how the significance of the Paris Clinical School was commonly interpreted. "The clinic" and "the gaze" acquired currency as fashionable terms in the late seventies and eighties, but were sometimes used with little reference to their meaning in Foucault. In the longer term, Foucault's view of medicine as a replacement for religion and his interest in issues of social control and the power of the expert, medical and otherwise, developed more fully in his later works on prisons and sexuality, have been more influential than his views on medical change in the clinic.[160]

Erwin H. Ackerknecht is one of the history of medicine's most distinguished representatives and a prolific author. In 1967 he published the book that, amongst his generous output, he and others have liked the most, namely *Medicine at the Paris Hospital, 1794–1848*. A synthetic work displaying many Ackerknechtian writing trademarks – telegraphic style, ability to coin a catchy label, and trenchant comments *inter alia* – this book has been the standard text on the subject of the Paris School for historians of medicine for more than twenty-five years.

The topic of the book was of longstanding interest for the author. Ackerknecht's classic papers on hygiene and anticontagionism in France, both published in 1948, led on to twenty papers on aspects of the Paris Clinical School before the book was published.[161] By 1950 Ackerknecht had coined his widely popular phrase "hospital medicine" to distinguish Paris Medicine from what he termed the "library" or "bedside medicine" that had preceded it and the "laboratory medicine" that followed.[162] In his article on Elisha Bartlett and the philosophy of the Paris Clinical School, published in 1950, he noted that the school was composed of "strong individualities" and that "far from being united in itself, – impressed contemporaries rather as anarchy and chaos". Yet, despite this, he stated his belief that:

> Today we are nevertheless entitled to regard this school medically as a unit, as in the perspective of history all differences among the Paris clinicians have become irrelevant as compared to the common principle underlying the practice of all of them: that is to study disease by relating the findings of clinical observation and examination (especially the new methods of percussion and auscultation) to the changes found in organs on the autopsy table as the most positive element of medical information.[163]

Ackerknecht, like Bouillaud, believed unity could be imposed on diversity. The story was complex, as his papers and book demonstrate, but he portrayed all those involved in Paris Medicine as motivated by the same agenda. In a sense this strategy was helpful to Ackerknecht in coming to grips with a large and somewhat unwieldy literature.

Ackerknecht's coverage of the Paris Clinical School is governed by certain constraints. He does not discuss in detail the work of the physiologists, microscopists, chemists, or other French scientists of the period. The reason, he explained, was that he was writing a medical history, and the philosophy or prejudices of the Paris clinicians effectively prevented their incorporating the discoveries of other branches of science into medicine. The largest gap created by this decision is the lack of discussion of Magendie and experimental physiology. His periodization also changed over time. In 1950 the School had four decades of influence from 1800 to 1840, by 1958 this had been extended ten years to 1850,[164] then for the book he settled on the period 1794–1848. This latter choice was determined by events in French political and cultural history as well as medical history. The political framework is from after the death of Robespierre and the reforms in medical education until the end of Louis Philippe's reign. Ackerknecht charts the coincidence between political and medical change. The year 1848 is more than a date to end his study of the Paris Clinical School. Ackerknecht claims that by this date "hospital medicine" had come to a "dead end", his phrase, its momentum spent. German predominance in medicine is on the horizon.

Ackerknecht was a clinician trained in Germany in the 1920s. Moving to Paris in the 1930s, he was, as he says himself, impressed by the "practicality and directness of French medicine", perhaps because it contrasted with his own training.[165] Ackerknecht admired the Paris clinicians' advocacy of the importance of sense impressions and direct experience in the acquisition of medical knowledge. He believed this gave medicine a concreteness and a freedom from abstraction that has subsequently been lost because of medicine's linkage with other sciences. In Ackerknecht's view "hospital medicine" was born not only out of political and social turmoil but also out of the coming of the Industrial Revolution. His detailed work on the French public health movement had made him fully aware of the health and social consequences of the growth of urbanization and industrialization in France.[166] In one of his vivid descriptions he refers to the hospitals of Paris as "medical factories filled with the waste products of the young industrial society and its peasant-absorbing great cities".[167]

In the case of both Foucault and Ackerknecht, their personal agendas are central to the approach they took to Paris Medicine. Both men felt a rapport with the Paris School. In a letter written to Henry Sigerist in the early 1950s, Ackerknecht commented: "I feel rather at home in Paris in 1830."[168] Both sought to use their vision of Paris Medicine as a model, in Foucault's case for how to study systems of thought and discourses, and in Ackerknecht's case for what he considered the best kind of medicine.

7. After Ackerknecht and Foucault

After the publication of Ackerknecht and Foucault's books in the 1960s, there was a hiatus until new book-length studies relating to the Paris Clinical School appeared in 1975.[169] David Vess in *Medical Revolution in France, 1789–1796*, using an Ackerknechtian framework, had the goal of expanding on part of the "myth". He sought to emphasize the role of military medicine in the Revolutionary restructuring of French medicine and medical education. Vess perpetuated the "bleak" view of eighteenth-century medicine and accepted *in toto* Ackerknecht's division of medicine's development into "library", "hospital", and "laboratory" phases.[170]

In 1979 Othmar Keel, a student of Canguilhem, published *La Généalogie de l'histopathologie: une révision déchirante: Philippe Pinel, lecteur discret de J.-C. Smyth (1741–1821)*, the first work in what would become a sustained effort (still ongoing) to offer a fundamental critique of the received view of Paris Medicine.[171] Using close textual analysis, Keel questioned the originality of the French contributions in tissue pathology by contending that Pinel took many of his ideas from the English physician Smyth, and then Bichat got his ideas from Pinel. This was part of Keel's larger project to "de-privilege" the Paris School. He embarked upon a massive comparative study of the origins of clinical teaching throughout Europe in the eighteenth century. He concluded that the birth of the clinic in France, the heart of Foucault's treatment, was only one among many and was neither the first nor the most distinguished.[172] Keel has offered the most serious critique of the distinctiveness of Paris Medicine. His work forces historians to ask how much of the reputation of the Paris School was the result of particular, partisan constructions and to what extent Paris Medicine can be understood unless a comparative approach is taken seriously.[173]

Following on the heels of the publication of Keel's book, Toby Gelfand published his study, *Professionalizing Modern Medicine: Paris Surgeons and Medical Science and Institutions in the Eighteenth Century*, in 1980.[174] His work was inspired by Owsei Temkin's 1951 classic essay "On the Role of Surgery in the Rise of Modern Medical Thought" and was set within the context of studies of professionalization being pursued by both historians and sociologists.[175] Gelfand offered a new twist on an old story. He argued for the importance of a vital, progressive surgical profession in eighteenth-century France in bringing about change in French medicine. He contrasted the dynamic nature of eighteenth-century Parisian surgery with the static, retrograde nature of medicine. Gelfand claimed that the practical, hands-on training that Paris surgeons received in the late eighteenth century from Jean Desault became the model for the Revolutionary reform of medical education. He did not take issue with Foucault's and Ackerknecht's belief that a new type of clinic appeared in Revolutionary Paris, but in his attention to the role of surgery in the reform of French medicine, he initiated a reconsideration of the origins of the Paris School.[176]

Also in 1980, Martin S. Staum published the first intellectual biography in English of the physician and spokesman for the French Idéologues, Pierre-Jean-Georges Cabanis (1757–1808). In *Cabanis: Enlightenment and Medical Philosophy in the French Revolution*, Staum examined Cabanis's goal of establishing a "science of man" uniting physiology, "analysis of ideas", and ethics. His book assisted the understanding of the aims of the Idéologues, whose thinking influenced the protagonists of medical change in the Revolution. Physicians in the group of Idéologues wished to integrate man into nature and make him an object of science by rigorous study of physical and mental relations. In addition to illuminating Cabanis's philosophy and influence on the medical revolution, Staum's research showed that there were inaccuracies in Ackerknecht's account of Cabanis in the chapter on philosophy in *Medicine at the Paris Hospital*.[177]

In 1984 John Lesch published a study of the emergence of experimental physiology in France between 1790 and 1855. He demonstrated that neither the work of nor the positions held by scientists such as Magendie were as separate from the world and activities of the Paris clinicians as Ackerknecht had claimed.[178] Lesch challenged Ackerknecht's demarcation of Paris Medicine. Not only did Magendie's experimental physiology flourish within the Paris medical world, but Lesch argued that it was even nurtured by it. In a sense, Lesch agrees with nineteenth-century assessments of the Paris School in which Magendie plays a significant part in establishing the pre-eminence of French medicine and science. While accepting the general tenets of the Ackerknechtian and Foucaultian accounts, Lesch questioned Ackerknecht on a fundamental point.

In a 1987 study of the development of pathological anatomy, especially of Bichat's tissue pathology, Russell C. Maulitz compared in detail the reception of these ideas in France and England. He found that differences in medical cultures, including professional organization and institutions, affect the degree to which notions of diagnosis and disease can be transplanted from one locale to another. He wrote within the Ackerknechtian framework, assuming that in the main, French pathological anatomy crossed the Channel to Britain, not the other way around.[179]

Other studies focused on specific individuals within the Paris School, especially Bichat, Broussais and Laennec. In 1984 Elizabeth Haigh published *Xavier Bichat and the Medical Theory of the Eighteenth Century*.[180] Her aim was both to explain the significance of Bichat's vitalist thought and work in histology and to understand the background to his work. Her contribution was to make clearer the Montpellier roots of vitalist thinking in France, the development of ideas on irritability and sensibility, and the influence of ideology on medicine.

Jacalyn Duffin's doctoral thesis on Laennec, completed in 1985, and based on extensive research in the Laennec papers, resulted in several articles which reminded historians of the vitalistic tradition within Paris Medicine, and explored the dichotomy between Laennec's public and private patients as well as other aspects of his life and practice. Duffin's biography of Laennec, *To See With a Better Eye: A Life of R. T. H. Laennec* will assist further evaluation of his role in Paris Medicine.[181]

In his research George Weisz has focused on medical education, medical professionalization and specialization, and most recently, the Royal Academy of Medicine of Paris. His monograph of 1995 on the Academy, *The Medical Mandarins: The French Academy of Medicine in the Nineteenth and Twentieth Centuries*, illuminates the significance of this institution for the development of a national medical elite and the Academy's involvement in manifold aspects of French medical life. In 1987 Weisz published an influential essay, "Creating the Posthumous Laennec", in which he did for Laennec what this volume hopes to accomplish for Paris Medicine writ large: he showed how the reputation that Laennec had in the 1820s and 1830s was later evaluated differently in light of changing political and religious realities and the need for national medical heroes. Weisz's work has contributed to a renewed interest not only in particular aspects of the Paris School, but also in nineteenth- and twentieth-century French medicine more generally. For him, Paris Medicine constitutes only one part of a larger story.[182]

Jean-François Braunstein and Michel Valentin are two authors who have taken up the charge to resurrect François Broussais. In a 1986 study on Broussais and materialism, Braunstein treated Broussais within the broader context of French intellectual currents during the Restoration and the July Monarchy. Braunstein increases understanding of the philosophical context in which Broussais's ideas flourished, but his work poses no real challenge to accepted historiography of the Paris School.[183]

Valentin uses the same point of entry as did Ackerknecht in his 1953 article, "Broussais, or a Forgotten Medical Revolution". The charge is laid out in Jean Bernard's preface to Valentin's book: "A century after his death Broussais was forgotten." Valentin provides a biographical account which enriches understanding of Broussais the man, but does not challenge received views of his significance for medicine. The metaphor of a duel figures prominently in Valentin's picture of Broussais, becoming almost a leitmotif in his life.[184] Valentin's is a traditional biography attempting to rescue a man that the author feels has been maligned and to show Broussais's personal/human side.[185]

In 1989, coinciding with the celebration of the bicentennial of the French Revolution, French historian of medicine Jean-Charles Sournia published *La Médecine révolutionnaire (1789–1799)*, a thorough coverage of the "rupture" of the Revolution and the creation of the Paris School. Sournia uses the work of both Ackerknecht and Foucault, responds to their interpretations, but offers a basically traditional account of the medical reforms of the Revolution. His work is done within the context of French Revolutionary historiography and he notes that none of the great chroniclers from Lamartine to Mathiez covered medicine in this period. He takes up the charge issued by the nineteenth-century historian of the Revolution Alphonse Aulard that "there is a book to be done on the history of medicine during the Revolution".[186]

Sournia argues for the disruption of medicine by the Revolution followed by the reconstitution of the Ecole de Paris, which then guides Western medicine for the next half-century. His account privileges the revolutionary changes in medicine, maintaining that "No human activity sustained such an overturning in the Revolution."[187] It was not only medicine but also the social and professional role of physicians that underwent a major transformation. After the Revolution, physicians functioned as civil servants and expert advisers to the government. French medicine was state medicine.

The Paris School, according to Sournia, was important as a precursor to experimental medicine. "Without the new anatomo-clinical medicine the experimental medicine of Magendie and Claude Bernard would never have seen the light of day."[188] This is a grand positivistic account with one stage in the progressive evolution following another. Sournia resents Foucault, although he tries to maintain a moderate position toward his work. He accuses Foucault of historical errors, but acknowledges Foucault's originality and influence.[189] Sournia gives short shrift to Broussais. In his account the good guys, Claude Bernard, Louis Pasteur, and Rudolph Virchow, won, and Broussais lost.

Paris Medicine: Perspectives Past and Present

Two recent works have enriched the history of the Paris School. The first is the book by Dora Weiner, *The Citizen-Patient in Revolutionary and Imperial Paris*.[190] Weiner approaches Paris Medicine from the patient's point of view. Her boldest move is to reconceptualize the idea of the patient. What the Revolution did, she argues, was to create a new kind of patient: the citizen-patient. This citizen-patient became one of the essential features of Paris Medicine – the raw material for clinical examination and autopsy. Weiner is also working on a biography of Philippe Pinel, one of the founding fathers of the Paris School, in which she plans to emphasize Pinel's contributions as a clinician as well as his role in the development of psychiatry.

Another recent book that is important in a reconsideration of Paris Medicine is Elizabeth Williams's *The Physical and the Moral: Anthropology, Physiology, and Philosophical Medicine in France, 1750–1850*, published in 1994. It is primarily focused on Montpellier.[191] One way of coming to terms with Paris Medicine is to determine what it was not. Montpellier physicians in the early nineteenth century were fighting to preserve their traditions and autonomy, indeed, to preserve their Faculty of Medicine, in the face of the Paris onslaught. They were opposed to many of the things for which Paris Medicine – at least one tradition within Paris Medicine – stood. They also described Paris Medicine in such a way as to make their own quest distinct. Williams's book gives the view from the provinces, that of a competitor that feared being swallowed up, and broadens understanding of the Paris enterprise by offering another perspective on it.

An important analysis of developments in Paris Medicine in the second half of the nineteenth century, especially in the area of the growth of medical specialities, is the book by Christopher G. Goetz, Michel Bonduelle, and Toby Gelfand, *Charcot: Constructing Neurology* (1995). This examination of the man and his milieu gives substance to one of Ackerknecht's components and highlights new areas of investigation by the anatomico-clinical method.[192]

Finally, to conclude this survey of post-Ackerknecht and Foucault studies, the extensive research conducted by John Harley Warner on the impact of the Paris Clinical School on medicine in the United States has received a full exploration in his book titled *Against the Spirit of System: The French Impulse in Nineteenth-Century American Medicine*.[193]

8. Reinterpreting Paris Medicine

As the essays in this volume show, challenges to accepted historiography can be made on several fronts. An element in the development of Paris Medicine has been the transformation of medical education wrought by the abolition of the pre-Revolutionary institutions and the founding of new ones. The "fossil" faculty of medicine of Paris was replaced by a new school where students were trained on the wards from day one. Laurence Brockliss's thorough examination of medical teaching in France before the Revolution shows that education in French medical faculties was neither antediluvian nor impractical. The impression that it was comes out of the rhetoric of medical reformers and their political allies in the 1790s, who were hardly lacking in self-interest. Toby Gelfand's historical investigation heralding French surgery as the source of the tendency to localism and the *Ecole de Chirurgie* as the institutional precursor of the post-Revolutionary clinic has helped to make firmer the negative view of pre-Revolutionary education for physicians.[194]

As Brockliss shows, charges of professional negligence and outdated curriculum are not supported by examination of such sources as faculty records, student notebooks and dissertations, course announcements, letters, autobiographies and journals. Faculty teaching did reflect current medical debates and courses in ancillary medical sciences were taught. In addition other institutions and private individuals offered educational resources.[195] The currently held notion that a medical school incorporates all aspects of medical training has blinded historians to the range of possibilities for education available to a prospective practitioner in late eighteenth-century Paris. Moreover, even if there was little formal faculty training in patient care, evidence exists that there was a working unofficial network of hospital instruction. Medical students gained experience by taking private courses with individual physicians. The frequently mentioned clinical course established at the Charité hospital by Desbois de Rochefort and Corvisart on the eve of the Revolution can be seen not as an attempt to emulate the surgeons, but as the formalization of a longstanding medical tradition. Much points to continuity rather than change.

Research also suggests that the claim for the rise of pathological anatomy based on tissues being uniquely associated with the clinical school of Paris should be closely assessed. Is this claim in some way a French artefact? Othmar Keel would argue that other nations have not received their due. He has found that after Morgagni the British took up the study of pathological anatomy and tissue pathology. Challenging the belief of both Foucault and Ackerknecht that tissue pathology was only developed at the beginning of the nineteenth century and also Foucault's claim that Bichat's conception of pathology based on tissues was the fundamental turning point in the birth of clinical medicine, Keel demonstrates the significance of the work of the Hunterian school in London, especially of John Hunter and Matthew Baillie.

Extensive autopsies had already displaced the seat of disease from organs to tissues at the end of the eighteenth century. Moreover Pinel and Bichat were familiar with and acknowledged the British research. Seeing the Paris Clinical School's emphasis on the importance of sense experience as stemming only from the ideology of Condillac, Keel argues, limits appreciation of how clinical observation developed in the eighteenth century. Paris Medicine received cross-fertilization from British influences in pathological anatomy from the 1790s on. In a sense, the excitement over Paris as a medical centre, fuelled by the reports of visiting British and other foreign students, has helped to overshadow British contributions.

As already indicated, both Ackerknecht and Foucault have argued, for different reasons, that the Paris clinicians should be regarded as a coherent group; Ackerknecht bases his linkage of individuals on their agreement that the clinical observation–autopsy equation was the only way to medical knowledge, Foucault, on the group's new way of seeing and of conducting discourse on disease. These approaches are useful historical strategies, but may also undercut what can be learned from a closer analysis of disagreement. And controversy abounded amongst figures associated with the Paris Clinical School. The celebrated quarrel of Laennec and Broussais was characterized by charges of poor pathology, plagiarism, and personal ill-will. Beyond the polemics, such disputes, as Jacalyn Duffin has found, illuminate the dynamic interaction taking place within the School on approaches to disease, diagnosis, and therapeutics. Seeing lesions did not assist understanding of the causes of disease. The same professional and cognitive environment, in fact, allowed for the development of more than one option in medical theory. In addition, the tensions displayed in the Laennec–Broussais dispute reveal that the "clinic", despite Foucault's conception of a new commonly shared set of rules for medical discourse, had not produced an acceptable language in which criticism of another's theories could be expressed.

Historians of medicine have frequently abstracted Foucault's idea of the clinical "gaze" from the other elements with which it is linked in the well-known opening sentence of *The Birth of the Clinic*: "This book is about space, about language, and about death; it is about the act of seeing, the gaze."[196] But Foucault's emphasis was on the reorganization of the relationship among these elements rather than on treating one in isolation. It was this that opened the way for clinical experience and "scientifically structured discourse about an individual".[197] With Foucault's aim in mind, W. R. Albury has studied Corvisart and Broussais's understanding of human individuality in relationship to death and disease. In a complex argument Albury demonstrates that these two clinicians hold a strikingly different view of the matter from that characterizing the Hippocratic-Galenic tradition extending from antiquity to the eighteenth century. Albury examines how the new medical perception was linked to Corvisart's and Broussais's professional ambitions and the status of medicine in general in the post-Revolutionary era. Thus, he brings together Foucault's analysis of the new perception of disease with the growth of medical power, fundamental themes throughout Foucault's *oeuvre*.

Inadequacies of the accepted model of Paris Medicine appear upon closer examination of its clinicians. Take Jean-Louis Alibert, on the face of it an exemplary practitioner of the Paris School. Educated in the 1790s in Paris, he had a career as a hospital doctor devoting himself primarily to the treatment of skin diseases, that is, he specialized in the manner deemed characteristic of the School by Ackerknecht. He used his institution, the Saint-Louis hospital, as a "clinic" where he instructed colleagues and students. In his works, the cases he discussed were vividly illustrated so that what was seen could be communicated to others. But, as L. S. Jacyna has found, analysis of Alibert's writings shows that he did not maintain a purely objective attitude to disease. He described his own affective responses to his patients' disfiguring ailments and sought to invoke such responses on the part of his readers. Nor did Alibert dismiss the patients' perception and description of their illnesses as a Paris clinician should. He reproduced lay beliefs about illness and described the often tragic effects of deformity on the personal lives of individuals. Alibert did not subscribe to a rigorously secular discourse on illness and healing either. A discursive religious element is to be found in his pathology. The example of Alibert demonstrates the difficulties of imposing a unitary point of view on early nineteenth-century French medicine. It poses a challenge to the notion of a unilinear transformation in medical outlook and action.

Paris Medicine: Perspectives Past and Present

Other essays examine Ackerknecht's contention on what was lacking in Paris Medicine that brought its glory days to an end. The weakness of French clinicians according to Ackerknecht was that they distanced themselves from the sciences, and by their failure to embrace laboratory medicine lost out to their neighbours to the north. John Lesch has already challenged the supposed gap between clinicians and physiologists. Now the alleged shortsightedness of Parisian pathological anatomists in failing to deploy the microscope comes under scrutiny. Ann La Berge has found that not only was there a microscopy community in Paris in the 1830s and later, but that leading physicians of the Paris School in the 1840s believed that the microscope was relevant to their work. Technical improvements in the instrument in the 1820s and a willingness to go beyond the unaided data of the senses helped bring this about. Advocates of microscopy promoted the value of the instrument for observation of bodily fluids and morbid tissue. Ambivalence about the utility of microscopy was certainly expressed in France, just as it was in other European countries, but, by 1850, the instrument had gained an accepted place in Paris Medicine as an adjunct to clinical observation and pathological anatomy.

The concept of the "dead end" itself has also come under scrutiny, as well as Ackerknecht's use of the changing destination of foreign students as an index of the rise and fall of the Paris School. By analyzing what American physicians sought in Paris and why later they favoured Germany and Austria, John Harley Warner counters the discontinuity implied by Ackerknecht's assertion. It was the promise of practical experience at the bedside and at the dissecting table that attracted American physicians to the French capital after 1815. Access to hospitals with large numbers of patients, seeing and touching the sick, and the possibilities of doing autopsies were the lures of Paris Medicine. The large numbers of students who followed famous professors on ward rounds made participation in such clinical performances difficult, but private clinical instruction in hospitals in small groups led by *internes* gave the Americans the bedside experience they sought. In addition, private lecture courses gave them facility in anatomical dissection, operative surgery, diagnostic techniques, and knowledge of particular subjects such as infantile, ocular, and skin diseases.

American migration to Paris continued undiminished after 1848, Ackerknecht's cut-off point, right through the 1850s and into the 1860s. In fact the commonness of such French experience made it lose its cachet as a source of professional distinction back home.

But the 1855 edict of the Dean of the Paris Faculty of Medicine suppressing teaching of private clinical courses by *internes* helped galvanize American interest in other European locations. It was not laboratory medicine, Warner argues, that attracted American students elsewhere, nor better therapeutics or patient care. It was the greater possibility that Vienna and Berlin began to offer for ready access to practical instruction at the patients' bedside.

In imposing categories on medicine's historical development, Ackerknecht had divided it – like Gaul – into three parts: the Paris School he labelled "hospital medicine" to distinguish it from its predecessor, "bedside medicine", that is, before 1794, and from "laboratory medicine" after 1848, when the torch passed from France to Germany. The rise of positivism, the neglect of the medical history of the Second Empire, the rebirth of republican sentiment after 1870, and the Pasteurian Revolution have overshadowed the continuation of a very strong clinical tradition in French medicine throughout the nineteenth century. Joy Harvey challenges Ackerknecht and the earlier studies written in the 1840s, by arguing that the clinical tradition continued much as before in Paris in parallel and complementary development with the laboratory approach. The clinical tradition remained so strong that many Parisian physicians refused to be "pasteurized".[198] If some American students started going elsewhere after 1855 because of reduced access to clinical experience in Paris, there was no hint of such a problem in the letters of Mary Putnam Jacobi, who studied in Paris in the 1860s and 1870s.[199] The focus on the Paris School by later French historians eager to perpetuate the "myth" has resulted in neglect of the clinical tradition in the period between the heyday of the Paris School and the Pasteurian Revolution.

These essays taken together allow us to suggest the following themes in a reinterpretation of Paris Medicine:

> (1) the role of rhetoric in Paris Medicine; (2) reconsideration of its boundaries; (3) dynamic tension; (4) the role of private and public courses; (5) the political nature of Paris Medicine; (6) reconsiderations of continuity/discontinuity; (7) the monolithic vision of Paris Medicine; and (8) medical theatre and medical iconography.

Some of these are overlapping categories, defying in themselves the distinctions proposed. Nevertheless, for the sake of clarity, the components of a reinterpretation are outlined in this way.

The Role of Rhetoric in Paris Medicine

Several of the essays show that calling attention to the reality behind the rhetoric is a way of re-examining the entity of Paris Medicine. Thus Brockliss's counter to the accepted view of the sterile, bookish nature of Old Régime medical instruction challenges claims for the discontinuity of Paris Medicine. He suggests that reformers' pamphlets cannot be taken at face value as an accurate assessment of French medical education. Rather, there is a need to understand how such texts were used: as rhetoric, to make the Old Régime seem worse than it really was. The pamphlet writers are social revolutionaries rather than professional reformers.

Likewise, Warner asks what is to be found behind the rhetoric of clinical training, the idea that in Paris students could get hands-on training at the bedsides of the sick. He challenges us to look at the actual nature of clinical instruction: who learned what, and where? One answer is found in Harvey's paper, in which Mary Putnam Jacobi is quoted as describing one of the official surgical clinics at the Charité hospital as very crowded. Jacobi was lucky in that both the *interne* and the other students gave her a place near the professor. Thus, unlike most of the students assembled that day, she was able both to see and to hear. La Berge also wants historians to look beyond the rhetoric of scientific debate to ask which physicians used the microscope and which did not, and for what reasons.

The rhetoric of decline dated from the 1840s, Ackerknecht's "dead end".[200] By the 1860s decline in medical and scientific prowess was accompanied by the more all-encompassing rhetoric of degeneration. Leading physicians and reformers declared French society to be pathological, as exemplified by the prevalence of tuberculosis, alcoholism, syphilis, and especially by the fall in marital fertility.[201] After the stunning French defeat in the Franco-Prussian War, French morale sank to an all-time low. This was precisely the period in which Bernard, Béclard and Axenfeld, Daremberg, and Rochard put forward their versions of Paris Medicine. French medicine and science emerged from this period with the work of Pasteur. From the 1880s on, the Pasteurian Revolution restored French faith in their medical and scientific prowess and was cause for national celebration – along with, for those of positivist sympathies, the restoration of republicanism and the liberal-radical agenda in the Third Republic. Historians at the time emphasized their links with the Paris Medicine of the first third of the century, as has been indicated above. What needs to be asked is, was decline real? Or did French medicine continue along much the same lines, as Harvey's paper suggests, and was only perceived to be in decline when compared with the take-off in German medicine?[202]

Further, Warner's paper challenges the whole notion of decline. For Ackerknecht and others, an influx of foreign students is equated with a dynamic medicine offering distinctive training available nowhere else. Conversely, a slowing down in the number of students coupled with a concomitant increase of students going elsewhere (Germany, Austria) indicates decline. Warner's argument is that the change was simply a reflection of changing access to clinical, practical instruction. When the teaching that Americans valued the most dried up following the law of 1855, they sought the same training elsewhere.

Historians of French science and medicine, who have written primarily from a positivistic perspective, have, with some exceptions, ignored the period from about 1840 to the 1870s. This lack of attention has reinforced the rhetoric of decline. Was it a useful strategy employed by the likes of Claude Bernard, Paul Broca, and other luminaries of the time to gain professional recognition and much-needed funding for research facilities? Just as Warner, La Berge, and Brockliss have asked us to go beyond the rhetoric to examine the reality of teaching resources so should this be done for the mid-nineteenth century as well.

Demarcating Paris Medicine

Various criteria have been used to determine what counts as Paris Medicine, and what approaches and areas are to be included. Some authors, such as Bouillaud and Delaunay, see no sharp break between the so-called accessory sciences, physiology, and medicine. Others, especially Ackerknecht, keep the accessory sciences outside and count experimental physiology as a science, distinct from clinical medicine. Although Ackerknecht privileged clinical medicine above all else, in general, demarcation has not been superimposed to fit particular agendas. Rather, certain limits existed in the constructions of the earliest commentators, depending on each author's differentiation of science and clinical medicine. Those favouring a *rapprochement* between the two tended to see Paris Medicine as representing a broad spectrum of approaches. Those wanting a sharp demarcation aimed at preserving the glory of Paris Medicine and at preventing the clinical tradition from being transformed into the laboratory tradition associated with German medicine. La Berge has argued that to exclude the so-called accessory sciences conveys a false sense of the nature of medicine in Paris. Nor is it accurate to set experimental physiology apart from medicine during this era. To move beyond the divisions set up by Ackerknecht, science must be put back into Paris Medicine.

Dynamic Tension

Dynamic tension is one of the major elements in a reinterpretation of Paris Medicine. Virtually all commentators have noted polarities and polemics as a dominant characteristic: either internal to medicine, as in the Laennec–Broussais rivalry, or external, as in the larger political divisions of the time, which in turn fuelled rivalries in medicine. There is, however, a striking difference between the approaches taken to this phenomenon. Many see the tensions as a problem to explain. The Paris School would have been even more influential if its participants could have spoken with one voice. The suggestion in this volume is that Paris Medicine is a recognizable entity not in spite of its polarities, but because of them. This tension created the charged atmosphere in which Parisian physicians functioned. The dialectic gave Paris Medicine its strength and its balance. As Bouillaud, and later Rochard, said, tension encouraged activity, growth, and response. Jacalyn Duffin's essay on the Laennec–Broussais "duel" is the best example of this point of view, but it is also demonstrated in Jacyna's paper on Alibert. Alibert, like Laennec, was an exemplar of the Catholic, royalist, and vitalist tradition which existed in tension with the dominant materialist, secular tradition of Broussais and others. The traditions were larger than the men themselves. The tensions between different approaches in Paris Medicine were not detrimental to the enterprise but instead worked to create a dynamic interaction among practitioners.

Role of Public and Private Courses

The role of public and private courses figures prominently in a reinterpretation. By this is meant the complementary education offered by the courses taught outside the formal institutional structure. Again, it is a question of emphasis. Most of the chroniclers have recognized the existence and some the importance of these courses, taught by luminaries such as Bichat, Laennec, Broussais, and Cruveilhier.[203] The argument now is that these courses were more than supplemental; they were integral and fundamental. Thus, while the crowded lectures of the likes of

Broussais and Andral are remembered as great performances, for hands-on clinical training, it was the private courses offered, not only by the luminaries, but also by the interns at the hospitals.

Medical guidebooks, such as Henri Meding's *Paris Médical* (1853) listed the courses, instructors, locations, and fees, if any.[204] Brockliss suggests that looking only at the activities of the official Faculty misses much of the education taking place in Paris. Private courses were not new in the nineteenth century. Antoine Petit, for example, gave courses from 1750 to 1780 in his private amphitheatre in Paris. So Brockliss argues that it was easy for students to get experience in practical patient care if they took advantage of the private courses. La Berge's essay shows how new subjects like microscopy, and new courses like pathological anatomy in its early years, were first taught in public and private settings. Only later were these subjects incorporated into the official medical curriculum. The huge variety of private courses at hospital clinics and institutions made Paris a smorgasbord of medical delights – to such an extent that medical tourism prevailed. Private courses were one of the factors that contributed the most to making Paris the medical centre of the Western world during the first several decades of the nineteenth century.[205] For many foreign students, who often already had an M.D. degree, as Warner demonstrates, private courses were the principal source of medical instruction in Paris. Thus the interplay between the formal and informal structures of medical education needs to be emphasized, while noting that the education offered in the private and public courses was later institutionalized and became an integral part of Paris medical education. The argument here is not one of uniqueness for Paris, but rather for recognition of the multifaceted nature of the educational facilities available.

The Political Nature of Paris Medicine

All who are familiar with the history of French medicine and science are aware of the political nature of Paris Medicine, but this point deserves clarification and emphasis, especially for non-French scholars. The French Revolution politicized medicine and centralized French medicine in Paris. As Sournia has pointed out, the Revolution not only transformed medical education and the practice of medicine, but also redefined the social and professional roles of physicians. Physicians working at the hospitals and the various teaching and research institutions were state employees. They could be hired and fired at the discretion of the state. The closing of the Faculty of Medicine in 1822, the firing of the physicians who taught there and the hiring of royalist physicians with much less clout, Laennec excepted, is the principal political story told about Paris Medicine after 1794. Most of the Parisian hospitals were public – state – institutions. The political discourse constrained Paris Medicine.[206] For the proponents of the various approaches that characterized Paris Medicine the underlying question was not only what was the best medicine, but also what kind of society/body politic did they want to live in?[207] The French have understood the political factors impinging on their science and medicine and acknowledge them tacitly in their accounts. But this should be made explicit, because it is easy for those from Anglo-American traditions to forget that French medicine was statist.

Continuity/Discontinuity

New research challenges whether Paris Medicine is a continuation or not of previous medicine. The debate over continuity/discontinuity of the French Revolution has been the main historiographic problem of French Revolutionary studies since de Tocqueville and Michelet. That discussion experienced a resurgence in recent years, especially when historians began to re-evaluate the Revolution in light of its bicentennial.[208] Brockliss and Keel both challenge Ackerknecht's claim for discontinuity in French medicine, while Keel mounts a fundamental critique of Foucault's epistemological rupture as well. Brockliss argues that students sought out hands-on clinical training in medicine – not just in surgery – before the Revolution. Keel challenges the uniqueness and distinctiveness of the Foucaultian gaze and of Paris Medicine itself. Were the claims for uniqueness a French artefact, constructed by the French themselves while they conveniently ignored similar work in pathological anatomy and tissue pathology going on elsewhere?[209]

Applying Foucaultian strategies to Paris Medicine has encouraged other significant departures from the "myth". The research of both Duffin and Albury shows the impact of Foucault. Duffin employs Foucault's notion of the underlying discourse, an episteme that constrains the systems of thought and practices of an era to show how the same professional and cognitive environment allowed for the development of more than one option in medical theory. What the research represented in this volume suggests is that there was no shared discourse among the Parisian physicians.

Albury, on the other hand, uses the notion of epistemological rupture that Foucault derived from Bachelard to suggest how in developing a new way of looking at health and disease, practitioners of Paris Medicine developed a theory which improved their professional position. The rupture that Albury sees is the abrupt shift from the eighteenth-century Hippocratic-Galenic focus on health and life to the orientation of Corvisart and Broussais which focused on disease and death. It was a changed view of nature from beneficent to destructive. This qualitatively different discourse, which Albury contends underlay pathological anatomy, allowed physicians to justify medical interventions. When the pathological became normal, the physician's expert knowledge was routinely needed. This orientation led to medicalization and provided a strategy for medical dominance. Nature could no longer be trusted, but doctors could.[210]

The Monolithic Nature of Paris Medicine

The new research challenges the "myth" of Paris Medicine as an entity characterized by the following: focus on disease, not patients; localism; materialism; detached objectivity, not involved subjectivity; a scientific orientation; secularism; and liberalism or republicanism. This was the model of Paris Medicine promulgated by Montpellier physicians, who sought to distance themselves from it. They tried to protect what they saw as the older, stronger tradition of Montpellier, characterized by vitalism, holism, Catholicism, and a humanistic, patient-oriented approach.[211] This was the model of Paris Medicine that had emerged by the twentieth century in great part, no doubt, because the chroniclers of the Third Republic wanted to write out the characteristics that did not fit into the positivist vision of what Paris Medicine had been. The research by Jacyna on Alibert and Duffin on Laennec is a reminder that other viewpoints did not disappear but remained an important part of medical thinking in the first three decades of the nineteenth century.

Medical Theatre and Medical Iconography

Two areas for further examination that have emerged from this research, but that are not addressed in detail in these essays are the theatrical nature of Paris Medicine and the importance of medical iconography. Medical theatre was a prominent theme of critics such as Peisse, outsiders such as the American students in Paris, and even Paul Broca, when writing on the microscopy debate in the Academy of Medicine. The lectures of the leading professors were great performances; classes taught in anatomy amphitheatres and the clinical rounds in hospitals were in their own way medical theatre.[212] Joy Harvey describes how the complex structure of the Parisian hospitals "resembled a piece of public theater". So too were the "great tournaments" that took place at the Academy of Medicine great performances of medical theatre. Lastly, although not discussed here, an important area for future research is the surgical theatres and the "animal theatre" of Magendie, replete with his performing dogs.[213]

Medical iconography as an important element in Paris Medicine is not new, but has not received the attention it deserves.[214] Daremberg stressed it, and in this volume it is central to the work of Jacyna on Alibert and underlies that of La Berge on medical microscopy. Contemporaries and later historians recognized the beauty and importance of the atlases of pathological anatomy of Cruveilhier, as well as the large folios of the microscopists and proto-dermatologists: Donné, Lebert, and Alibert. The illustrations of Ambroise Tardieu exemplify this tradition as well.[215] Furthermore, this was the period when Daguerre introduced photography to the Parisian scientific and medical community, and Donné, for one, was quick to apply the new technology to microscopy, introducing the technique of photomicrography.[216] Medical iconography is a potentially rich area for further study and may well lead to new insights into Paris Medicine.

Medicine and Religion and Medicine and Gender

Finally, research in this volume does not address two areas of investigation that hold some promise. The first would be a detailed exploration of religious themes in Paris Medicine. Once the blinders are removed, scholars are in a position to take seriously the relationship of religious thought and practices, and spirituality to medicine. Jacalyn Duffin's biography of Laennec shows how religious concerns played an important role in Paris Medicine.[217]

Nor have gender considerations figured much in the research represented. With few exceptions, women have not been a part of the construction of Paris Medicine. The tensions between the objectives of the religious sisters who nursed the patients in hospitals and those of the physicians pursuing clinical teaching have been the subject of some attention.[218] But both nurses and midwives merit more investigation as well as female patients. Weiner's research on nun-administrators of hospitals and on female patients, both citizens and insane, is a start. Joy Harvey shows us women as medical students, although in a later period than in the one under discussion.[219] Even a more traditional approach to women patients as perceived by practising physicians is still missing. Jacyna's paper is a beginning for this kind of study, since much of Alibert's "pious pathology" concerned his very personal assessment of female patients.[220]

Conclusion

In the effort to understand both modernity and science, Paris Medicine looms large. If Paris was the birthplace of a medicine that is labelled modern and scientific, then Paris Medicine is of interest to all when grappling with competing visions of medicine, culture, and society in the late twentieth century.

As those who have previously constructed Paris Medicine applied their own vision, and used history to their own ends, so do we. We hope that this volume will stimulate a dialogue, and will encourage other historians reconsidering classic episodes in the history of medicine and science to challenge the "myths" we have lived with and work towards constructing new ones. We believe that this collaborative work has opened up new areas of historical investigation and should encourage new interpretive strategies.

As we try to make sense out of our times, we reinvent and reinterpret the past as a way of coming to grips with – and sometimes escaping – the present, not just in terms of practical problem solving, but as a way of retrieving a vision that has been lost, or of understanding the visions we accept, or of finding visions as yet unimagined.

Paris Medicine: Perspectives Past and Present

Notes

1. The exact number of old Régime faculties that were awarding doctorates of medicine is difficult to ascertain. Different sources give different figures. Jules Rochard, *Histoire de la chirurgie française au XIXe siècle* (Paris: Baillière, 1875), 1, says that there were eighteen.
2. Virtually all accounts emphasize the importance of 1794. See Toby Gelfand, *Professionalizing Modern Medicine: Paris Surgeons and Medical Science and Institutions in the Eighteenth Century* (Westport, Connecticut: Greenwood Press, 1980); Jean-Charles Sournia, *La Médecine révolutionnaire (1789-1799)* (Paris: Payot, 1989); and Charles Coury, *L'Enseignement de la médecine en France des origines à nos jours* (Paris: Expansion Scientifique Française, 1968). For a recent endeavour to approach French developments and medical education from a larger comparative perspective, see Thomas Neville Bonner, *Becoming a Physician: Medical Education in Great Britain, France, Germany, and the United States, 1745-1945* (Oxford and New York: Oxford University Press, 1995), esp. chs. 4, 5, and 6.
3. Paul Delaunay, *D'une Révolution à l'autre, 1789-1848: l'évolution des théories et de la pratique médicale* (Paris: Editions Hippocrate, 1949); Erwin Ackerknecht, "La Médecine à Paris entre 1800 et 1850", *Les Conférences du Palais de la Découverte*, Série D, No. 58 (Paris: 1958); Michel Foucault, *La Naissance de la clinique: Une archéologie du regard médical* (Paris: Presses universitaires de France, 1963); Erwin Ackerknecht, *Medicine at the Paris Hospital, 1794-1848* (Baltimore: Johns Hopkins Press, 1967).
4. Erwin Ackerknecht, "Broussais, or a Forgotten Medical Revolution", *Bull. Hist. Med.* 27 (1953): 320. On mythology in medical history, see Owsei Temkin, "An Essay on the Usefulness of Medical History for Medicine", *Bull. Hist. Med.* 19 (1946): 14. For recent discussions of "myth" in history, or historical myths in general, see Peter Novick, *That Noble Dream: The Objectivity Question and the American Historical Profession* (New York: Cambridge University Press, 1988). For specific reference to the question of myths in French history, see Chantal Grell, *L'Histoire entre érudition et philosophie: Etude sur la connaissance historique à l'âge des Lumières* (Paris: Presses universitaires de France, 1993), esp. part 4, "L'Histoire de France", ch. 7, "L'élaboration d'une mythologie nationale", 195-219.
5. Robert Gildea, *The Past in French History* (New Haven, Connecticut: Yale University Press, 1994), 10.
6. Richard Shryock, *The Development of Modern Medicine: An Interpretation of the Social and Scientific Factors Involved* (London:

Oxford University Press, 1936; New York: Alfred A. Knopf, 1947), 151.
7. Erwin Ackerknecht, *A Short History of Medicine* (New York: Ronald Press, 1955), 145, 146.
8. See W. F. Bynum, *Science and the Practice of Medicine in the Nineteenth Century* (Cambridge: Cambridge University Press, 1994), ch. 2, "Medicine in the Hospital", 25-54. A recent general history of medicine discusses the Paris School only briefly, but refers to the accomplishments cited in the text. See Lois Magner, *A History of Medicine* (New York and Basel: Marcel Dekker, 1992), 336-41.
9. Quoted in Henry Sigerist, *The Great Doctors: A Biographical History of Medicine* (New York: W. W. Norton, 1933), 291.
10. *Ibid.*, 266.
11. The sources consulted were only concerned with France. It is not that writers thought the French situation with regard to the relationship of medicine and surgery was unique; they just did not address non-French medicine.
12. Sigerist, *Great Doctors*, 268.
13. *Ibid.*
14. Knud Faber, *Nosography, The Evolution of Clinical Medicine in Modern Times*, 2nd edn. (New York: P. S. Hoeber, 1930), 54.
15. Jean-Charles Sournia, *Histoire de la médecine* (Paris: Editions La Découverte, 1992), 219.
16. Antoine Fourcroy, *Rapport du projet du décret sur l'enseignement d'une Ecole centrale de santé à Paris*. Speech given on behalf of the Comités de Santé et d'Instruction Publique. 7 frimaire, l'an III (Paris, 1794), 17-18.
17. Antoine Fourcroy, *Exposé des motifs du projet de loi sur l'exercice de la médecine*, 19 ventôse, an 11 (Paris, March 1803), 350-1.
18. Pierre Rayer, *Sommaire d'une histoire abrégée de l'anatomie pathologique* (Paris: Gabon et Méquignon-Marvis, 1818), 128.
19. Erwin Ackerknecht, "Elisha Bartlett and the Philosophy of the Paris Clinical School", *Bull. Hist. Med.* 24 (1950): 43-60.
20. Charles Daremberg, *Histoire des sciences médicales*, 2 vols. (Paris: Baillière, 1870), 2: 1296-7.
21. Rayer, *Sommaire*, 134-5.
22. Philippe Pinel had pointed out already in 1793 in an unpublished essay that clinical teaching had been developed elsewhere than France. See Philippe Pinel, *The Clinical Training of Doctors: An Essay of 1793*, ed. and trans. and with an introduction by Dora B. Weiner (Baltimore, Maryland: Johns Hopkins University Press, 1980), 74-9.
23. Jean-Baptiste Bouillaud, *Essai sur la philosophie médicale et sur les généralités de la clinique médicale* (Paris: Rouvier et le Bouvier, 1836), 114.

24. *Ibid.*, 114-15.
25. Louis Desbois de Rochefort founded the *clinique médicale* at the Charité hospital in 1780. He was succeeded in 1788 by Jean Nicolas Corvisart. Jean Desault founded the *clinique chirurgicale* at the Paris Hôtel-Dieu, where he was chief physician. See Paul Triaire, *Récamier et ses contemporains (1774-1852): Etudes d'histoire de la médecine aux XVIIIe et XIXe siècles* (Paris: Baillière, 1899), 105-107; Toby Gelfand, "A Clinical Ideal: Paris, 1789", *Bull. Hist. Med.* 51 (1977): 397-411.
26. Dupuytren, cited in Bouillaud, *Essai*, 115-16.
27. Bouillaud, *Essai*, 115.
28. *Ibid.*, 117.
29. See John Harley Warner, "The Selective Transport of Medical Knowledge: Antebellum American Physicians and Parisian Medical Therapeutics", *Bull. Hist. Med.* 59 (1985): 213-31.
30. Pierre Louis, *Pathological Researches on Phthisis*, trans. and with an introduction by Charles Cowan (London: Sherwood, Gilbert, and Piper, 1836), xix.
31. F. Campbell Stewart, *Eminent French Surgeons, with a Historical and Statistical Account of the Hospitals of Paris* (Buffalo: A. Burke, 1843), xvi.
32. Pathological anatomy, for example, was taught outside the Faculty until a chair was established in 1835, as were microscopy courses dating from 1837. Sometimes private courses were taught within the physical facilities of the Faculty.
33. Stewart, *Eminent French Surgeons*, 139.
34. On Enlightenment discourse, see Jean Starobinski, *The Invention of Liberty, 1700-1789* (Skira, 1962) and his *Blessing in Disguise, or, the Morality of Evil* (Cambridge, Massachusetts: Harvard University Press, 1993), ch. 1. See also Keith Baker, *Condorcet: From Natural Philosophy to Social Mathematics* (Chicago, Illinois: University of Chicago Press, 1975); Sergio Moravia, "Philosophie et médecine en France à la fin du XVIIIe siècle", *Studies on Voltaire and the Eighteenth Century* 89 (1972):1089-151; Georges Gusdorf, *Dieu, la nature, l'homme au siècle des lumières* (Paris, 1972); George Rosen, "The Philosophy of Ideology and the Emergence of Modern Medicine in France", *Bull. Hist. Med.* 20 (1946): 328-39.
35. At least this was the case in the *Encyclopédie* tradition. As Nellie Schargo pointed out in her treatment of history in the *Encyclopédie*: "The role assigned to the individual in the development of science is very important and for the Encyclopedists the history of science is clearly tied together with that of good scientists." Nellie N. Schargo, *History in the Encyclopédie* (New York: Columbia University Press,

1947), 142. See also pp. 173-9 for her discussion of the role that Encyclopedists assigned to individuals in shaping the course of history. On p. 173, she cites D'Alembert in the preliminary discourse of the *Encyclopédie*, 247, as commenting "The history of science is naturally bound up with that of the small number of great geniuses." See also on Enlightenment historiography, Benedetto Croce, *History: Its Theory and Practice* (New York: Russell and Russell, 1960), 243-263. See J. H. Brumfitt, *Voltaire Historian* (London: Oxford University Press, 1970; first published 1958), 124, on the importance of great men in Voltaire's history.
36. Bouillaud, *Essai*, 104-109.
37. *Ibid.*, xi.
38. *Ibid.*, 215.
39. *Ibid.*
40. *Ibid.*, 110. For an example of this tension at the end of the nineteenth century, see Martha Hildreth, *Doctors, Bureaucrats, and Public Health in France, 1888-1902* (New York: Garland, 1987).
41. Bouillaud, *Essai*, 79.
42. *Ibid.* On eclectics and medical eclecticism, see Eugène Bouchut, *Histoire de la médecine et des doctrines médicales*, 2 vols. (Paris: Germer-Baillière, 1873), 2: 582-585; Triaire, *Récamier et ses contemporains, 1774-1852*, 342-347; Jacalyn Duffin, "The Medical Philosophy of R. T. H. Laennec (1781-1826)", *History and Philosophy of the Life Sciences* 8 (1956): 209-10; Ackerknecht, *Medicine at the Paris Hospital*, 101-13.
43. Bouillaud, *Essai*, 26.
44. *Ibid.*, 113-18.
45. *Ibid.*, 67-8.
46. *Ibid.*, 70-1.
47. *Ibid.*, 96.
48. See n. 42 on eclectics. Jacalyn Duffin notes that Broussais brought out the third edition of the *Examen* in 1834 and devoted most of the volume to attacking Laennec. The quarrel did not end until both men were dead. Only then did the Academy of Medicine read Laennec's eulogy (1839). Laennec had been dead for twelve years. See also George Weisz, "Creating the Posthumous Laennec", *Bull. Hist. Med.* 61 (1987): 541-62.
49. Bouillaud, *Essai*, 101.
50. Bouillaud, *Essai*, 45, 71; Ackerknecht, in "Broussais, or a Forgotten Medical Revolution", also uses the phrase "medical revolution" of 1816.
51. Bouillaud, *Essai*, 85. See also Weisz, "Creating the Posthumous Laennec".

52. Bouillaud, *Essai*, 84.
53. *Ibid.*, 90, note #1. Bouillaud did not discuss Laennec's Catholicism or vitalism except to say that Laennec was not "completely free of the spirit of party", and to imply that Laennec had not been "entirely impartial and fair" in his attitude towards Broussais's mortality statistics. See *ibid.*, 92-3.
54. Bouillaud, *Essai*, vii. On the rhetoric of Hippocratic medicine, see Louis Peisse, *La Médecine et les médecins: philosophie, doctrines, institutions*, 2 vols. (Paris: Baillière, 1857), 1: 236. Ann La Berge is publishing an article on the rhetoric of Hippocrates at the Paris School.
55. On the "cult of Hippocrates", see the discussion by Elizabeth Williams, *The Physical and the Moral: Anthropology, Physiology, and Philosophical Medicine in France, 1750-1850* (New York: Cambridge University Press, 1994), 65-6, 79. For illustration, see Pinel, ed. Weiner, *Clinical Training of Doctors*.
56. Bouillaud sees Paris Medicine as the direct heir of Hippocratic medicine which had been restored to the West in the Middle Ages by the Paris Faculty of Medicine: "it is to the Paris Faculty of Medicine that the honour belongs of the definitive restoration of Greek medicine". Bouillaud, *Essai*, 4-9.
57. Bouillaud, *Essai*, 101.
58. For biographical information on Peisse, see Jules Guérin, "Obsèques de M. Peisse", *Bulletin de l'Académie de Médecine* 9 (1880): 1055-9. In addition to his writings on medicine, Peisse was known as a translator of philosophical texts from English by William Hamilton and Dugald Stewart, and from Italian by P. Galuppi. He also added notes and a biographical notice on the life and works of P. J. G. Cabanis to the eighth edition of Cabanis's *Rapport du physique et du moral de l'homme* (Paris, 1844). For his work as an editor and translator of contemporary philosophical works, he was also elected to membership in the Académie des sciences morales et politiques as the successor to Cabanis.
59. Louis Peisse, *Sketches of the Character and History of Eminent Living Surgeons and Physicians of Paris,* trans. Elisha Bartlett (Boston: Carter, Hendee, and Babcock, 1831). Originally published in French in two volumes in 1827-8 as *Les Médecins français contemporains*.
60. It was this two-volume work of 1857 that secured his reputation and earned him election to the Academy of Medicine. See Guérin, "Obsèques de M. Peisse", 1057-1058.
61. Peisse, *Sketches*, xi.
62. *Ibid.*

63. *Ibid.*, 32-3. Quote, 32.
64. *Ibid.*, 39.
65. *Ibid.*
66. It brings to mind Robert Nye's recent study of male codes of honour and their influence on French medical discourse in the nineteenth century. See Robert Nye, *Masculinity and Male Codes of Honor in Modern France* (New York: Oxford University Press, 1993).
67. Peisse, *Sketches*, 39.
68. *Ibid.*, 89.
69. *Ibid.*, 51.
70. *Ibid.*, 52-3.
71. *Ibid.*, 58.
72. *Ibid.*, 82.
73. *Ibid.*, 79.
74. *Ibid.*, 40.
75. *Ibid.*, 84. Antoine Dubois (1756-1832), a pupil of Desault, taught surgery and obstetrics, and was Dean of the Paris Faculty of Medicine in 1830. Ackerknecht, *Medicine at the Paris Hospital*, 41.
76. Peisse, *Sketches*, 93.
77. *Ibid.*, xiii.
78. *Ibid.*, xii.
79. Jules Guérin, "La médecine en 1840", *Gazette médicale de Paris*, 9 janvier 1841, 17. Quoted in Paul Delaunay, *D'une Révolution à l'autre*.
80. Rochard, *Histoire de la chirurgie française au XIXe siècle*, 269-70. He cited as his source Réveillé-Parise in the *Gazette médicale*, 23 December 1843.
81. Paul Broca, "Séance de l'Académie de Médecine", *Moniteur des hôpitaux*, 5 Oct. 1854, 945.
82. Paul Broca, *Moniteur des hôpitaux*, 17 Oct. 1854, 986.
83. Paul Broca, *Moniteur des hôpitaux*, 25 Nov. 1854, 1110.
84. Erwin Ackerknecht, *Rudolf Virchow: Doctor, Statesman, Anthropologist* (Madison: University of Wisconsin Press, 1953). The changed tone of the writings of Rudolf Virchow who had earlier had close and most cordial relations with the Paris School is a good example.
85. Robert Nye, *Crime, Madness and Politics: The Medical Causes of National Decline* (Princeton, New Jersey: Princeton University Press, 1984).
86. Claude Bernard, *Rapport sur le progrès et la marche de la physiologie générale en France* (Paris: Imprimerie impériale, 1867).
87. *Ibid.*, 7.
88. French inferiority is inferred from German superiority. Thus Bernard

noted: "Nowhere besides in Germany does there exist as many universities, as many eminent physiologists, as many beautiful and good laboratories, as many national and foreign students who cultivate experimental physiology." Bernard, *Rapport sur la physiologie générale en France*, 237, no. 238.
89. *Ibid.*
90. *Ibid.*
91. Jules Béclard and Alexandre Axenfeld, *Rapport sur le progrès de la médecine en France* (Paris: Imprimerie impériale, 1867), 2.
92. *Ibid.*, 3.
93. Bouchut, *Histoire de la médecine*, 1:2; 2: 310.
94. *Ibid.*
95. *Ibid.*, 1: v-vi.
96. Henry I. Bowditch, *Brief Memoirs of Louis and Some of His Contemporaries in the Paris School of Medicine of Forty Years Ago* (Boston: John Wilson Press, 1872), 8.
97. *Ibid.*, 21-2.
98. *Ibid.*, 30.
99. Charles Daremberg, *La Médecine: Histoire et doctrines* (Paris: Didier et Cie., 1865), 290-304. Daremberg applauded Lebert's integrative approach, which he saw as a felicitous combination of the German research/laboratory method with the French clinical orientation.
100. *Ibid.*, 293-4.
101. *Ibid.*, 297-9. Quote, 297-8.
102. *Ibid.*, 302-3. For a historical overview of medical iconography, see Jacalyn Duffin, "Imaging Disease: The Illustration and Non-illustration of Medical Texts, 1650-1850", in B. Castel, J. A. Leith, and A. W. Riley, eds, *Muse and Reason: The Relation of Arts and Sciences, 1650-1850*, Royal Society of Canada Symposium, *Queen's Quarterly*, 1994, 79-108.
103. Daremberg, *La Médecine*, 299.
104. Daremberg, *Histoire des sciences médicales*.
105. Jules Rochard (1819-96) was a naval physician who, in his earlier career, published extensively on naval medicine. Believing that progress in surgery was the result of achievements in anatomy, physiology, and the natural sciences, as well as in medical institutions, in the 1870s he wrote his *Histoire de la chirurgie française*. This substantial work, whose literary merit equalled its knowledgeable critique according to contemporaries, brought him to the attention of the learned world and earned him membership of the Academy of Medicine in 1877. In 1894, he became president of the Academy. For details on Rochard's career and writings, see P.

Lereboullet, "Obsèques de M. J. Rochard", *Bulletin de l'Académie de Médecine* 36 (1896): 325-9.
106. Paul Triaire was a physician from Tours, who published on questions relating to hygiene. In the 1890s he turned to history of medicine, publishing not only on Récamier, but also on Bretonneau (*Bretonneau et ses contemporains*). Later he published an edition of the letters of Larrey and was working on an edition of the letters of Gui Patin at the time of his death. For his death notice, see C. Gariel, "Décès de M. Triaire, correspondant nationale", *Bulletin de l'Académie de Médecine* 67 (1912): 176-177.
107. Rochard, *Histoire de la chirurgie*, ix.
108. *Ibid.*, x. Quoted from Rudolf Virchow, *Discours prononcé au congrès des naturalistes allemands*, held in Rostock in 1872.
109. *Ibid.*, x.
110. *Ibid.*, xii.
111. *Ibid.*, xi.
112. *Ibid.*, quotes, 11, 13.
113. *Ibid.*, 13.
114. *Ibid.*, 91.
115. *Ibid.*, 96.
116. *Ibid.*
117. *Ibid.*, 111.
118. *Ibid.*
119. *Ibid.*, 399-410. Rochard's source for the priority of Raspail and Royer-Collard is Paul Broca, *Traité des tumeurs* (Paris: Asselin, 1866). Broca's influence on medical microscopy is discussed in Ann La Berge's essay in this volume.
120. Triaire, *Récamier et ses contemporains, 1774-1852*, x, xiv.
121. *Ibid.*, 102.
122. *Ibid.*, 364.
123. There is a growing literature on this era of French medicine. A good recent account of the Pasteurian Revolution and the origins of the Pasteur Institute is Anne Marie Moulin, "Bacteriological Research and Medical Practice in and out of the Pastorian School", in Ann La Berge and Mordechai Feingold, eds, *French Medical Culture in the Nineteenth Century* (Amsterdam, Atlanta: Rodopi, 1994), 327-349. See also Claire Salomon-Bayet, ed., *Pasteur et la révolution pastorienne* (Paris: Payot, 1986).
124. Triaire, *Récamier et ses contemporains*, 94-95.
125. *Ibid.*, 96. Both quotes on p. 96. Michel Thouret (1748-1810) became dean of the new *Ecole de Santé* and François Chaussier (1746-1828) was professor of anatomy and physiology.

126. *Ibid.*, 98.
127. *Ibid.*
128. *Ibid.*, 102.
129. *Ibid.*
130. *Ibid.*, 110-112.
131. *Ibid.*, 114.
132. *Ibid.*, 126.
133. *Ibid.*, 127.
134. *Ibid.*, 128.
135. *Ibid.*, 133.
136. *Ibid.*, 138, note 1.
137. *Ibid.*, 135-137, 170-171.
138. *Ibid.*, 245-250, 272-276, 346.
139. *Ibid.*, 272-276.
140. *Ibid.*, 361.
141. *Ibid.*, 362-364. Quote, p. 364.
142. *Ibid.*, 364.
143. These were largely published as articles. But book-length studies of individuals were also produced. For example, Alfred Rouxeau wrote two books on Laennec: *L'enfance et la jeunesse d'un grand homme: Laennec avant 1806* (Paris, 1912) and *Laennec après 1806* (Paris, 1920). Paul Ganière wrote *Corvisart: médecin de Napoléon (1755-1821)* (Paris, 1951). François Magendie was the subject of a book-length biography in the 1940s: J. M. D. Olmsted, *François Magendie: Pioneer in Experimental Physiology and Scientific Medicine in XIX Century France* (New York: Schuman's, 1944).
144. Delaunay, *D'une Révolution à l'autre.*
145. *Ibid.*, 14.
146. *Ibid.*, 17.
147. *Ibid.*, quote, p. 70.
148. The biographical details of Foucault's life come from two recent biographies: Didier Eribon, *Michel Foucault*, trans. Betsy Wing (Cambridge, Mass.: Harvard University Press, 1991) and James Miller, *The Passion of Michel Foucault* (New York: Simon and Schuster, 1993). See also the biography by David Macey, *The Lives of Michel Foucault: A Biography* (New York: Pantheon, 1993), especially his contextualization and account of *The Birth of the Clinic* in ch. 6.
149. Paris: Presses universitaires de France, 1963.
150. London: Tavistock, 1973; New York: Vintage, 1975.
151. *The Order of Things: An Archaeology of the Human Sciences* (New York: Random House, 1973).
152. Trans. Richard Howard. New York: Pantheon, 1965.

153. Quoted in Eribon, *Michel Foucault*, 215.
154. Miller, *Passion of Michel Foucault*.
155. See on Broussais, Jean-François Braunstein, *Broussais et le matérialisme: Médecine et philosophie au XIXe siècle* (Paris: Méridiens-Klincksieck, 1986).
156. Jean Starobinski, review of *The Birth of the Clinic* in *New York Review of Books*, 26 Jan. 1973, 18-22.
157. Foucault, "Truth and Power", in *Power/Knowledge: Selected Interviews and Other Writings, 1972-1977* (New York: Pantheon, 1980), 115. See also Colin Jones and Roy Porter, eds, *Reassessing Foucault: Power, Medicine and the Body* (London and New York: Routledge, 1994).
158. For recent analysis of the impact of *The Birth of the Clinic* on modes of biomedical thought, see Thomas Osborne, "On Anti-Medicine and Clinical Reason", in Jones and Porter, eds, *Reassessing Foucault*, 28-47, and also David Armstrong, "Bodies of Knowledge/Knowledge of Bodies", in *idem*, 17-27.
159. Ackerknecht, *Medicine at the Paris Hospital*, 7.
160. *Discipline and Punish: The Birth of the Prison*, trans. Alan Sheridan (New York: Vintage, 1979); *Histoire de la sexualité*. 3 vols. (Paris: Gallimard, 1976-84).
161. These are listed in the bibliography at the end of *Medicine at the Paris Hospital*. Ackerknecht, "Anticontagionism between 1821 and 1867", *Bull. Hist. Med.* 22 (1948): 562-93; Ackerknecht, "Hygiene in France, 1815-1848", *Bull. Hist. Med.* 22 (1948): 117-55.
162. For the use of Ackerknecht's characterizations in the sociological analysis of medicine and hospitals, see Ian Waddington, "The Role of the Hospital in the Development of Modern Medicine: A Sociological Analysis", *Sociology* 7 (1973): 211-24 and N. Jewson, "The Disappearance of the Sick Man from Medical Cosmologies, 1770-1870", *Sociology* 10 (1976): 225-44.
163. Ackerknecht, "Elisha Bartlett", *Bull. Hist. Med.* 24 (1950): 50.
164. Ackerknecht, "Elisha Bartlett"; Ackerknecht, "La Médecine à Paris".
165. Ackerknecht, *Medicine at the Paris Hospital*, 201.
166. Ackerknecht, "Hygiene in France".
167. Ackerknecht, "Elisha Bartlett", 49.
168. John Harley Warner found this quote in the Sigerist Papers at the Yale Archives.
169. In 1970, Pierre Huard and Mirko Grmek published *Sciences, médecine et pharmacie de la Révolution à l'Empire* (Paris: Dacosta). This very well-illustrated book is primarily descriptive and does not analyze the origins or assess the significance of the Paris School. It does describe military medicine in the Revolutionary wars and under

Napoleon.
170. David M. Vess, *Medical Revolution in France, 1789-1796* (Gainesville: University Presses of Florida, 1975).
171. Paris: Vrin, 1979.
172. Othmar Keel, "The Politics of Health and the Institutionalisation of Clinical Practices in Europe in the Second Half of the Eighteenth Century", in W. F. Bynum and Roy Porter, eds, *William Hunter and the Eighteenth-Century Medical World* (Cambridge: Cambridge University Press, 1985), 207-258.
173. Keel is not the only scholar to have investigated the development of the clinic. See, for example, Toby Gelfand, "Gestation of the Clinic", *Medical History* 25 (1981): 169-180; Guenter B. Risse, "Clinical Instruction in Hospitals: The Boerhaavian Tradition in Leyden, Edinburgh, Vienna, and Pavia", in "Clinical Teaching Past and Present", symposium no., *Clio Medica* 21 (1987/1988): 1-19.
174. Westport, Connecticut: Greenwood Press, 1980.
175. Owsei Temkin, "On the Role of Surgery in the Rise of Modern Medical Thought", *Bull. Hist. Med.* 25 (1951): 248-59. See also L. W. B. Brockliss, "Medical Reform in Late Eighteenth-Century France", in Roy Porter, ed., *Medicine in the Enlightenment* (Amsterdam and Atlanta: Rodopi, 1995), 69-70, and n. 24. For important examples of work set within the context of studies of professionalization, see Matthew Ramsey, *Professional and Popular Medicine in France, 1770-1830: The Social World of Medical Practice* (New York: Cambridge University Press, 1988) and *idem*, "The Politics of Professional Monopoly in Nineteenth-Century Medicine: The French Model and its Rivals", in Gerald L. Geison, ed., *Professions and the French State, 1700-1900* (Philadelphia: University of Pennsylvania Press, 1984), 225-305.
176. Gelfand now proposes to investigate the Paris School in the second half of the nineteenth century.
177. Martin S. Staum, *Cabanis: Enlightenment and Medical Philosophy in the French Revolution* (Princeton, New Jersey: Princeton University Press, 1980). See also Ludmilla Jordanova, "Reflections on Medical Reform: Cabanis' *Coup d'Oeil*", in Roy Porter, ed., *Medicine in the Enlightenment* (Amsterdam and Atlanta: Editions Rodopi, 1995), 166-180.
178. John E. Lesch, *Science and Medicine in France: The Emergence of Experimental Physiology, 1790-1855* (Cambridge, Mass.: Harvard University Press, 1984).
179. Russell C. Maulitz, *Morbid Appearances: The Anatomy of Pathology in the Early Nineteenth Century* (New York: Cambridge University Press, 1987).

180. *Medical History*, Supplement no. 4, 1984.
181. Jacalyn Duffin, "Vitalism and Organicism in the Philosophy of R. T. H. Laennec", *Bull. Hist. Med.* 62 (1988): 525-45; "Private Practice and Public Research: The Patients of R. T. H. Laennec", in La Berge and Feingold, eds, *French Medical Culture*, 118-148; "The Medical Philosophy of R. T. H. Laennec (1781-1826)", *History and Philosophy of the Life Sciences* 8 (1986): 195-219. Duffin's new biography of Laennec has recently been published by Princeton University Press.
182. Weisz, *The Medical Mandarins: The French Academy of Medicine in the Nineteenth and Early Twentieth Centuries* (New York and Oxford: Oxford University Press, 1995); Weisz, "Creating the Posthumous Laennec"; George Weisz, "The Medical Elite in France in the Early Nineteenth Century", *Minerva* 25 (1987): 150-70; "The Self-Made Mandarin: The Eloges of the French Academy of Medicine, 1824-47", *History of Science* 26 (1988): 13-39; and "The Development of Medical Specialization in Nineteenth-Century Paris", in La Berge and Feingold, eds, *French Medical Culture*, 149-188.
183. Braunstein, *Broussais et le matérialisme*.
184. Michel Valentin, *François Broussais, Empereur de la Médecine* (Dinard: Association des Amis du Musée du Pays de Dinard, 1988).
185. Broussais has also been discussed at some length in Georges Canguilhem, *The Normal and the Pathological* (New York: Zone Books, 1991), esp. 47-64; Foucault, *Birth of the Clinic*, 174-194; and Williams, *Physical and the Moral*, 166-175.
186. Jean-Charles Sournia, *La Médecine révolutionnaire (1789-1799)* (Paris: Payot, 1989), 7. Russell Maulitz is also exploring aspects of the history of medicine in France during the Revolutionary period and shortly after.
187. Sournia, *La Médecine révolutionnaire*, 8.
188. *Ibid.*, 252.
189. *Ibid.*, 150, 158.
190. Baltimore: Johns Hopkins University Press, 1993.
191. New York: Cambridge University Press, 1994.
192. Christopher G. Goetz, Michel Bonduelle, and Toby Gelfand, *Charcot: Constructing Neurology* (Oxford and New York: Oxford University Press, 1995).
193. Princeton University Press, 1998. See, for example, John Harley Warner, "The Selective Transport of Medical Knowledge: Antebellum American Physicians and Parisian Medical Therapeutics", *Bull. Hist. Med.* 59 (1985): 213-231; and "Remembering Paris: Memory and the American Disciples of French Medicine in the Nineteenth

Century", *Bull. Hist. Med.* 65 (1991): 301-25.
194. Gelfand, *Professionalizing Modern Medicine*. In her review of Gelfand's book, Caroline Hannaway suggested that surgery had been emphasized at the expense of medicine: *Bull. Hist. Med.* 58 (1984): 596-8.
195. See also L. W. B. Brockliss, "L'enseignement médical et la Révolution: essai de reévaluation", *Histoire de l'Education* 42 (1989): 79-110 and *idem*, "Medical Reform, the Enlightenment and Physician-Power in Late Eighteenth-Century France", in Roy Porter, ed., *Medicine in the Enlightenment* (Amsterdam and Atlanta: Rodcpi, 1995), 64-112. The extensive social and cultural history of French medicine from the sixteenth century to the French Revolution published by Laurence Brockliss and Colin Jones, *The Medical World of Early Modern France* (Oxford: Oxford University Press, 1997) further illuminates the background to nineteenth-century developments in French medicine.
196. Foucault, *Birth of the Clinic*, 9.
197. *Ibid.*, xiv.
198. See Moulin, "Bacteriological Research and Medical Practice".
199. See also Joy Harvey, "La Visite: Mary Putnam Jacobi and the Paris Medical Clinics", in La Berge and Feingold, eds, *French Medical Culture*, 350-371. Joy Harvey is working on a biography of Mary Putnam Jacobi.
200. On the rhetoric of decline, see Robert Fox and George Weisz, "Introduction", in Robert Fox and George Weisz, eds, *The Organization of Science and Technology in France, 1808-1914* (Cambridge: Cambridge University Press; Paris: Editions de la Maison des Sciences de l'Homme, 1980), 22-28; Harry Paul, "The Issue of Decline in French Science", *French Historical Studies* 7 (1972): 416-50; and also Robert Fox, "Scientific Enterprise and the Patronage of Research in France, 1800-70", in Robert Fox, *The Culture of Science in France* (London: Variorum, 1992), 442-73. This article was originally published in 1973 in *Minerva*.
201. Nye, *Medical Causes of National Decline*; see also Daniel Pick, *Faces of Degeneration: A European Disorder, 1848-1918* (Cambridge: Cambridge University Press, 1989).
202. On the notion of decline in French science and medicine, see Paul, "Issue of Decline in Nineteenth-Century French Science", 416-50. See also Fox and Weisz, "Introduction: The Institutional Basis of French Science in the Nineteenth Century", in Fox and Weisz, eds, *Organization of Science and Technology in France, 1808-1914*, 1-28.
203. See, for example, Pierre Huard and Marie-José Imbault-Huart,

"L'Enseignement libre de la médecine à Paris au XIXe siècle", *Revue d'histoire des sciences* 37 (1974): 45-62. Ackerknecht, *Medicine at the Paris Hospital*, pays considerable attention to them. See also George Weisz, "Reform and Conflict in French Medical Science", in Fox and Weisz, eds, *Organization of Science and Technology in France*, 62-9, and Ann La Berge's essay in this volume.

204. Henri Meding, *Paris Médical* (Paris: Baillière, 1853). For discussion of these guidebooks as a historical source for understanding medical specialization, see George Weisz, "The Development of Medical Specialization in Nineteenth-Century Paris", in La Berge and Feingold, eds, *French Medical Culture*, 149-188.

205. For the role of private courses in English medical instruction, see Susan Lawrence, *Charitable Knowledge: Hospital Pupils and Practitioners in Eighteenth-Century London* (New York: Cambridge University Press, 1996), esp. ch. 5. Extramural courses were a common and important component of medical education in nineteenth-century Edinburgh as well.

206. See Jacques Léonard, *La Médecine entre les savoirs et les pouvoirs: histoire intellectuelle et politique de la médecine française au XIXe siècle* (Paris: Aubier Montaigne, 1981).

207. For an analysis of the effects of the French Revolution on the political and human body, see Dorinda Outram, *The Body and the French Revolution: Sex, Class, and Political Culture* (New Haven and London: Yale University Press, 1989).

208. See, for example, Keith Michael Baker, Colin Lucas, *et al.*, *The French Revolution and the Creation of Modern Political Culture*, 3 vols. (New York: Pergamon Press, 1987) and Roger Chartier, *The Cultural Origins of the French Revolution*, trans. Lydia G. Cochrane (Durham, North Carolina: Duke University Press, 1991).

209. See chapter 3 in Gildea, *The Past in French History* for the centrality of grandeur in French reconstructions of the past.

210. Albury's interpretation fits nicely with Roger Cooter's analysis of how anticontagionism could be used as a strategy for medical dominance in just the same period. See Roger Cooter, "Anticontagionism and History's Medical Record", in *The Problem of Medical Knowledge*, ed. P. Wright and A. Treacher (Edinburgh: Edinburgh University Press, 1983), 87-108.

211. See Williams, *Physical and the Moral*, 21.

212. See Goetz, Bonduelle, and Gelfand, *Charcot*, ch. 5, for the theatricality of Charcot's neurological practice.

213. This term comes from the title of a talk by Anita Guerrini at the annual meeting of the History of Science Society in 1993, in which

she was discussing an aspect of the history of animal experimentation. Such a term may well have been used in nineteenth-century Paris although no reference has yet been found.
214. For an overview, see Duffin, "Imaging Disease". For a discussion of medical iconography in the Enlightenment, see Barbara Maria Stafford, *Body Criticism: Imaging the Unseen in Enlightenment Art and Medicine* (Cambridge, Mass.: MIT Press, 1992).
215. Ambroise Tardieu was a leading public hygienist during the Second Empire. He was also a well-known medical illustrator. See, for example, Ann La Berge, *Mission and Method: The Early Nineteenth-Century French Public Health Movement* (New York: Cambridge University Press, 1992), 210, 212, 214.
216. On Donné's introduction of photomicrography, see Ann La Berge, "Medical Microscopy in Paris, 1830-1855", in La Berge and Feingold, eds, *French Medical Culture*, 302-3.
217. Duffin, *Laennec*. Although not dealing with clinical medicine, Catherine Kudlick's recent book on cholera in nineteenth-century Paris also provides an example of the integration of religious and medical concerns. See Catherine Kudlick, *Cholera in Post-Revolutionary Paris: A Cultural History* (Berkeley and Los Angeles: University of California Press, 1996).
218. Toby Gelfand, for example, has discussed this issue in the 1790s with regard to Desault's course. See his "A Confrontation over Clinical Instruction at the Hôtel-Dieu of Paris During the French Revolution", *J. Hist. Med.* 28 (1973): 268-82. See also Pierre Huard and M. J. Imbault-Huart, "L'enseignement de la chirurgie à l'Hôtel-Dieu d'après lettre inédite de Desault à l'Assemblée Nationale (1791)", *Revue d'histoire des sciences* 25(1) (1972): 55-63. See also, Dora B. Weiner, "The French Revolution, Napoleon, and the nursing profession", *Bull. Hist. Med.* 46 (1972): 274-305.
219. Thomas Neville Bonner discusses the entry of women into medicine in Paris in his book *To the Ends of the Earth: Women's Search for Education in Medicine* (Cambridge, Mass.: Harvard University Press, 1992), 48-54.
220. As a further suggestion the case studies of Armand Velpeau on breast cancer patients promise to be a fruitful area for research on woman patients. See Armand Velpeau, *Traité des maladies du sein* (Paris: Masson, 1854). Outram, *The Body and the French Revolution*, has pioneered the investigation of the effects of this political change on perceptions of the female body.

2

Before the Clinic: French Medical Teaching in the Eighteenth Century

L. W. B. Brockliss

I

In the period 1770–1793, a number of French physicians and other interested parties produced radical proposals for the reformation of the country's system of medical education.[1] The most detailed and most influential programme was the one presented by the Société Royale de Médecine to the French National Assembly in November 1790 and generally attributed to the Société's secretary, Félix Vicq d'Azyr (1748–94).[2] The reformers offered a variety of viewpoints as to the best way of restructuring medical education, but they were unanimous in their contempt for the system that pertained.[3] This system, based on the medical faculties of the French universities,[4] was found wanting in two major respects. On the one hand, the system was marred by corruption in that professors were lazy and degrees were awarded without a proper examination of the candidate's knowledge. On the other, and the two were not unconnected, the curriculum of the medical faculties was completely inadequate as a training for medical practice. Vicq d'Azyr's splenetic dismissal of the ineffectiveness of faculty teaching was representative:

> Indeed, what can be expected from a few years of study passed in taking down dictations or reading medical prolegomena, uniquely consisting of definitions and sterile divisions. What can be expected of schools where, in the majority of cases, there is no teaching of either human anatomy in its entirety, or the art of dissection, or botany, or medical chemistry in its full scope, or pharmacy, or the art of writing prescriptions, or nosology, or the history of medicine, or pathology; where not one word is said of the public functions of medicine; where no-one has taught his art at the bedside of the sick;

Before the Clinic

and whence finally one leaves without having learnt anything that a medical practitioner should know?'[5]

Consequently, young graduates had no choice but to learn their profession by trial and error. 'A young physician', wrote the *philosophe* Diderot, 'therefore makes his first essays [at his art] on us, and only becomes skilful by dint of assassination'.[6]

In the course of the 1790s, as the several Revolutionary assemblies debated the regeneration of French education *tout court*, the reformers' critique of the deficiencies of the ancien-régime medical faculties went unquestioned. A number of the medical reformers found themselves on key educational committees and in key administrative posts with the result that their verdict became a common currency.[7] According to the 1707 Edict of Marly all medical practitioners in France had to have a doctor's degree from a French university.[8] From March 1791 this requirement no longer pertained, and in September 1793 the faculties themselves were abolished with the rest of the university system. In Frimaire of the Year III the Thermidorians decided to establish a completely new system of medical education, one which would give special emphasis to clinical instruction. Their spokesman before the Convention, the chemist A.-F. de Fourcroy (1755–1809), pointedly contrasted the utility of the curriculum of the proposed *écoles de santé* with the inadequacy of the defunct faculties. Before 1789, he insisted, no faculty had taught a proper course of medicine. 'Prolegomena stuffed with sterile definitions were the sole base [of the curriculum]. The physical and exact sciences, which are the only source of a solid instruction, were forgotten.' So too had been hands-on experience in the laboratory and the hospital. 'Reading little, seeing and doing much: this will be the basis of the new teaching.'[9]

Nine years later when Fourcroy proposed that the *écoles de santé* should be changed into degree-giving *écoles de médecine*, his attitude towards the faculties of the ancien régime had scarcely mellowed. He accepted that the revolutionaries had made a mistake in deregulating medical practice, for the abolition of the royal decree of 1707 that medical practitioners had to be faculty graduates had proved a charlatans' charter. If nothing else, the faculties had played a useful role in controlling access to the medical profession. Nevertheless, most had not proved worthy of their trust. Apart from Montpellier and Paris the examination of candidates had been scandalously lax, 'the title of doctor being conferred on absentees, and degree certificates sent by post'.[10]

In the present century this unflattering picture of the ancien-régime medical faculties has become a historical commonplace. Historians of nineteenth-century France – be they historians of higher education, such as Liard, or historians of medicine, such as Ackerknecht – have swallowed the rhetoric of the reformers and their revolutionary allies uncritically.[11] Indeed, they have added to the myth by insisting that the education given in the medical faculties was not only impractical, but also antediluvian. Courses in theoretical medicine were presented in a scholastic format and based on outmoded classical authors whose conclusions were dogmatically accepted. Thus, as late as 1978, Léonard could write that in the faculties 'Galen and Hippocrates were deemed infallible'.[12] Historians' of French medicine and medical teaching before the Revolution have been seldom more charitable. Delaunay in the early decades of this century was ready to grant some intellectual vitality to the Paris faculty, but at the same time he accepted that its teaching was largely impractical.[13] The recent work of Gelfand on Paris surgical education has only hardened the traditional orthodoxy. Gelfand's desire to promote the eighteenth-century Paris *Ecole de chirurgie* as the institutional precursor of the post-Revolutionary clinic has done nothing to promote a re-evaluation of the role of the faculties. In his published work, their somnambulance has always been deliberately contrasted to the vitality and practicality of Parisian surgical education.[14]

The present essay sets out to challenge the reality of this stereotyped image. The traditional assumption is almost entirely based on the accounts to be found in the pamphlets and speeches of the medical reformers and their revolutionary allies. Such self-interested witnesses are unlikely to provide reliable testimony, all the more that the 1790s was a peculiar era in which political rhetoric was organized around a discourse of absolute judgements whose veracity was deemed unimpeachable. People and institutions were either good or bad, virtuous or wicked, useful or useless. There was no half-way house. Revolutionaries like Fourcroy, if not reformers like Vicq d'Azyr, belonged to a Manichean political culture which always thought in polar opposites. Their statements about ancien-régime medical education cannot be taken as objective fact.[15] Fortunately, there are many, less suspect, sources for the study of eighteenth-century French medical education: faculty matriculation and graduation records, faculty minutes and memoranda, professorial and student notebooks, student dissertations, course advertisements, student letters, and medical autobiographies and journals.[16]

Admittedly, these sources are not as full as one would like, but once they are carefully perused, then a much more positive picture of medical training in the ancien régime appears.[17] Although the present chapter does not claim to provide a complete account of medical training in the ancien régime, it does throw further light on the context out of which the Paris medical school emerged. Ultimately, it adds cautious support to the view of Othmar Keel that, *pace* Gelfand, the nineteenth-century clinical school had its antecedents in the eighteenth-century training of physicians rather than surgeons.[18]

II

The claim that faculty professors frequently neglected their teaching duties definitely has little substance. Had professors really been negligent, then references to the fact would surely exist in the surviving faculty archives. Concern about the maintenance of corporate duties was strong in the eighteenth century, and if the faculties themselves had done nothing to enforce their statutes, they would have been quickly leant upon by the local courts. The virtual absence of contemporary complaints about professorial assiduity suggests that this was not a problem. The only evidence of negligence comes from Montpellier in the second quarter of the century, where on several occasions students protested that individual professors were failing to lecture. A particular target was the head of the faculty in the 1730s, J. François Chicoyneau (1702–40), who was said to prefer wine and women to teaching.

These complaints, however, were not heard after 1740 when older men were replaced by respected teachers, such as the nosologist, François Boissier de Sauvages (1707–67). Although the students continued to find fault with the lecturing provision, their protest was now levelled at the faculty's habit of appointing substitutes for professors out of town.[19] Professors in the eighteenth century wore many hats. Their medical practice could take them all over the country and include spells at court, while in wartime they might be expected to go to the front. Moreover, in an age when the crown was taking a novel interest in the health of its subjects, Montpellier's professors were frequently called on to serve on government committees or as medical administrators.[20] Their presence then could never be guaranteed. It was clearly galling for students who came to hear the renowned vitalist, Paul-Joseph Barthez (1734–1806), to find that this medical star was elsewhere, but this was hardly the faculty's fault, which in fact was doing its best to maintain the lecturing provision.[21]

Admittedly, there were a number of medical faculties in the eighteenth century where there was no teaching given at all, but this reflects the structure of the country's medical education, not professorial negligence. There were twenty-four French universities in 1789 and all but four possessed faculties of medicine. Only a minority of the faculties, however, received and taught a significant number of students: Montpellier, Paris, Strasbourg, Besançon and Toulouse.[22] Others, such as Caen, had a small, regionally recruited, clientele, but perhaps as many as half a dozen of the faculties had no students at all. Faculties like Bourges, Poitiers and Nantes were simply faculty boards that awarded degrees.[23] The existence of non-teaching faculties should not be blamed on professorial negligence. It rather reflected the size of the medical market. There were just not enough medical students in France in the early-modern period to justify the existence of so many faculties, and teaching by tradition had tended to become concentrated in a handful of centres.[24]

Of course many professors of medicine may not have been particularly stimulating. Many may have coveted the position for the honour it brought, not out of a love of teaching.[25] On the other hand, the method of appointing professors in most faculties should have ensured at least some competence. Chairs were awarded primarily as the result of an open *concours*, where candidates had to demonstrate their lecturing as well as their debating skills.[26] Even if candidates were ultimately selected on the basis of their contacts and not their ability, they still had to perform in public first of all. It was perhaps for this reason that, especially in the second half of the eighteenth century, few chairs were inherited.[27] The *concours* system, however actually operated, made it difficult for chairs to become family fiefs in the way that they did at eighteenth-century Edinburgh.[28] The one significant faculty where professors might well have been indifferent performers was Paris. Here the professors were not appointed for life after a competitive *concours*, but were elected for a period of two years by the resident body of Paris graduates, known as the doctors regent.[29] Theoretically complete incompetents could be selected, but it seems more likely that the faculty officials rigged the ballot to ensure that willing and able candidates emerged.[30] In fact, if eighteenth-century medical professors were boring, this reflected not the inadequacy of the teachers but the method of teaching. Lectures were very formalized. Professors were expected to lecture for an hour a day, six days a week. The first part of the lecture consisted of a dictation from a prepared *cahier*. The rest of the time was taken up by a more detailed viva voce exposition of the subject.

No time seems to have been set aside for informal discussion or the interrogation of students.³¹ Professors, then, were scarcely likely to be sparkling. Nor were they likely to teach a highly original course.³² Chairs seem to have been allotted according to generalist criteria of sufficiency, and experts in particular disciplines were not always to be found teaching their speciality. When Chaptal studied at Montpellier in the mid-1770s, he found *inter alia* the chemist Venel giving his faculty lectures not on chemistry but hygiene.³³

III

Once attention is concentrated on the faculties which actually received and taught students, the accusation levelled against the curriculum is also found to be false or at least greatly exaggerated.³⁴ In the first place, the theoretical core of the course was not antediluvian in its inspiration, but reflected contemporary debates and developments. Nothing could be further from the truth than the claim that the professors were dyed-in-the-wool Galenists. In the first part of the eighteenth century the professors were divided into two, often mutually hostile, camps. The first comprised supporters of iatrochemical theories of physiology and pathology, who attempted to explain health and disease largely in terms of benign or malign chemical reactions. One of the leading members of the group was the Montpellier professor, Antoine Deidier, whose medical teaching was published in textbook form shortly before he died in 1732.³⁵ The other camp consisted of iatromechanists who tried to explain health and disease in terms of the fibrous tension of the solids. The physiological process of chilification, for instance, was thought to be caused simply by the pummelling and shaking to which ingested food was subject as it passed through the stomach and the gut. Triturationists, as they were called, ultimately drew their inspiration from the works of Baglivi and Boerhaave. Inside France their great champion in the early eighteenth century was the Paris doctor and Jansenist, Philippe Hecquet (1661–1737), who waged a bitter pamphlet war against iatrochemical theories until his death.³⁶ Much of the intensity of the quarrel between the two groups sprang from the therapeutic implications of the triturationist philosophy. The iatromechanists attacked chemical drugs and in the eyes of their opponents became dependent on a single remedy: phlebotomy.

> They [the iatromechanists] say that purgatives and emetics are almost always harmful and that frequent phlebotomies are much more useful[,] because [phlebotomy] is uniquely advised for the

elasticity of the solids[,] and because so much of the motion of the fluids is primarily produced by this said elasticity[.] It is absurd [they go on] to fight to the end the saline constitution of the blood with solvents and other suitable [to the iatrochemists] remedies, to trample on a too great expansion of sulphur with acids, [or] absorb superfluous watery particles with earthy matter.[37]

Despite the energies of its supporters, triturationism never became the dominant medical philosophy in the faculties. It put at risk too many professional livelihoods. Patients always preferred drugs to phlebotomy.[38] It also threatened the cosy, often familial relationship between many physicians and apothecaries. It was no coincidence that one of Hecquet's opponents in the Paris faculty was the academician, E.-F. Geoffroy (1672–1731), whose father and brother were both wealthy pharmacists.[39] The quarrel, moreover, quickly died down once the major protagonists on either side had departed, and professors in the mid-eighteenth century seem to have taught an eclectic medical philosophy that combined chemical and mechanist elements. This reflected a new belief that medical theory was an uncertain science and that prudence was the better part of valour.[40] By 1760 members of the Montpellier faculty were beginning to wonder whether the physical sciences were appropriate tools for the explanation of life at all. Influenced by Haller's work on irritability and German vitalists, Montpellier under Barthez became the centre of a new medical school that asserted that matter was sentient and self-moving.[41] Vitalist ideas seem to have been introduced to Montpellier by Boissier de Sauvages as early as the 1740s.[42] By the time that Barthez was promoted to his chair in 1760, they commanded general respect. Although the dissertations that Barthez himself sustained in the *concours* of that year made no overt vitalist references, this was not true of those of his competitors. One Pierre-Etienne Crassous, for instance, in examining the phenomenon of 'convulsive motion', declared that even such a minor physiological process as sternuation could never be wholly explained mechanically or chemically. Dusty particles on their own could not produce such a dramatic effect: they must somehow trigger a moving or sentient power in the nostrils.[43]

Vitalism, however, was very much the philosophical fad of the Montpellier faculty. Until the very end of the ancien régime it received little support elsewhere, especially in the north. Professors were highly unwilling to jettison the Cartesian idea that all matter was inert, at least as a guiding assumption if not a dogmatic fact. Even the concept of irritability as a distinctive and common organic property was slow to gain acceptance. As late as 1778, the idea was attacked in a dissertation at Caen sustained under the professor H. F. A. Roussel (1748–1812). *Pace* Haller, it was claimed, irritability and sensitivity were not separate phenomena. Experiments intended to demonstrate that insensitive tissues could be irritated were all flawed.[44] In the majority of faculties after 1760 the most common position was one of philosophical scepticism. Professors and their students evinced profound opposition to all forms of system-building. Medicine ceased to be seen as a rational, deductive science based on incontrovertible first principles, wherein the role of experiment and observation was the essentially rhetorical one of finding evidential support (however thin) for what were really biological stories.[45] Instead, medicine was perceived as the Baconian science par excellence, a corpus of knowledge defined, compiled and controlled by accumulated experience.[46]

This growth of medical scepticism, it should be stressed, did not lead to a new philosophical polarization within the medical professoriate. The vitalists were not system-builders in the manner of their iatrochemical and iatromechanical predecessors. Vitalism was an emotional conviction, more than a carefully worked-out logical philosophy.[47] Vitalists asserted that it was impossible to reduce life to a mechanism, but they could say little about the sentient force which they believed was present in organic matter. As much as the sceptics, they were interested in the promotion of a medical science based on observation and experiment. As the Caen student Jacques-François Denise made clear in 1786, the sentient powers of matter were only activated through the medium of investigable mechanical and chemical forces:

> This irritability, this organic *erectio*, this principle of life must never be confounded with mechanical forces. Nevertheless, while these are barriers by which it may not be attenuated, they are [the means] through which it is extended, grows and truly blossoms.[48]

In the final decades of the ancien régime, therefore, the concept of the science of medicine promoted in the faculties experienced a general, radical shift. Furthermore, this epistemological development had a profound effect on the way theoretical medicine came to be taught. In the first part of the century the five parts of the course – physiology, hygiene, semiology, pathology and therapeutics – had all been interconnected, held together by a common philosophical thread. In the last decades of the ancien régime each tended to become a discrete medical science.

As a result, physiology was reduced to an account (albeit sometimes critical) of the experimental discoveries of contemporary *mécaniciens* and chemists as they related to processes such as sensation and respiration. At Reims in 1787, for instance, the professor L.-H. Raussin presided over a thesis which discussed the mechanics and role of the lungs. In the thesis the candidate betrayed both a detailed knowledge of the work done on the connection between air and life since the time of Stephen Hales, and of the most recent developments in gas chemistry, citing in particular the discoveries of Priestley and Lavoisier.[49] The scope of a course in hygiene was similarly circumscribed, as it ceased to be the casual study of the non-naturals *tout court* and became principally an account of the relationship between disease and the environment, as this was gradually becoming understood through the work of the Société Royale de Médecine.[50] The content of semiology, in contrast, remained little changed but the course placed a much greater emphasis on the 'proper' (in the contemporary sense) classification and identification of diseases and provided for the first time a detailed account of their individual biological history. Throughout reference was made to the observational work of contemporary *clinici* who had perfected or rectified many of the received conclusions of the ancients. When the Paris student, C. N. Beauvais de Preau, discussed the character of puerperal fever in a dissertation in 1785 he particularly singled out for praise the observational work of British physicians, such as Thomas Denman, John Millar, Nathaniel Hulme, John Leake and Thomas Kirkland.[51]

The greatest changes occurred in the teaching of pathology and therapeutics. In studying the cause of disease, professors ceased to concentrate their attention on locating and relating the proximate (internal) and remote (external) cause of disease, and à la Morgagni focused on describing its seat in the body. Thus, according to Beauvais de Preau, autoptic evidence demonstrated conclusively that puerperal fever could be connected to an abdominal lesion. Victims of the disease 'exhibited a manifest milky congestion diffused through the abdominal cavity, by the presence of which the natural state and consistency of the solid parts of this organ are more or less altered'. What had caused the lesion, however, was a matter for pure speculation.[52] Such novel humility inevitably cut therapeutics adrift from pathology. Information about the seat of the disease could only provide limited assistance to the art of healing. Barthez for one was sceptical about its having any practical value:

> Practical anatomy is useful, but it has many inconveniences. Dissecting bodies only reveals the end point of the effects of the disease, and does not permit us to know the first lesions that it has produced. Indeed, often, it does not let us know the end point.[53]

Therapeutics, then, became primarily an empirical science. There had always been a tendency to accept the autonomy of experience in the art of healing, for doctors continually prescribed drugs whose action they found difficult to explain. Witness the difficulties the early eighteenth-century Caen iatrochemist, Jean-François Le Court, had in explaining the utility of cortex peruvianus in fever therapy. In his opinion fever was caused by an acid coagulation in the blood, but it was impossible to show that quinine was an alkali.[54] The dogmatists of the first part of the century, however, had always been embarrassed by their failure to attribute a rationale to successful therapies. After 1760 empirically-based healing became totally respectable. Courses on the treatment of particular diseases had little to say henceforth about the way a favoured remedy worked and concentrated instead on its application and likely effect. Thus François Broussonet at Montpellier in 1785 was quite candid in admitting his ignorance as to how mercury acted in the cure of venereal disease. As a good vitalist, he simply concluded that mercury rubs merely helped nature to help herself.[55] What interested Broussonet was the preparation of the patient and the methods of alleviating the worst effects of the treatment. He was unimpressed, for instance, with the introduction of gold leaf into the mouth to check a stubborn salivation.[56]

The professors, however, did not preach a laissez-faire empiricism. They lambasted the quacks and empirics who deployed drugs untested or without a properly conducted trial. Barthez wanted therapeutics to become a 'corpus of rationalized empirical knowledge' ('corps d'empiricisme raisonnée'). It might be impossible to know how a remedy worked, but by building up a store of case histories of its use, it was possible to predict the probabilities of success or failure. Medicine's problem was that its data-base was so small compared with, say, astronomy's. Physicians were too quick to hypothesize when the facts were lacking. As a result (and here Barthez revealed his Rousseauist credentials), 'savages, who have none of their faculties enfeebled by art [i.e., an inherited body of practical knowledge], have resources themselves which are natural and surer than ours'.[57] Admittedly, a rigorous empiricist therapeutics, on the other hand, would not necessarily guarantee success in every case. Ultimately recuperation depended on the vital principle in each individual. 'It happens that in the same circumstances, and the same illnesses, the principle of life makes up its mind in different ways.'[58] Nevertheless, Barthez was optimistic. Now that the new conception of therapeutics had been popularized, mankind was on the brink of a medical revolution (his term). Although French physicians had made no obvious contribution to the collection of data, this was not the case elsewhere. The true authors of this revolution, he told his audience, were John Huxham, Sir John Pringle and William Cullen in Britain (he said England); A. de Haen, A. Störck, S. T. Vogel and J. G. Zimmerman in Germany (and Austria); and M. Sarcone in Italy.[59]

IV

From what has been said above, the traditional conception of the faculty curriculum as antediluvian is clearly absurd. Rather, after 1760 the professors had embraced a conception of medical science which in major respects anticipated the philosophy propounded in the Paris school of the early nineteenth century as described by Ackerknecht.[60] Nor was the curriculum as narrowly theoretical as has always been supposed. By 1789 the leading faculties all offered regular practical courses in the ancillary medical sciences, and some had done so for a considerable time.[61] Professors at Montpellier were expected to perform four dissections each year as early as 1550, while by the late 1590s the faculty possessed specialist chairs in anatomy and botany and pharmacy and surgery. Other faculties, notably Paris, followed Montpellier's lead in the course of the seventeenth century, pre-empting by many decades the crown's decision of 1707 that courses in anatomy, botany and pharmacy (Galenic and chemical) were to become a standard part of the medical curriculum.[62] The major innovation of the eighteenth century lay in the foundation of independent courses in obstetrics and chemistry. The first course in obstetrics seems to have been founded at Strasbourg under J. J. Fried in 1728; others were later created at Paris in 1745 and at Reims and Montpellier in the 1780s.[63] On the eve of the Revolution seven faculties (Montpellier, Paris, Caen, Toulouse, Nancy, Reims, and Perpignan) offered students the opportunity of learning not only the art of preparing drugs but also the science of their chemical structure. Indeed, in the second half of the eighteenth century, in an age of growing therapeutic empiricism, chemistry came to be seen as the key to the reconstitution of a rational medical science. According to the royal letters-patent which established the Caen chair in 1757, without the aid of chemistry, 'medicine would see itself as perpetually enveloped in the deepest darkness of scepticism, and could explain neither the connection between medicaments and the maladies they destroyed, nor predict their effects'.[64]

It is possible that in the seventeenth century courses in the ancillary medical sciences were poorly attended and given little weight by professors and students. Unfortunately, there is no way of knowing, as records do not survive of attendance at individual courses. Towards the end of the ancien régime, however, it is quite clear that the practical courses were an integral part of the curriculum. In December 1773 the Toulouse faculty was the first in France to lay down a specific syllabus for its students to follow. In the first year they were expected to assist 'at anatomical, chemical and botanical demonstrations' ['aux démonstrations d'anatomie, de chimie et de botanique'] alongside attending lectures in physiology and hygiene. In the second, while studying pathology and therapeutics, they had to attend lectures on materia medica and then to take 'the treatise which will be dictated by the professor of surgery' ['le traité qui sera dicté par le professeur de chirurgie']. Materia medica and surgery also was a compulsory component of the third and final year's course.[65]

The quality of the teaching in these practical ancillary courses is difficult to gauge. Much, it must be admitted, depended on the resources of the individual faculty. A number of medical schools (and this included Strasbourg) only contained two or three professors, so that the expansion of the curriculum led to a heavier, and perhaps insuperable teaching load. François Lorry at Aix in the early eighteenth century was teaching three different courses concurrently: physiology, anatomy and pharmacy.[66] Only Paris and Montpellier were well endowed with chairs at the end of the ancien régime, having eight respectively. In the capital there were individual faculty professors in surgery (two), pharmacy, *matière médicale*, midwifery and chemistry.[67] However, even when individual chairs were established, the incumbents were not always paid. Robert Toussaint Deschamps (1750–1815), the first holder of the Caen chair of chemistry, was threatening to abandon his post in 1774 because he had not been paid for ten years.[68]

Another problem was dilapidated facilities. Even well-frequented faculties did not always have a sturdy, purpose-built anatomical theatre before the second half of the eighteenth century. Paris only had a purpose-built, stone amphitheatre from 1749 while the Toulouse faculty had to await a municipal benefaction in 1770.

Prior to this anatomies had taken place in the residential Collège de Périgord.[69] Moreover, cadavers were not always easy to obtain in an age when hospital administrators were unwilling to hand over the bodies of the poor for dissection. Even at Montpellier courses had to be sometimes suspended for lack of subjects.[70] Botanical gardens were another luxury. The Montpellier garden dated from 1593, but Caen only acquired one in 1718 and at least until 1765 it was maintained largely at the professor of botany's own expense.[71] Toulouse and Paris, on the other hand, never had a garden at all. In many provincial faculties, if professors of botany wanted to show their pupils living plants, then they had to organize periodic herborizations.

Despite these provisos, the impression remains that the situation was improving as the century progressed. Moreover, students in the chief medical faculties had other resources to fall back on if they found the official courses in the practical medical sciences inadequate. At Paris quality tuition in the ancillary medical sciences was given at the independent Collège Royal and the Jardin du Roi, where the chairs were staffed throughout the century by the country's leading anatomists, chemists and botanists.[72] Furthermore, alongside the official curriculum there was a network of private, supplementary courses that the assiduous could and did attend. The existence of a large number of private courses of anatomy and surgery in the capital in the eighteenth century has been well documented by historians. It has always been assumed, however, that these were given by surgeons like H. F. Le Dran (1685–1770), for the benefit of apprentice surgeons and foreign visitors who wanted to learn the latest surgical techniques from the Continent's most innovative operators.[73] Historians have failed to notice that from the middle of the century at least private courses in the ancillary medical sciences were also given by physicians and attended by medical students.

The number of private courses available in the capital towards the end of the ancien régime was legion. One particularly assiduous faculty student, Guillaume-François Laennec, followed perhaps as many as ten in the years 1769–72.[74] Their value for the medical student was obvious. Private courses in anatomy especially often gave the student the opportunity to perform dissections himself, something that the faculty courses certainly did not permit. Favoured students, too, could get to know the professors personally and benefit from their private conversation. The Avignon professor, Esprit Calvet (1728–1810), who took the private anatomy course of the physician, Antoine Petit (1718–94), in the early 1750s claimed that he had been able to talk with Petit for two hours a day, often privately in his cabinet.[75] Sometimes students could even board with the private teachers. Two Scottish medical graduates, who went to Paris in 1772, boarded with the recently appointed professor at the Collège Royal, Antoine Portal (1749–1832).[76]

The private courses in the capital were not just attended by students of the Paris faculty. Many like Calvet must have been graduates from provincial faculties who had received their initial medical training elsewhere and wanted to find out more about the ancillary sciences. Paris, however, was not the only centre of private medical teaching in the second half of the century. Many graduates, like Calvet again, must have been drawn, if only for economic reasons, to the similar, if less extensive, facilities offered by Montpellier.[77] The possibilities for extracurricular study in the latter town are made abundantly clear in the autobiography of Pierre-Joseph Amoreux, who studied in the faculty in the early 1760s. Amoreux was born in 1741, the son of Guillaume (1714–90), a physician at Beaucaire. Having studied his humanities and philosophy at a local Doctrinaire college, his father sent him to Montpellier in 1759. There he applied himself particularly to the study of anatomy. While following the faculty course given by Jean-François Imbert (1722–85), he also attended the private lessons of two surgeons, Joseph Sarrau (1727–83) and J. B. Laborie (1730–96).[78] 'There one saw increasingly [anatomical] objects, one touched them, one freely questioned the demonstrator.'[79] Leaving this course, he moved on to another private anatomy class given by a Montpellier physician, called Avézard, where he helped prepare anatomical specimens and performed several dissections with another pupil. 'Thus we ran through again all the parts of anatomy, scalpel in hand, and we were soon convinced that through dissection anatomy is learnt more accurately than through being a simple listener or spectator in an amphitheatre.'[80] Amoreux also had time to study privately other ancillary medical sciences. While at Montpellier he lodged with the physician, Pierre Cusson (1722–83), who acted as his tutor and introduced him to Linnaean botany. This proved the beginning of a lifetime's enthusiasm and Amoreux spent many hours on trips to the countryside with another Montpellier physician, Antoine Gouan (1733–1801).[81] Finally, he attended a private course in chemistry given by the professor Gabriel-François Venel in the amphitheatre of the pharmacist, Jacques Montet (1722–82).[82] Montpellier, however, did not exhaust Amoreux's interest in extracurricular tuition. After graduation he too journeyed to the capital, where he indulged in his passion for herborization with Bernard de Jussieu (1699–1777), professor at the Jardin du Roi, and attended courses in anatomy, obstetrics and 'maladies' in the amphitheatre of Antoine Petit.[83]

Medical graduates in the second half of the eighteenth century, then, had no excuse for neglecting the study of the practical ancillary medical sciences. On the other hand, at first sight it would seem (just as the reformers maintained) that there was little opportunity during their training for them to learn about and experience patient care: a vital lacuna. While a number of faculties outside France – notably Leiden, Edinburgh, Vienna and Pavia – pioneered the development of hospital-based patient study as a compulsory part of the curriculum, no French faculty followed suit.[84] A clinical chair was established at Strasbourg in 1756 under the influence of J. J. Sachs (1686–1762), but the Alsatian faculty, it must be stressed, was not, although well attended, a significant part of the system of French medical education. Most of the students there came from the German bank of the Rhine.[85]

However, even in this respect the situation was not as depressing as the critics claimed. In the first place, there was some move towards the study of patient care in the leading ancien-régime faculties. At Montpellier from 1634 bachelors and licentiates were supposed to make twice-monthly visits to the city's hospitals, while locally domiciled licentiates had to spend six months in the field before taking their doctorate. At Paris a similar requirement was laid down in 1696: bachelors and licentiates were expected thereafter to attend the faculty's twice-weekly out-patient clinic, and doctorands to serve a two-year practical apprenticeship, by either attending a hospital physician or accompanying a physician in private practice.[86] At Montpellier a further important development occurred in 1715 with the foundation of a chair 'for visiting and serving the poor' ['pour la visite et le service des pauvres']. Thereafter part of the official curriculum consisted of a course built around an out-patients' clinic. From 1769, moreover, the Languedocien faculty provided teaching visits for its students in the army's Hôpital de Saint-Louis, albeit an institution limited to patients with venereal and skin diseases.[87] Elsewhere, admittedly, official patient-based training of any kind was never evolved for students. There again several faculties on the eve of the Revolution had established chairs in a new discipline: *medicina practica*. Although little is known about the course that their incumbents offered, it is difficult to believe that it was built completely around hypothetical patients. There can be no doubt that the faculties considered this new course of crucial importance. According to the Toulouse statutes of 1773 the study of practical medicine was to be the fundamental component of the third and final year of the course.[88]

In the second place, even if there was little official training in patient care, it was not difficult for medical students to gain experience privately. Many 'apprenticed' themselves to hospital physicians or doctors in private practice during or after their studies. Pierre Amoreux began his training in patient care in his second year at Montpellier by accompanying the physician, Pierre Fournier (1703–66), on his visits to the Hôtel-Dieu (Saint-Eloi).[89] But it was only after graduation, as he confesses, that he really applied himself to bedside learning. For the next two years he continued attending the Hôtel-Dieu, while also following the physician, Jacques Farjon (1719–*an* IX), at the Miséricorde and assisting his father who had now moved to Montpellier from Beaucaire.[90] Of course, it could be argued that Amoreux was peculiarly privileged through his father's contacts and that his practical preparation for a medical career was exceptional. Nevertheless, there are many other examples of a similar, if less intensive cursus. Hospitals were legion in France (some 2,000) and many hospital physicians accepted paying *élèves*. Few Montpellier students may have enjoyed Amoreux's easy access to the city's Hôtel-Dieu, but many must have gained their medical spurs in the hospitals of other towns in the Midi. All that was required in an age of patronage was an effusive letter of recommendation from an established practitioner, like the one written by the Montélimar physician, Salamon, to his friend Calvet, on behalf of a Montpellier graduate, Joseph de Boissieu (called Bellegarde de Boissieu) in 1778. Calvet was the physician at the Avignon Hôpital de Sainte-Marthe and Bellegarde was seeking to become a paying *élève* there, drawn, if we believe Salamon, by Calvet's great celebrity.[91] Indeed, the existence of a working unofficial network of hospital instruction may well have retarded the development of official clinical courses. Hospital physicians in university towns who were not professors may well have felt their income threatened by the possible establishment of formal hospital instruction. The opposition of hospital authorities to hordes of students on the wards on the grounds that their presence would harm the patients is well documented.[92] It would be interesting to know how far the material fears of attendant physicians lay behind such concern.

The significance of private medical training in the hospitals of the ancien régime is not to be underestimated. On the eve of the Revolution, as is well known, two Paris hospital physicians, Louis Desbois de Rochefort (1750–86) and Jean-Nicolas Corvisart (1755–1821), established a clinical course for paying students at La Charité. This move has usually been seen as an attempt to provide for physicians the kind of practical facilities in hospitals already available for apprentice surgeons and to have been largely inspired by the clinical teaching at the hospice of the Paris Ecole de Chirurgie.[93] Once it has been established, however, that practical hospital training for physicians existed throughout the century, then the 'pioneering' efforts of the two Parisians, one of whom would later become a professor at the Revolutionary Paris Ecole de Santé, looks more like the formalization of a long-standing medical tradition.[94]

V

The one real weak link in the system of French medical education in the eighteenth century lay in the examination procedures. To practise medicine legally it was necessary to possess a doctorate from one of the country's medical faculties. In most cases, this was a relatively easy process. Under the provisions of the 1707 edict students had to have studied medicine in a faculty for three years (but not necessarily in the faculty in which the doctorate was sought), and then to have gained the degrees of bachelor and licentiate. These could be obtained merely after undergoing two viva-voce examinations before the faculty board and sustaining two public dissertations.[95] There was no question of students demonstrating any acquaintance with the practical ancillary sciences or patient care. Only two faculties – Paris and Montpellier – required evidence from all doctorands of practical knowledge.[96] As we have seen, both faculties expected their graduates to have some knowledge of patient care by the time they took the doctorate, and they also tested their students on their knowledge of the ancillary sciences. At Montpellier, students for the licence had to undergo a two-hour examination in practical therapy and from 1734 to perform three anatomical dissections. At Paris the demands were tougher still. From 1724 students had to sustain a dissertation on surgery, and from 1733 and 1735 they had to demonstrate their practical experience in anatomy and surgery in two week-long examinations on a cadaver.[97]

This discrepancy between Paris and Montpellier and faculties elsewhere would not have been so marked, had the majority of students both attended these two faculties and also graduated there. In fact, this was not the case. Probably at least 60 per cent of French physicians did train in the schools of Paris and Montpellier, but only 35–40 per cent actually took a degree there. The Paris faculty was particularly shunned. While welcoming some forty-five new students per year in the second half of the century, the faculty seldom bestowed ten doctorates per annum. Instead Paris students took their degrees in other faculties: Reims, Nancy, or sometimes Caen. The reason for this was financial. Paris doctorates were inordinately expensive (for reasons that will be explained below). On the eve of the French Revolution they may have cost as much as 7,000 livres, while other faculties (including Montpellier) charged only 3–500 livres. The faculty, then, which demanded the most of its graduates played hardly any part in assessing the capacity of prospective physicians.[98] Moreover, a number of faculties which specialized in graduating students were known to show little zeal even in testing their knowledge of theoretical medicine. Reims, where often twenty to thirty doctorates per annum were bestowed every year after 1750, was notorious for its venality. The university was continually the butt of satirical comment, including this epigram by the poet de Piis:

> For one hundred écus placed in a bowl,
> You are adopted on the right side as Cujas's child
> [a lawyer].
> But if by chance you went to the left,
> You would find yourself a physician.[99]

Nevertheless, before castigating the ancien-régime faculties too severely for their laxity in respect of examinations, several points need to be made in their defence. The corruption, although not to be dismissed altogether, should not be exaggerated. A study of the *academia peregrinatio* of French medical students suggests that those who did take medical degrees in venal faculties had usually studied elsewhere for the appropriate length of time.[100] Also, the sheer number of printed dissertations which survive from Reims emphasizes that if the Champagne faculty bestowed degrees regardless of the calibre of the candidate, there was at least one venal faculty where applicants still had to go through the motions.[101] Furthermore, the decision to graduate at an easy-going faculty was not a necessary sign of ignorance at the end of the ancien régime. Graduates of Reims included the botanist, Antoine-Laurent de Jussieu (1748–1836), for example.[102] Some candidates sought an easy path to the doctorate because they were insufficiently qualified in Latin, the language in which the examinations were supposed to be conducted. Thus, in 1765 Antoine Petit wrote to his old pupil Calvet, now professor at Avignon, asking his aid in the graduation of an unnamed surgeon. The surgeon was negotiating for a position as *médecin* in the royal household and needed a medical degree. Unfortunately, he only had attestations from Petit (i.e., he had attended the Paris doctor's private courses), was a poor Latin speaker, and had not got the time to get the proper qualifications. Petit assured Calvet that his client was a suitable candidate, who was too worthy to be a surgeon and deserved to be a physician.[103]

In addition, where faculties did uphold the demands of the 1707 decree and followed their own statutes, then the examination in theoretical medicine was quite challenging. Next to nothing is known about the way that the viva-voce examinations were conducted, but they were not mere charades. At Toulouse, according to the revision of the statutes in 1773, the examination for the baccalaureate lasted two hours at least and covered 'all the lessons that [the students] have taken during the entire course of their medical studies'. Students at Toulouse were also expected to undergo an examination of two hours in length at the end of each year.[104] Much more, on the other hand, can be said about the dissertations sustained as public *actes*. In the past the quality of student theses has been heavily criticized on the grounds that most were unoriginal, many were prepared with the help of the presiding professor, and not a few were copied from dissertations sustained in other faculties or at an earlier date.[105] All the comments are true. But the critics have missed the point. The theses were not dissertations in the modern sense of the word; nor were they dissertations of the kind sustained in the eighteenth century at Edinburgh and certain German faculties where students wrote a detailed account of a particular medical problem, often demonstrating at least some evidence of independent research.[106] Rather, they were merely a series of notes, drawn from the lecture-courses and private reading which served as the starting-point for a lengthy public debate.[107] For three to four hours, sometimes longer, a candidate had to hold his ground against the faculty board, fellow graduands and students.[108] The experience may not have helped create a good physician, but it certainly required stamina.

Finally, it must be realized that the doctorate was not always the final hurdle the aspirant physician had to leap. Doctors of medicine who wanted to set up in the most populous towns of France (and it was here that a living could be most easily made) had to become affiliated to one of the forty-odd medical colleges that had a monopoly of medical practice in the large cities.[109] Entrance to the colleges was largely determined by money and patronage. But the venal basis to the system was disguised, like the bases to so many other corporate monopolies in ancien-régime France, by the demand that the applicant demonstrate his capacity for the honour. By the second half of the eighteenth century this meant that candidates had to prove not only that they had studied at an approved faculty (usually Montpellier), but also that they had acquired a reasonable level of practical knowledge and experience. Thus, according to the statutes of the new college established at Nancy in 1752, nobody was to be admitted who had not spent three years exercising their profession in the countryside. In addition, candidates were to be examined for three hours on medical practice, *matière médicale*, chemistry, pharmacy and surgery.[110] The existence of the medical colleges explains the high cost of graduation and the level of competence demanded at Paris. Usually, a medical degree was not a passport to practise in the local faculty town. However, doctors of the Paris faculty were automatically members of the Paris college. A Paris degree then gave the graduate an entrée into the lucrative medical market of the capital. A similar situation pertained in certain other faculties, too, but elsewhere more than one kind of degree was given. At Reims, for instance, a candidate who wished to practise in the city took a special degree known as a *grand ordinaire*, which was both more demanding and more expensive.[111]

VI

Enough has been said thus far to demonstrate that the traditional picture of French medical education before the Revolution is a fiction, created in the first instance by the medical reformers of the last decades of the ancien régime. Once this is understood, it becomes possible in turn to read the polemic against the old medical faculties more sensitively. What is striking on closer acquaintance is that the rhetoric of disgust, properly attuned to the Manichean needs of late-Enlightenment and Revolutionary polemic, was never the only manner in which the educational provision of the ancien régime is discussed. Bisecting the narrative from time to time there was a more nuanced form of discourse which reveals that the authors were well aware that faculty education was not always inadequate. Thus Vicq d'Azyr ended the opening section to his programme in which he had castigated the existing medical system at length by begging the indulgence of his readers. In charting the abuses of the ancien régime, he had not meant to offend. There were some faculties (not named) where 'diverse teaching assignments may be usefully and faithfully carried out' ['divers enseignements soient utilement et fidèlement exécutés'], and where good doctors were formed. All was not darkness.[112]

It might be argued that such provisos were an essential part of the polemic. After all, unless it were possible somewhere and somehow to become a proficient doctor on the eve of the Revolution, the authoritative testimony of the reformers could be immediately called into question. They themselves were products of the ancien-régime faculties and had achieved the status of experts, deserving attention, because of their prominence within the profession whose training they derided.[113] The intrusion of a more restrained voice in the polemic, however, suggests that the real target of the reformers' ire was not faculty education *tout court* but its decentralized, inegalitarian, corporate features. As we have seen, it was relatively easy to acquire a solid theoretical and practical medical education if one attended the right faculty, invested in private courses, and had a patron who could open hospital doors. The medical reformers disliked the structureless informality of the system, which in their eyes ensured that only the wealthy gained a sound education.[114] Furthermore, they disliked the way in which a medical degree, even from a prestigious faculty like Montpellier, did not allow its holder to practise anywhere in France. Ideally, the ambitious physician would have liked to have practised in the capital, but Paris was closed to all but the rich and connected.[115] Medical colleges throughout the country could be just as exclusive. Sometimes it was not even possible to practise anywhere in a particular province unless a degree had been obtained from a local university.[116] The reformers wanted to end this complex web of privilege and localism and replace it by a uniform system of medical education, where the standard of teaching would be the same in each faculty/medical school, the opportunity for practical studies would be available to all, and a properly examined degree would be the only passport to medical practice.[117] Thereby the polemicists reveal themselves to be social revolutionaries rather than professional reformers. The system of medical education was judged inadequate because it was a part of ancien-régime society. The medical reformers belonged to that group of enlightened Frenchmen on the eve of the Revolution who wanted to take France by the scruff of its neck and create an open, meritocratic, unitary state. It was irrelevant whether or not the faculties had taken on board the new, empirically orientated conception of medicine or developed practical courses. The developments had all occurred within the context of the ancien-régime system and to doctrinaire egalitarians this was not enough. One suspects that reformers would have been just as incensed by the even more ad hoc method of medical instruction in the British Isles. What they wanted was to institutionalize the eighteenth-century developments in medical education within a new social context. The deficiencies in the existing system were exaggerated and pilloried as a way of proving to themselves and their audience that contemporary medical education was dangerous as well as unjust. In Enlightenment discourse the just and the useful were indistinguishable, so it was incumbent on all promoters of reform in the second half of the eighteenth century to demonstrate that institutions to which they morally objected were also corrupt.

If the reformers' programme was ultimately determined by a wider, egalitarian impulse, then the foundation of the *Ecoles de santé* in the Year III may be a less significant moment in the history of French medical teaching than has been traditionally thought. At least as far as the basic components of the medical curriculum were concerned, the establishment of what was to become the Paris school and its provincial sisters was not a new departure, the creation of a new type of medical education hitherto unknown in France. Rather, the new medical schools provided a medical education little different from that available before the Revolution to serious students. The eighteenth-century developments in medical training were merely formally incorporated within the faculty curriculum, so that (in theory at least) all students could gain a good knowledge of the ancillary medical sciences and practical patient care. The importance of the introduction of proper clinical courses in medicine and surgery is not to be underestimated, but the ancien-régime tradition of hospital training must not be forgotten. The only two apparently novel curricular subjects introduced in the Year III were medical jurisprudence and the history of medicine. As neither are subjects in which historians have shown interest, their course-content remains unexplored and their genuine novelty impossible to judge.[118]

In fact, what was undisputably revolutionary about the *Ecoles de santé* was not their curriculum, but the new conception of the role of a medical school that lay behind their inception. In the immediate term, the *écoles* were founded to supply deficiencies in the army medical corps; 600 *officiers de santé* had apparently died in the previous eighteen months.[119] But Fourcroy made clear that his intention was to create the best medical schools in Europe, which would be engaged in research as well as teaching. 'Their function is not to be limited to teaching what is known; they have as their further purpose the most extensive research into all the branches of the art of healing; [they have] as their aim the advancement of all the sciences which can shed light on the physics of life.'[120]

This requirement, actually stipulated in the Convention's decree, was completely novel. It suggested that a medical professorship was a full-time occupation and that a professor need not (perhaps even should not) be a medical practitioner.[121] It was the one innovation in the establishment of the *Ecoles de santé* which definitely gave birth to the Paris school as a distinctive medical enterprise. On the other hand, even this novel stipulation was perfectly in keeping with the general drift of the reform of medical education. Medical research in France was not suddenly born as a result of the creation of the *Ecoles de santé*. It was a long-established tradition, but one, like the system of medical education, which was unorganized and dependent on personal initiative. The Société Royale de Médecine certainly promoted research in medicine by offering a forum for publication in the 1780s but it scarcely gave research an institutional focus. Fourcroy, doubtless out of a Baconian belief in the value of state-run research institutes, aimed to bring a uniformity and coherence to medical research as well as to medical education. His goal was crudely nationalistic: 'French genius was to be commanded to surpass all the deeds in that branch of human knowledge, just as it already surpasses them in a great number of arts.'[122]

The most important innovation in the organization of medical teaching actually came in 1803 not 1794, when medicine was reconstituted as a profession and it was decided to join together under one institutional umbrella the formation of physicians and surgeons. This was something the reformers had called for on the grounds that the two professions were so mutually dependent that their traditional separation was ridiculous.[123] While recognizing that medical students might wish to specialize eventually in one or other discipline, it was decreed that henceforth the elite of the two professions should be trained together.[124] This decision clearly confirmed the eighteenth-century rise in status of the surgeon, but whether it should be viewed as a totally new departure is another question. It was not as if surgery was absent from the faculty curriculum in the eighteenth century. Nor had surgeons and physicians always been trained separately. In many faculties courses in surgery were attended by both apprentice surgeons and medical students, while Montpellier in 1728 had established a specialist and relatively popular doctorate in surgery, surely the precursor of the 1803 decree.[125] What had happened in the eighteenth century in effect was that the surgeons had sought to raise their status *vis-à-vis* the physicians by providing detailed formal instruction for their apprentices independent of the faculties: hence the establishment of the separate *Ecoles de chirurgie* in large towns. Whether these institutions provided better surgical instruction than the faculties is difficult to decide. Arguably they did, especially at Paris.[126] But it would be very wrong to see (as Gelfand does) the developments of 1794–1803 as the result of a *putsch* by the surgeons to take control of medical training *tout court* and impose the effective, practically orientated curriculum of the *écoles* in the place of the antedeluvian faculties. Rather the 1803 reform could be interpreted in an entirely different way. The medical reformers were all physicians and in their polemics they were just as cutting about the education of surgeons as of members of their own profession. Indeed, an essential plank in the programme was to improve the education of rural surgeons. To combine the training of the two professions, then, was to do surgeons as much of a favour as physicians, probably more. Nothing should be made of the fact that the Paris Ecole de Chirurgie became the location of the new Ecole de Santé. It was a recently erected, magnificent building of the kind needed to house the best medical school in France, but it was deemed inadequate as it stood. Fourcroy in announcing its appropriation was dismissive of its immediate utility: 'Despotism and vanity, which caused this monument to be erected, had not bothered to furnish it.'[127]

Yet if it can be argued that continuity not change was the keynote to the reform of medical education between 1794 and 1803, this need not detract from the importance of the new medical schools. It remains quite possible that the medical education purveyed by the new schools, while largely based on the pre-Revolutionary system, was still greatly superior (at least in terms of the Enlightenment ideal of a medical education).[128]

There are certainly several reasons for believing that there was an improvement in the standard of teaching. In the first place, lectures were more professionally delivered. Professors (appointed initially by nomination, subsequently by *concours*) were experts in their discipline; French became the normal language of the classroom; the *dictée* was abandoned in favour of a less ponderous form of presentation; and student understanding in lectures on theoretical medicine was aided by illustrative material. Thus, when Alphonse

Le Roy lectured on the physiological basis to a healthy mind and body in 1800, he did so in the manner of Hamlet, constantly addressing the five skulls on the table before him.[129] Also, the facilities for teaching practical medicine were greatly improved. Above all, now that cadavers were readily released from local hospitals, the courses in surgery and anatomy must have been far better regulated.[130]

Nevertheless, it is difficult to agree totally with Fourcroy's verdict in 1803 that 'the art of healing has never been taught with more care, nor in a more evolutionary and integral manner'.[131] However practically orientated the new curriculum might have been, it still remained the case that the official course offered little opportunity for hands-on experience. If a student wanted to gain a personal acquaintance with the art of dissection or surgical operations, he had to attend a private course just as before. Fortunate students could win a place at the newly formed Ecole pratique de dissection (opened in 1797).[132] But only forty places were on offer each year while the Paris school had 1000 students in 1800 and 2000 by 1820.[133] Most students then still had to pay to attend a private amphitheatre, like Poumiès de la Siboutie, studying in the capital in the 1810s.[134] Similarly, if a student wanted to become experienced in diagnosis and prescription he had generally to become an 'apprentice' to a practising physician.[135] Access to hospitals remained restricted. The wheels of patronage may have no longer controlled who was admitted to assist the resident physicians and surgeons, but entrance to the coveted extern- and internships (which were established in 1802) was by examination and the number of places was few. In 1812 – the year that Poumiès de la Siboutie gained an internship at the Salpêtrière – the Paris hospitals only offered eighteen such posts.[136] Few students, therefore, could have benefited from what was certainly an ideal form of practical training.[137]

The large numbers attending the Paris school – the result of the decision to establish only three *Ecoles de médecine* inside the 1789 boundaries of France and to educate physicians and surgeons together – also had a deleterious effect on the value to students of parts of the official course. Clinical study was supposed to be the centrepiece of the curriculum and students were intended to spend four months of each of the three years of the course attending a clinic. But it is difficult to believe that students gained a great deal from the experience when the numbers were so large and there were initially only three clinical professors.[138] By 1815 Chambon de Montaux, an erstwhile reformer, had no doubts that the teaching of clinical medicine (the flagship of the Paris faculty) was wholly inadequate:

> three clinical chairs are insufficient in France for the instruction of students; those to be found at Paris are too numerous to profit from the lessons. Even if few in number, they are crowded around each bed; [one day] some see the face of the patient [and] recognize the signs of the morbid complaint from the remarks of the professor; but the day after, they are kept away from the bedside by their peers, with the result that it is impossible to obtain a continual series of observations relating to one and the same disease, [which is so] necessary to gain a solid understanding.[139]

The vast numbers equally affected the structure of the examinations in the early nineteenth century. If there was now a uniform system of validation throughout the country, it was scarcely demanding. At the end of their three-year course students had to undergo five public viva-voce examinations (two in Latin) whose content matched the different parts of the official course. After this they had to sustain a thesis written in either Latin or French. Not surprisingly, given the number of graduates – some 300 per annum at Paris – the viva-voce examinations were rapidly concluded, lasting seldom more than fifteen minutes. If they had lasted longer then the twelve professors and their understudies would have been examining all year. The examinations were clearly little different in structure from those derided under the ancien régime. Noticeably, there was no practical element.[140]

The reality of the new medical schools was a long way from the vision of the reformers. Vicq d'Azyr had envisaged a course which would last six years rather than three and wherein students would have the opportunity to gain real hands-on experience.[141] He had also been anxious to ensure that medical graduates would be examined at length, calling for the total abolition of the traditional methods of verification and the establishment in their stead of a gruelling series of written examinations and practicals.[142] Had Vicq lived to see the Paris school, he would have been very disappointed. Indeed, in many respects the traditional system with its mixture of public and private courses and its provision for a rigorous examination of physicians who wished to practise in major towns was the better guarantor of Enlightenment medical standards. Doubtless by the mid-nineteenth century the post-Revolutionary system of medical education had improved manifold.[143] However, in its first decades, one might conclude that it deserves to be remembered more for its contribution to medical research than for the quality of its medical teaching.[144]

Admittedly, it is unjust to judge the Paris school simply in terms of the access that it provided to practical medical instruction. The concept of experiential learning is not unproblematic, whatever its champions in the eighteenth and early nineteenth centuries might have maintained. A just comparison between the practical tuition available in the Paris school and the ad hoc provision which existed before the Revolution must also take into account the underlying *raison d'être* for its promotion. The historian of medicine needs to know in what ways experiential learning was intended to relate to medical theory and how precisely a practical acquaintance with anatomy and bedside care was to aid the physician to diagnose and cure disease. It might be the case that the purpose of experiential learning was understood differently in the Paris school from the way it had been viewed in the eighteenth century. The medical reformers of the 1780s and early 1790s might indeed merely have wished to institutionalize the developments of the eighteenth century in such a way that access was more open and provision more certain. The professors and physicians who came to dominate the Paris school in the early nineteenth century, however, may have deployed the new institutions for practical tuition in a completely new way. There again, the reformers' failure to recognize the extent of practical tuition already available, may not just be a reflection of their egalitarianism but also of their disillusionment with the uses to which contemporary experiential learning were put.

Foucault and his followers would undoubtedly embrace the first hypothesis.[145] In his classic study of the Paris school, Foucault emphasized that its originality lay not in its stress on the importance of practical, even hospital-based, learning *per se*, but in its novel concept of the medical 'gaze'. Foucault accepted that clinical teaching existed before the Paris school, even if he understandably failed to grasp that ad hoc hospital tuition was widely available in pre-Revolutionary France. Nevertheless, he insisted that the eighteenth-century clinic was no more than a pedagogical tool, whereby physicians could demonstrate, after the event, the validity of the theoretical nosology taught in the classroom. The individual malady was merely viewed as an imperfect representation of an ideal disease-type. In the course of the Revolution, however, this demonstrative concept of experiential learning was replaced by an active and creative one, where knowledge and experience, professor and pupil, were not diametrically divided. As a result of the abolition of the faculties and the use of hospitals for ad hoc medical instruction, a new concept of the possibilities of experiential learning developed in the 1790s which was formalized in the Paris school. The clinic became an institution for the creation of knowledge, the individual malady in all its chaotic idiosyncracy came to be taken seriously, and pathological anatomy (the invisible made visible) came to be seen as the key to medical progress.[146]

Whether Foucault is correct in his delineation of the Paris school will become clearer in the following essays, as their authors compare and contrast the theoretical assumptions underpinning the work of a number of its leading figures: Alibert, Corvisart, Laennec, Broussais, and so on. As a result, it should become clearer, too, how far the professors of the Paris school were genuine medical revolutionaries or pygmies standing on the shoulders of eighteenth-century giants, such as Morgagni and Cullen. However, much more work will need to be done before we know the real relationship between the Paris school and its specifically French eighteenth-century antecedents. Gelfand's work on the development of French surgery is clearly a significant contribution, but it only explores one part of the story. Further, much-needed light will be thrown on the problem when Caroline Hannaway completes her study of dissection and anatomy teaching in pre-Revolutionary France, especially as her work is focused around the pivotal figure of Vicq d'Azyr.[147] Sadly, it seems unlikely that it will be possible to get beyond the activities of the leading proponents of experiential learning in the second half of the eighteenth century and obtain a rounded picture of the rationale of the plethora of private courses in the practical medicine. Few sets of course notes survive, and medical autobiographies or letters home only reveal the courses attended, not the content.[148] Information about bedside instruction is particularly difficult to find, so what eighteenth-century physicians taught their pupils to 'see' may never be known. Perhaps they merely instructed them in the right bedside manner and did not use patients as vehicles for instruction about disease at all.[149]

For these reasons, then, it is impossible at present to offer a complete account of French medical teaching in the eighteenth century before the 'age of the clinic', and assess its relationship with the Paris school. This essay has concluded that the chief ingredients of the Paris school were all in place before the Revolution, but this is obviously a conclusion based on a superficial exploration of the available tuition in practical medicine. Future research may well reveal that the claim is premature. On the other hand, the essay has definitely shown that eighteenth-century French medical education was far more vibrant and practically orientated (whatever that exactly meant) than has traditionally been thought. At the very least, it has made the assertion that the history of medical teaching before and after the Revolution was one of continuity rather than change – a plausible hypothesis worthy of further exploration.

Notes

1. The period also saw reform plans published in many other countries: e.g., Samuel Tissot, *Essai sur les moyens de perfectionner les études de médecine* (Lausanne, 1785); Johann P. Frank, *Plan d'école clinique ou méthode d'enseigner la pratique de la médecine dans un hôpital académique* (Vienna, 1790). Tissot's work was also published in Paris in 1785.
2. 'Nouveau Plan de constitution pour la médecine en France', in *Histoire et mémoires de la Société royale de médecine, 1787-1788*, vol. ix (Paris, 1790), 1-201. A number of other programmes are summarized, *ibid.*, pp. 157-71. The *Société Royale de Médecine*, founded in 1776, was a society of elite physicians patronized by the government and dedicated to the collection and organization of medical data: see esp. Caroline Hannaway, 'Medicine, Public Welfare and the State in Eighteenth-Century France: The Société Royale de Médecine de Paris (1776-1793)', Ph.D. dissertation, Johns Hopkins University, 1974. See also Caroline Hannaway, 'Caring for the Constitution: Medical Planning in Revolutionary France', *Transactions and Studies of the College of Physicians of Philadelphia* 14 (1992): 147-66.
3. In addition to Vicq d'Azyr's 'Plan', I have consulted: D. Diderot, 'Plan d'une université pour le gouvernement de la Russie' [1775-6], in *idem, Oeuvres complètes*, ed.,J. Azzézat, iii, 438-9, 497-505; G. C. Wurtz, *Mémoires sur l'établissement des écoles de médecine pratique à former dans les principaux hôpitaux civils de France à l'instar de celle de Vienne* (Paris, 1784); Dulaurens, *Essai sur les établissemens nécessaires et les moins dispendieux pour rendre le service des malades dans les hôpitaux vraiment utiles à l'humanité* (Paris, 1787); Nicolas Chambon de Montaux, *Moyens de rendre les hôpitaux plus utiles à la nation* (Paris, 1787); Antoine Petit, *Projet de réforme de l'exercice de la médecine en France* (Paris, 1791); Pinel, 'Mémoire' (1793), in D. B. Weiner, ed., and trans., *The Clinical Training of Doctors: An Essay of 1793* (Baltimore: Johns Hopkins University Press, 1980).
4. The number of medical faculties in France on the eve of the French Revolution will be discussed below.
5. 'Plan', 3. 'Que peut-on attendre, en effet, de quelques années d'étude,

qui se passent à dicter ou à lire des Prolégomènes de Médecine, uniquement formés de définitions & de divisions stériles? Que peut-on attendre d'Ecoles dans la pluspart desquelles on n'enseigne ni l'Anatomie complette de l'homme, ni l'art de dissection, ni la Botanique, ni la chimie médicale dans toutes son étendue, ni la Pharmacie, ni l'Art de formuler, ni la Nosologie, ni l'Histoire de la Médecine, ni la traité des maladies; où l'on ne dit pas un mot des fonctions publiques du Médecine; où nul encore n'a professé son Art près du lit des malades; & d'où l'on sort enfin sans avoir rien appris de ce qu'un Médecin practicien doit savoir?' The lack of assiduity of the professors supposedly reflected their recognition that the knowledge that they imparted was practically useless.

6. Diderot, 'Plan d'une université', 439. 'Un jeune médecin fait donc ses premiers essais sur nous, et ne devient un homme habile qu'à force d'assassinats.'
7. Chambon de Montaux was mayor of Paris, 1792-3.
8. For the Edict of Marly, see A.-J.-L. Jourdan, Decrusy and F. Isambert, eds, *Recueil général des anciennes lois françaises depuis 1420 jusqu'à la Révolution* (29 vols.; Paris, 1821-33), xx, 508-17. Many medical practitioners, of course, exercised the profession of physic illegally in the eighteenth century; this was particularly true of surgeons: see Matthew Ramsey, *Professional and Popular Medicine in France, 1770-1830: The Social World of Medical Practice* (Cambridge and New York: Cambridge University Press, 1988), ch.1.
9. A.-F. de Fourcroy, *Rapport et projet de décret sur l'établissement d'une Ecole centrale de santé à Paris* (Paris, Year III), pp. 5 and 9; speech delivered 7 Frimaire; on 14 Frimaire the Convention agreed to the foundation of three medical schools. See British Library, Dept. of Printed Books (hereafter BL), R 405, no. 16. 'Des prolégomènes chargés de définitions stériles en faisoient l'unique base. Les sciences physiques & exactes, seule source d'un enseignement solide, y étoient oubliées. ... Peu lire, beaucoup voir & beaucoup faire, telle sera la base du nouvel enseignement.' Fourcroy was a doctor of medicine of the Paris faculty but was never officially a doctor regent (for this distinction, see below, note 29), and was in bad odour with the faculty for belonging to the Société Royale. The faculty saw the Société as an interloper which was usurping its traditional role as the policeman of French medicine and the medical profession: see Hannaway, 'Medicine, Public Welfare and the State', ch. 7.
10. A.-F. de Fourcroy, 'Exposé des motifs du projet de loi sur l'exercice de la médecine' (1803), in *Recueil des loix et règlements concernant l'instruction publique, depuis l'édit de Henri IV en 1598 jusqu'à ce jour.*

Publié par ordre de son Excellence le Grand-Maître de l'université de France (8 vols.; Paris, 1814-27), ii, 349. '... [L]e titre de docteur conféré à des absens, et des lettres de réception envoyées par la poste.'
11. L. Liard, *L'Enseignement supérieur en France 1789-1889* (2 vols.; Paris, 1888-94), i, 75-82; Erwin H. Ackerknecht, *Medicine at the Paris Hospital, 1794-1848* (Baltimore: Johns Hopkins Press, 1967), ch. 1.
12. Jacques Léonard, *Les Médecins de l'ouest au XIXe siècle* (3 vols.; Lille, 1978), i, 132-5. 'Galen et Hippocrate passent pour infallible'. See also the particularly caustic remarks in David M. Vess, *Medical Revolution in France, 1789-1796* (Gainesville, Florida: University Presses of Florida, 1975).
13. Paul Delaunay, *Le Monde médical parisien au dix-huitième siècle* (Paris: Librairie Jules Rousset, 1906), esp. ch. 1. The picture remains unaltered in Charles Coury, 'The Teaching of Medicine in France from the Beginning of the Seventeenth Century', in C. D. O'Malley, ed., *The History of Medical Education* (Los Angeles: University of California Press, 1970), 121-73 (particularly the concluding remarks).
14. Esp. Toby Gelfand, *Professionalizing Modern Medicine. Paris Surgeons and Medical Science and Institutions in the Eighteenth Century* (Westport, Conn.: Greenwood Press, 1980). Gelfand's work, it must be said, is an outstanding contribution to our understanding of the development of surgical medicine.
15. The best introduction to the Revolutionaries' mentality is François Furet, *Pensée la Révolution française* (Paris, 1978), pt. ii, ch. 3. In important respects Manicheanism was also a characteristic of Enlightenment thinking in eighteenth-century France.
16. Least useful are faculty statutes, for these were revised so seldom and often provide little detail about the curriculum and examinations. A reliance on the statutes is the fundamental weakness of A. Finot, *Les Facultés de médecine de province avant la Révolution* (Paris, 1958). The only faculty whose history has been carefully, if not always critically, studied in recent years is Montpellier thanks to the efforts of Louis Dulieu: see esp. his *La Médecine à Montpellier: L'Age classique* (2 vols.; Avignon, 1973).
17. This paper refines and develops earlier accounts of French eighteenth-century medical education: see L. W. B. Brockliss, *French Higher Education in the Seventeenth and Eighteenth Centuries: A Cultural History* (Oxford: Oxford University Press, 1987), ch. 8; and *idem*, 'L'Enseignement médical et la Révolution: Essai de réévaluation', in D. Julia, *Les Enfants de la Patrie: Education et enseignement sous la Révolution française*, spec. no. of *Histoire de*

l'Education 42 (1989), 79-110.
18. Othmar Keel, 'The Politics of Health and the Institutionalization of Clinical Practices in Europe in the Second Half of the Eighteenth Century', in W. F. Bynum and Roy Porter, eds, *William Hunter and the Eighteenth-Century Medical World* (Cambridge: Cambridge University Press, 1985), 207-56.
19. Colin Jones, 'Montpellier Medical Students and the Medicalization of Eighteenth-Century France', in Roy Porter and Andrew Wear, eds, *Problems and Methods in the History of Medicine* (London, 1987), 67-69. At Montpellier student complaints were articulated through elected councillors. Basic biographical information about Chicoyneau, Boissier de Sauvages, and other Montpellier professors and physicians mentioned below can generally be found in Dulieu, *La Médecine à Montpellier*, ii, *sub nomine*.
20. E.g., Gabriel-François Venel (1723-75), professor at Montpellier from 1759, was continually on the move in the 1760s preparing a report for the Académie des Sciences on French mineral waters.
21. Paul-Joseph Barthez was a Montpellier professor from 1761 to1793. He never taught at all after 1781.
22. In the context of the study of the education of physicians in pre-Revolutionary France, Strasbourg, although well attended, is of little importance for reasons that will be explained below.
23. Brockliss, *French Higher Education*, 13-19; Dominique Julia and Jacques Revel, 'Les Etudiants et leurs études dans la France moderne', in *idem*, *Les Universités européennes du XVIe au XVIIIe siècle: Histoire sociale des populations étudiantes*, vol. II (Paris, 1989), 260-4. Information about matriculands is missing for a number of medical faculties in the 18th century but there can be no doubt which were the leading five in terms of the annual number of students registering for the first time. An account of geographical recruitment is given on pp. 327-35.
24. There were c. 500 medical students in France in 1789: see R. Chartier, M. M. Compère and D. Julia, *L'Education en France du XVIe au XVIIIe siècle* (Paris, 1975), 274. Julia and Revel, 'Les Etudiants', 291, suggests c. 160 doctorates in medicine each year.
25. E.g., professors at Reims were placed on the nobles' *vingtième* role.
26. In the case of Montpellier many of the dissertations candidates sustained as part of the *concours* have survived.
27. The *concours* system was subverted to a certain extent at Montpellier through the habit of appointing a *survivancier* to chairs held by permanent absentees. Boissier de Sauvages was a beneficiary of this system of patronage when appointed to his first faculty post in 1734.

28. Unfortunately nothing is known about the way candidates to French chairs were ultimately selected. At Edinburgh professors were appointed by the Town Council. Some professors who inherited their posts, such as Alexander Monro III, were notoriously bad teachers: see Lisa Rosner, *Medical Education in the Age of Improvement: Edinburgh Students and Apprentices 1760-1826* (Edinburgh: Edinburgh University Press, 1991), 59.
29. Some one hundred in number. Paris doctors only became doctors regent and eligible to enjoy the benefits of faculty membership after a probationary period and a specific faculty vote.
30. On the other hand, the evidence from the faculty minutes recording professorial elections suggests that doctors regent seldom served twice. See Bibliothèque de la Faculté de Médecine, Paris (hereafter BMP), MS 17-24: elections were held at the beginning of the academic year; the minutes have been published in part: see G. Steinheil, ed., *Commentaires de la Faculté de Médecine de Paris, 1777 à 1786* (2 vols.; Paris, 1903). One Paris chair was permanent.
31. This system was universal but outside France the teaching in other faculties could be more informal: cf. the situation at Edinburgh described in Rosner, *Medical Education*, ch. 3. When the Austrian government promulgated new statutes for the University of Louvain in 1788, it was specifically laid down that one day a week should be spent on interrogating the students: see 'Directio pro facultate medica ... 30 Septembris 1788 praescripta', in Jean Molanus, *Les Quatorze livres sur l'histoire de la ville de Louvain*, ed., P. F. X. de Ram, pt. ii (Brussels, 1861), 1085.
32. The most original courses were probably given by professors of medicine attached to the Paris Collège Royal. This was not part of the University of Paris but an independent institution founded by Francis I in the 1530s. Anyone could attend the lectures. These were sometimes highly informal. Cf. the comments on the teaching of the physician, Jean Astruc (1684-1766), in J. Astruc, *Mémoires pour servir à l'histoire de la faculté de médecine de Montpellier*, ed., Lorry (Paris, 1766), p. xliv (from the editor's *éloge* of Astruc). The standard history of the Collège Royal is still Abel Lefranc, *Histoire du Collège de France* (Paris, 1893).
33. Comte Chaptal, *Mes souvenirs*, ed., A. Chaptal (Paris, 1893), 15.
34. In writing this section I have used student notebooks, professorial *cahiers*, and student dissertations composed as part of their examination for the doctorate: see below, sect. v. Student dissertations survive in abundance and are a particularly good source for the study of developments in faculty teaching. I have used collections from Paris,

Montpellier, Caen, Reims, Toulouse and Angers. Collections also exist for Strasbourg but these have not been consulted for the reason cited above. The collections I have chiefly used are Bibliothèque de la Faculté de Médecine, Paris, *Theses medicae Parisiensis* (hereafter TMP), 9 vols. in fo., and 16 vols. in 4o; Bibliothèque de la Faculté de Médecine, Montpellier (hereafter BFMM), nos. 275005 (6 vols.), and 275010 (6 vols.); Bibliothèque Municipale (hereafter BM) Reims, no. CRII MM 725 (6 vols.); Archives Départmentales (hereafter AD) Calvados [Caen], 1D 986-9, 991, 996; Archives Municipales Toulouse, GG 844; AD Maine-et-Loire [Angers], 4D 9.

35. A. Deidier, *Institutiones medicinae theoricae, physiologiam et pathologiam complectentes* (Paris, 1731). Cf. also the undated MS course of his colleague, Pierre Chirac (1650-1732): BM Montpellier, MS 213, 'Institutiones medicarum tentamen primum phisiologicumm seu de hominis oeconomia'.

36. See L. W. B. Brockliss, 'The Medico-Religious Universe of an Early Eighteenth-Century Parisian Doctor: the Case of Philippe Hecquet', in Roger French and Andrew Wear, eds, *The Medical Revolution of the Seventeenth Century* (Cambridge: Cambridge University Press, 1989), esp. 196-201.

37. J. B. Ravix Dumas, 'An nova de fluidorum et solidorum, vi mutua et reciproca hypothesis, excludens fermentationes, secretiones, etc, sit oeconomiae animali magna congrua, et tam in theoria quam in praxi medica utilis magis? Negativus.' Student dissertation, Avignon, Aug. 1726: see BL, 1180 b. 11 (7). 'Inutiles sunt, inquiunt, fere semper purgationes et noxia vomitoria et utiles longe frequentes venae sectiones quia unice consulendum est elateri solidorum et per accidens tantum motus fluidorum a praedicto elatere primario producto[.] Absurdum est salinam sanguinis constitutionem diluentibus caeterisque opportunis remediis debellare, sulphurea nimis expansa acidis depromere[, aut] superfluas aqueas particulas terrenis absorbere.'

38. Iatromechanical therapeutics became the butt of contemporary satirists. Hecquet was satirized in Le Sage's *Gil Blas* as the bloodthirsty doctor Sangrado.

39. Geoffroy's iatrochemical allegiance was made clear in the theses that he sustained for his doctorate : TMP in fo. IX, no. 1569a: 'An omnis morbus a coagulatione?' (1703).

40. E.g., the eclectic views on chilification expressed by a student at Caen in 1751 under the presidency of Jean-Guillaume de Mortreux: Bibliothèque de l'Arsenal, Paris, MS 824, fos. 241-3, Jacques Postel, 'Theses ex physiologia selectae'.

41. See esp. Bernard J. Gottlieb, 'Bedeutung und Auswirkungen des

Hallischen Professors ... Georg Ernst Stahl auf den Vitalismus des 18. Jahrhunderts insbesondere auf die Schule von Montpellier', *Nova Acta Leopoldina*, 12: 89 (1943), 470-87.

Barthez's complex medical philosophy is best approached through J. Lordat, *Exposition de la doctrine médicale de P. J. Barthez et mémoires sur la vie de ce médecin* (Paris, 1815). The best account of vitalism to date is contained in F. Duchesneau, *La Physiologie des lumières: empiricisme, modèles et théories* (The Hague, 1982).

42. Elizabeth Haigh, *Xavier Bichat and the Medical Theory of the Eighteenth Century*, Medical History Supplement no. 4 (London, 1984), 28-31. The first publication in which Sauvages displayed his vitalist sympathies only appeared in 1760, when he presided over the student dissertation of one J.-J. Dupont, entitled: 'De animae imperio in cor', BFMM, 275005, vol. ii, no. 2.
43. P.-E. Crassous, 'Nam motus convulsi sympathici, ut sternutatio, ex sola vi a stimulationibus impressa, sine potentiae sentientis et moventis concursu possent intelligi?' [Negative], in *idem, Quaestiones medicae 12*, 24-6 July 1760 (Montpellier, 1760), Q. 8, pp. 18-20.
44. AD Calvados, 1D 987, no. 13, F. V. Morin, 'An a nervis irritibilitas fibrae muscularis?' [Positive]. Morin was Paris-trained.
45. The idea that theoretical medicine in France before 1760 was little more than story-telling owes much to the argument in Andrew Wear, 'Medical Practice in Late Seventeenth and Early Eighteenth Century England', in French and Wear, eds, *Medical Revolution*, 294-320. Admittedly, the philosophical dogmatists did stress the role of experience. Thus J. B. Callard de La Ducquerie of Caen in 1696 declared that anatomy 'est enim totius medicinae basis et stabilimentum. Facem aliquam recte dixeris, cuius liminibus, in cognitionem morbis ou partis affectae deducimur'. BM Caen, MS 114, 'De anatome', p. 135.
46. I use the term 'Baconian' in the classic nineteenth-century sense. Eighteenth-century French *philosophes* did not specifically identify experientially-based science with Bacon, although his name was continually used as a totem of modernity: see M. Malherbe, 'Bacon, l'*Encyclopédie* et la Révolution', *Etudes philosophiques* (1985), 387-454.
47. This judgement may seem harsh. A more positive reading of French vitalism is contained in the forthcoming book of Roselyne Rey, to appear in *Studies on Voltaire and the Eighteenth Century*.
48. J.-F. Denise, 'An detectus ab Harvaeo sanguinis circuitus ad medicinae progressus fecerit?' [Negative], AD Calvados 1D 996, fos. 351-7. 'Neque haec irritibalitas, haec *organice* erectio, haec vis vitae cum potentiis mechanice umquam confudenda, quae, nedum verum

harum obicibus imminuatur, his e contra intenditur, increscit et revera germinatur.' The thesis is not obscurantist. Denise attacks the sufficiency of mechanist theories and praises the ancients for their reliance on observation. 'Quam longe praecellat pulchra, si ita loqui fas est, veterum ignorantia, sola observatione sincera, sola edocturum natura.'

49. BM Reims, CR II MM 725/5-6, no. 36, Pierre Antoine Petit, 'An respirationis et combustionis, eaedem causae, eadem phoenomena' [Positive]. Accounts of sensation dealt with the nature of nervous motion: was it a mechanical or was it an electrical phenomenon?
50. There was also an interest in diseases peculiar to children, the old and women.
51. 'An congestioni abdominali lacteae puerperarum acutae, vulgo febris puerperalis, dictae ipecacuanhae?' [Positive], BFMM 275010, vol. vi, no. 42. All the British physicians cited had published works on puerperal fever (sometimes in a general study of practical medicine).
52. *Ibid.*, '... congestionem manifesto lacteam, in abdominis cavitate propria diffusam, exhibeant, ex cujus praesentia, solidarum huius organi partium naturalis status et consistentia plus minus-ve alterantur'. The first Paris dissertation to claim that the physician need only know the internal site of the disease was sustained in 1776: see TMP in 4o, xvi, no. 96, F. de la Planche, 'An a sola observatione sympathiae doctrina' (p. 16).
53. BM Montpellier, MS 256, Barthez, 'cours de thérapeutique', no date, fo. 9 [no accents]: 'L'anatomie pratique est utile, mais elle a beaucoup d'inconveniens. L'ouverture des cadavres ne demontre que le dernier terme des effets de la maladie, a laquelle nous devions nous opposer, et ne nous fait pas connoitre les premieres laesion qu'elle a faites. Souvent meme, elle ne nous en fait pas connoitre le dernier terme.' Similar worries about the value of pathological anatomy were raised as early as 1760 by the Montpellier graduate Pierre Vigarous in the *concours* of that year: see *Quaestiones medicae 12*, 21-3 Aug. (Montpellier, 1760), Q. 7, 'An theoriae, an vero praxi medicae utiliores sint notiones anatomicae' (pp. 4-5) [BL, T 162 (8)]. In this and other quotations in French, cited below, the original orthography has been retained.
54. BM Caen, MS 476, 'Tractatus de febribus', no date, esp. p. 109. Le Court remained committed to the Galenic theory of curing by opposites.
55. BM Montpellier, MS 257, pt. vii, Broussonet, 'Tract. de morbis venereis', 1785, fos. 479-81. Broussonet had gained a chair at Montpellier in 1778.

56. *Idem*, fo. 494. The gold leaf was supposed to attract the mercury.
57. BM Montpellier, MS 256, fos. 12-16. '[L]es sauvages qui n'ayant aucune de leurs facultés affoiblies par l'art, ont eux-mêmes des resources naturelles et plus sures que les notres.'
58. *Ibid.*, fo. 23. 'Il arrive que dans les mesmes circonstances, et les mesmes maladies, le principe de la vie prend des determinations differentes.'
59. *Ibid.*, fos. 24-5.
60. Ackerknecht, *Medicine at the Paris Hospital*, esp. the sect. on therapeutics.
61. Details in Brockliss, *French Higher Education*, 392-5.
62. Edict of Marly (art. 22): see above, note 8. Many of these courses were also attended by surgeons and apothecaries.
63. These courses were for midwives, too.
64. Archives Nationales (hereafter AN), M 196, no. 71/7, letters-patent, 14 May 1765. '[L]a medecine se verroit aussi perpetuellement environnée de tenebres les [plus] profondes du s[c]epticisme, et ne pourrait expliquer ni le rapport des medicamens avec les maux qu'ils detruisait ni en prédire les effets.'
65. Doc. published in J. Barbot, *Les Chroniques de la faculté de médecine de Toulouse du XIIIe au XIXe siècle* (2 vols.; Toulouse, 1905), i, 270-2.
66. See Vicq d'Azyr, *Oeuvres*, sub Lorry, *éloge*. Of course Boerhaave also taught a number of courses at the same time at Leiden, so the quality of teaching need not necessarily have suffered.
67. A useful source for the number of chairs in the different faculties in 1789 is M. A. Baras, *L'Etat actuel des établissements destinés en Europe à l'instruction pratique et au progrès des connaissances humaines* (2 vols.; Paris, 1793), vol. ii, *sub département*. Dates of the foundation of separate chairs are given (fairly accurately) in Finot, *Les Facultés de médecine*.
68. AN M 196, no. 71/6, letter 23 Nov. 1774.
69. Barbot, i, 208, 275-82; J.-A. Hazon, *Eloge historique de la faculté de médecine* 16 Oct. 1770 (Paris, 1773), 63-64.
70. Chaptal, *Mémoires*, 16-17. Faculties generally relied on the bodies of executed felons. Obtaining female cadavers was particularly difficult.
71. A. Germain, *L'Ecole de médecine de Montpellier: ses origines, sa constitution, son enseignement* (Montpellier, 1880), 76-8; AD Calvados, 1D 963, no. 1 (gen. account of the Caen garden); AN M 196, no. 69: letter of 16 March 1765 by the professor, Charles-Nicolas Desmoueux (1728-1801): this, of course, was typical of the ancien régime where all office-holders were expected to finance their own office to a degree.

72. See esp. Y. Laissus, 'Le Jardin du Roi', in René Taton, ed., *L'Enseignement et diffusion des sciences au dix-huitième siècle* (Paris: Hermann, 1963), 287-341. For the Collège Royal, see above, note 32. Quality tuition in the surgical sciences was also given at the Ecole de Chirurgie, founded in the 1720s: details in Gelfand, *Professionalizing Modern Medicine*, ch. 5. Foreign medical students definitely attended lectures there, but it is doubtful that many French students did so. The Ecole de Chirurgie was set up by the Paris *communauté des chirurgiens* in defiance of the Paris faculty that believed that surgical education should be in its own hands.

73. There are many extant accounts of these private surgical courses in the first half of the century in the diaries of travellers: e.g. esp. *Johann Gessners Pariser Tagebuch 1727*, ed., U. Boschung (Berne, 1985).

74. A. Rouxeau, *Un étudiant en médecine quimpérois (Guillaume-François Laennec) aux derniers jours de l'ancien régime* (Nantes, 1926), chs. 2-6. Laennec also attended courses at the Jardin du Roi and the Collège Royal.

75. BM Avignon, MS 2349, fos. 113-23: Calvet to Petit, 16 March 1785. Petit in the third quarter of the century regularly gave private courses in anatomy, surgery, *matière médicale*, and surgical intervention: see the *annonces* in TMP, ix in fo., nos. 122-4. Laennec attended his courses in anatomy and obstetrics; Petit did not offer students the chance to practise themselves: see Rouxeau, *Un étudiant*, 38, 50.

76. Benjamin Bell, *The Life, Character and Writings of Benjamin Bell* (Edinburgh, 1868). The physician, Portal, gave private anatomy courses in the 1770s: see Rouxeau, *Un étudiant*, 37. He was Montpellier-trained and never became a member of the Paris faculty.

77. Joseph Guerin, *Vie d'Esprit Calvet* (Avignon, 1825), 13. Calvet graduated at Avignon in 1745 and then went to Montpellier to study *int. al.* under Sauvages. There were also private courses given at Strasbourg: see R. Steegmann, 'Le Milieu médical à Strasbourg au XVIIIe siècle' (Master's dissertation, University of Strasbourg II, 1977), 180 *et seq.* As has been pointed out, however, Strasbourg was not part of the French system of medical education.

78. Both were professors at the independent Montpellier *école de chirurgie*, founded in 1741: see L. Dulieu, *La Chirurgie à Montpellier: De ses origines au début du XIXe siècle* (Avignon, 1975), 110-27; the second half of this work is a biographical dictionary.

79. BM Avignon, MS 1269, p. 24. 'La on voyait de plus en plus les objets, on les touchoit, on questionnoit librement le démonstrateur.' The autobiography remains unedited.

80. *Ibid.*, 25-26. 'Nous repassâmes ainsi toutes les parties de l'anatomie le scalpel à la main et nous fûmes bientôt convaincus que par la dissection, on apprend l'anatomie plus exactement qu'en étant un simple auditeur or spectateur dans un ampithéâtre.'
81. Neither Cusson nor Gouan were ever permanent faculty professors during the ancien régime, although both acted on occasion as substitutes for absentees.
82. BM Avignon, MS 1269, pp. 23, 27, 29-30. Biog. details on Montet in L. Dulieu, *La Pharmacie à Montpellier de ses origines à nos jours* (Avignon, 1973), 266-68.
83. BM Avignon, MS 1269, pp. 32-38.
84. The best study of clinical training in the eighteenth century is Guenter Risse, *Hospital Life in Enlightenment Scotland* (Cambridge: Cambridge University Press, 1986), ch. 5. Also, for Pavia, see Antoinette Emch-Deriaz, *Tissot: Physician of the Enlightenment* (New York: Lang, 1992).
85. E. Wickersheimer, 'La clinique de l'hôpital de Strasbourg au XVIIIe siècle', *Archives internationales de l'histoire des sciences*, 16 (1963), 253-76. For the geographical origin of the faculty's recruitment, see G. Knod (ed.), *Matrikeln der Universität Strassburg (1621-1793)*, vol. II: *Die Matrikeln der medicinischen und juristischen Fakultät* (Strasbourg, 1897).
86. See Brockliss, *French Higher Education*, 395.
87. Dulieu, *La Médecine à Montpellier*, i, 15-27, 549-54; Jones, 'Montpellier medical students', 70. Saint-Louis had an eventual capacity of 180 beds.
88. Barbot, *La Faculté de médecine de Toulouse*, i, 270; for the foundation of the chair at Toulouse, *ibid.*, 265-9. At Caen in the late 1780s, the professor of practical medicine, J.-P. Chibourg (1725-1806), was also significantly the hospital physician: information from collections of Caen dissertations cited in note 34 above.
89. This was the principal hospital of the town, catering for 2-300 inmates.
90. BM Avignon, MS 1269, pp. 32, 34. The Miséricorde, also known as the Hôpital-Général, was the third Montpellier hospital (founded in 1687).
91. BM Avignon, MS 1050, fo. 714, Salamon to Calvet, 22 Jan. 1778. Bellegarde took his Montpellier doctorate in 1779.
92. E.g., Colin Jones, *Charity and 'Bienfaisance': The Treatment of the Poor in the Montpellier Region, 1740-1815* (Cambridge: Cambridge University Press, 1982), 124-8; Dulieu, *La Médecine à Montpellier*, ii, 746, 774. Imbert had attempted to get clinical teaching set up at the Montpellier Hôtel-Dieu in 1760 and 1774 but on both occasions he

had been defeated by the administration.
93. Notably Gelfand, *Professionalizing Modern Medicine*, esp. 144-5.
94. The medical reformer, Nicolas Chambon de Montaux (1748-1828) also seems to have been giving formal clinical instruction at the Paris hospital of La Salpetrière on the eve of the Revolution: see BFMP MS 5143, 'Remarques sur le mode de l'enseignement clinique' (nd), fo. 8v, separately foliated memo.
95. Edict of Marly: see note 8 above.
96. As will be explained below, some faculties did demand proof of practical expertise from doctorands who wished specifically to set up practice in the local town.
97. See Brockliss, *French Higher Education*, 74-75. The examinations in theoretical medicine were also harder in these two faculties.
98. Details in Revel and Julia, 'Les Etudiants de médecine', 260-81, and tables 460-86. Slightly different figures for the cost of a Paris degree are given in L. W. B. Brockliss, 'Patterns of Attendance at the University of Paris, 1400–1800', *Historical Journal*, 21: 3 (1978), 530. G.-F. Laennec took his degree at Montpellier which (as he recognized) was peculiar for a Paris student: see Rouxeau, *Un étudiant*, 58-59, 73-74, 86.
99. Quoted in O. Guelliot, *La Fin de la faculté de médecine de Reims* (Reims, 1909), 31.

'Moyennant cent écus dans un bassin,
Comme enfant de Cujas à droite on vous embauche.
Mais par hazard, si l'on donnait à gauche
On se trouverait médecin.'

This was why so many (often over half) of the graduates were students from the British Isles (mainly Irish) looking for a cheap and speedy qualification before they returned home. I have engaged in a study of English-speaking medical graduates from Reims.
100. Revel and Julia, 'Les Etudiants', 267-8, a study of Avignon graduates.
101. Cf. the collection cited in note 34 above.
102. Jussieu had a Paris MA. His bachelor's dissertation in 1769, 'An generatio naturae arcano', survives: see BM Reims, CR II MM 725, ii, no. 56.
103. BM Avignon, MS 2353, fos. 197-8, Petit to Calvet, 10 Oct. 1765. Petit claimed to write in ignorance as to whether Avignon did grant speedy degrees.
104. Barbot, *La Faculté de médecine de Toulouse*, i, 270: '... toutes les leçons qu'ils auront prises pendant le cours entiers de leurs études de médecine'. At Besançon the viva consisted of a half-hour discourse

followed by a question-and-answer session: see BM Avignon, MS 2825, fos. 33-41, letter from the Besançon faculty on its graduation procedures, 1749.
105. E.g., F. Gidon, 'Des thèses de l'ancienne faculté de médecine de Caen 1659-1740', *Bulletin de la Société de l'histoire de médecine* (1952), 21-40; O. Guelliot, 'Les Thèses de l'ancienne faculté de médecine de Reims', *Travaux de l'Académie de Reims*, 81 (1970), 198-263; N. Le Grand, *La Collection des thèses de l'ancienne faculté de médecine [de Paris] depuis 1539 et son catalogue inédit jusqu'en 1793* (Paris, 1913).
106. See Rosner, *Medical Education*, 72-8. Edinburgh theses were 20 to 50 pages long. French medical theses were seldom over 10 in quarto. Among Edinburgh graduates whose dissertations included personal research was the Philadelphian, Benjamin Rush: see *The Autobiography of Benjamin Rush: His Travels Through Life Together with his Commonplace Book for 1789-1813*, ed., G. W. Corner (Princeton, NJ, 1948), 43.
107. Hence their value as a source for studying faculty teaching.
108. At Montpellier doctorands had to sustain a series of theses which lasted three days. At Edinburgh students only sustained the one dissertation and the public interrogation was brief: Rosner, 84-85.
109. Most faculties of medicine constituted a college, formed by the professors and a number of *agrégés*. Caen c. 1780 had 4 profs. and 15 *agrégés*: see AN M 196, no. 90/3. In addition, there were *c.* 20 colleges in other towns; the exact number is a matter of dispute: see Julia and Revel, 'Les Etudiants', 296, n. 51.
110. TMP, IX in 4o., no. 156, royal letters patent (printed).
111. Candidates had to take a practical examination and pay 3,500 *livres* by 1789: see BM Reims, MS 1084, fos. 24-6, a description of its graduation procedures *c.* 1770; Julia and Revel, 'Les Etudiants', 280. Reims also offered a degree which brought no right to practise in France, called *le doctorat étranger*. Applicants had only to pass a viva-voce examination; hence the attraction of Reims to students from the British Isles; presumably it was in granting these degrees that most of the corruption occurred: see A. Jacquinet, *Le Centre universitaire médical de Reims (1550-1966): Son oeuvre, son rayonnement* (Reims, 1967), 12.
112. 'Plan', 7-8.
113. Most were graduates of Montpellier or Paris but Pinel had trained at Toulouse before moving to Montpellier.
114. Cf. Fourcroy on Paris medical education: in *Rapport*, 5. The less wealthy, he suggested, had to build on their faculty instruction by private, unstructured (and hence useless) reading.

115. Members of the Paris faculty in the eighteenth century were usually either the sons of Paris physicians or outsiders who had taken a first degree elsewhere and practised their profession in the provinces for many years. As an outsider Vicq d'Azyr was rather exceptional in becoming a faculty member at an early age.
116. E.g., according to the 1707 Edict of Marly (see note 8 above), physicians in French Artois and Flanders had to be graduates of Douai.
117. See esp. Vicq d'Azyr, 'Plan', 45-55 (on medical examinations), 94-102 (on clinical teaching), and 104-7 (on the structure of the profession).
118. If the history of medicine was taught as Vicq d'Azyr desired, then it should have consisted in part of a study of past medical schools and their deficiencies, and in part as a guide to reading and observation. Presumably the course was intended to emphasize the break with continuity in the new, empirically orientated medical schools: see 'Plan', 22.
119. Fourcroy, *Rapport*, 2.
120. Cited in a note to [A.-F. de Fourcroy], *Rapport et décret de la convention nationale sur les Ecoles de Santé de Paris, Montpellier et Strasbourg* 14 Frimaire, Year III (Paris, 1794), 17-18. 'Ce n'est pas seulement à l'enseignement de ce que l'on sait que se bornent leurs fonctions; elles ont encore pour objet les recherches les plus étendues sur toutes les branches de l'art de guérir; pour but l'avancement de toutes les sciences qui peuvent éclairer la physique animale.' Except for the notes and the text of the decree, this pamphlet is the same as Fourcroy's *Rapport* of 7 Frimaire on the establishment of the Paris school alone.
121. A development only really possible if the professors were paid a good enough salary.
122. *Rapport et décret*, 18 (cited above, note 120). 'C'étoit commander au génie français de surpasser toutes les actions dans cette partie de connaissances humaines, comme il les surpasse déjà dans un grand nombre des arts.'
123. E.g., Vicq d'Azyr, 'Plan', 5.
124. The 1803 decree established a slightly different examination procedure for those who wished to specialize in surgery. The fifth and final exam was an external rather than an internal clinical exam. 'Loi du 19 Ventôse an 11', cl. 6: see *Recueil des loix et règlements*, ii, 335.
125. Jones, 'Montpellier Medical Students', 70; Dulieu, *La Chirurgie*, 174-7. The degree was the inspiration of Pierre Chirac.
126. See note 72 above. For a general account of the spread of surgical

colleges, see Pierre Huard, 'L'Enseignement médico-chirurgical' in Taton, ed., *L'Enseignement et diffusion*, 194-209. For particular cases, besides Gelfand and Dulieu (cited in notes 72 and 78 above), see Barbot, *La Faculté de médecine de Toulouse*, i, 360-406; G. Péry, *Histoire de la faculté de médecine de Bordeaux et de l'enseignement médical dans cette ville 1441-1888* (Bordeaux, 1888), 176-209.

127. Fourcroy, *Rapport*, 8. 'Le despotisme & la vanité, qui avoient fait élever ce monument, ne s'étoient point occupés de le meubler.'
128. Before the eighteenth century the perfect physician was learned rather than experienced. To use Fourcroy's terms the emphasis was on reading not seeing.
129. Related by Amoreux who visited Paris in later life to experience the tuition given by the new *Ecole*: see BM Avignon, MS 1269, pp. 127-28.
130. The nursing sisters at Montpellier and Strasbourg, however, seem to have hindered the establishment of clinical courses in the two provincial faculties: see Colin Jones, 'Professionalizing Modern Medicine' in French Hospitals', *Medical History* (1982), 348 (essay review of Gelfand's book).
131. Fourcroy, 'Exposé des motifs du projet de loi sur l'exercice de la médecine', in *Recueil des loix et règlements*, ii, 350-1. 'Jamais l'art de guérir n'a été enseigné avec plus de soin, plus de développement et plus d'ensemble.'
132. M.-J. Imbault-Huarlt, *L'Ecole pratique de dissection ou l'influence du concept de médecine pratique et de médecine d'observation dans l'enseignement médical-chirurgical au XVIIIe siècle et au début du XIXe siècle*, reproduced dissertation (Lille, 1975), esp. 182 *et seq.* on the training offered at the Ecole pratique.
133. Ackerknecht, *Medicine at the Paris Hospital*, 36.
134. François-Louis Poumiès de la Siboutie, *Mémoires* (Paris, 1870), 90-120. Attendance at private courses in midwifery, like that given by Joseph Capuron at the Hôtel de Cluny, was essential for the art was not taught as part of the official curriculum.
135. Although this was supposedly difficult according to the reformers: patients did not like it: see Vicq d'Azyr, 'Plan', 102. Poumiès de la Siboutie spent two months with a Versailles physician called Texier: see *Mémoires*, 107.
136. Poumiès de la Siboutie, *Mémoires*, 107-8. Poumiès was also an intern at the Hôpital Saint-Louis (for venereal disease) and the Hôtel-Dieu. The creation of the *internat* seems to have been an extension of the ancien-régime practice of allowing a surgeon to qualify as a master without the customary examination in return for serving in a hospital for a number of years. Such *chirurgiens gagnant maîtrise* were

sometimes appointed as the result of a *concours*: see Dulieu, *La Chirurgie*, 151-61.

137. The surgeon Caron has left a good account of his time as intern at the Hôtel-Dieu: see BFMP, MS 5061, 'Journal de chirurgie de Caron...' (1808-12).

138. The numbers would have been even larger if the 'loi de ventôse' had not established an inferior category of *officiers de santé* (akin to the rural surgeons of the ancien régime), who would not need to train in the medical schools.

139. Chambon de Montaux, 'Projet de réforme dans l'enseignement de la médecine', fo. lv (Paris, 1815), separately foliated MS in BFMP, MS 5143: 'trois chaires de clinique sont insuffisantes en France pour l'instruction des étudiants; ceux qui abondent à Paris sont trop nombreux pour profiter des lecons. Entassés autour de chaque lit, quoi qu'en petit nombre, quelques uns voient la face du malade, reconnoissent d'après les remarques du professeur, les signes de l'affection morbifique; mais éloignés le lendemain par leurs camarades de la proximité du lit, il leur est impossible d'obtenir une continuité d'observations, propres a leur procurer des idées justes, sur une seule et même maladie.' Similar sentiments in C. Duchanoy, *Projet d'organisation médicale* (np, nd [c. 1800]). The situation presumably improved dramatically with the creation of a further five clinical chairs (including one for midwifery) in 1823. Admittedly, students could attend a number of privately-run clinics in the first two decades of the nineteenth century, such as Pinel's at La Salpêtrière.

140. 'Loi du 19 ventôse an 11', cl. 6 and 7 (see note 124 above).

141. Six years was the optimum length of the course; he objected to the ancien-régime practice of demanding *attestations* of attendance from doctoral candidates and was willing for graduands to have studied at home: 'Plan', 41-45.

142. 'Plan', 46-51. Written examinations were used before the Revolution in the Paris *agrégation*, an examination which created a pool of professors in the humanities and philosophy for the Paris *collèges de plein exercice*.

143. Not only were there more clinical chairs, but more attention was paid to surgery; students could pass the first part of their course in *écoles sécondaires* (13 existed by the end of the Empire); and from 1843 a fourth year was added to the course which was entirely hospital-based: see Léonard, *Les Médecins de l'ouest*, ii, 638-41.

144. There were many factors why the new medical schools failed to fulfil the reformers' ambitions. Weight of numbers does not explain everything, especially the fondness for Latin in the examinations.

Perhaps an important determining factor was the pressure exerted on the government by the medical profession at large which probably had a less rigorous conception of an adequate medical education. Ordinary practitioners must have thought a detailed knowledge of the practical medical sciences was a waste of time in an age when the art of healing was deemed an empirical science and interventionism frowned on. The research of the Paris school into pathological anatomy had no obvious therapeutic value: see the speculative remarks in Brockliss, 'L'Enseignement médical et la Révolution', 106-10.

145. I am indebted to Professor Jan Goldstein of the University of Chicago for making me think about the implications of my research into the eighteenth-century medical curriculum in the light of Foucault's theory of an epistemic change at the turn of the nineteenth century.

146. Michel Foucault, *Naissance de la clinique* (Paris, 1963). It is impossible to do justice to Foucault's complex and often arcane account of the Paris school in a few lines.

147. See, for example, Caroline Hannaway, 'Vicq d'Azyr, Anatomy, and a Vision of Medicine' in Ann La Berge and Mordechai Feingold, eds, *French Medical Culture in the Nineteenth Century* (Amsterdam and Atlanta: Editions Rodopi, 1994), 280-95.

148. The one person of importance (in terms of the number of physicians he trained), whose teaching could be explored, is Antoine Petit: see the series of lecture-notes contained in Library of the Wellcome Institute for the History of Medicine, London, MS 3842-51.

149. This may well have been the sum of a student's experience if he followed a physician on his rounds, which might explain the reformers' hostility to the practice and their insistence on the hospital as the site of bedside learning: the hostility was hidden under the claim that private patients did not like the physician to be accompanied: see note 135 above. When physicians allowed students to walk the wards with them, many may have offered no guidance at all: cf. the brief account given by G.F. Laennec of his clinical experience in Rouxeau, *Un étudiant*, 40. Chambon de Montaux at La Salpêtrière on the eve of the Revolution seems to have allowed students to diagnose and treat hospital patients, but, as a leading medical reformer, he was presumably exceptional: see BFMP MS 5143, 'Remarques sur le mode de l'enseignement de la médecine clinique', p. 8v.

3

Was Anatomical and Tissue Pathology a Product of the Paris Clinical School or Not?*

Othmar Keel

Anatomical and tissue pathology played a central role in the transformation of Western medicine that began in the last decades of the eighteenth century. To grasp fully the conditions of this medical revolution it is essential to define clearly the conceptual and institutional factors that permitted the development of this pathology at the time. This leads 1) to a better understanding of the state of European medicine at the end of the eighteenth century, 2) to a reinterpretation of the context of the medical revolution, that is, of the rise of anatomico-clinical medicine, and 3) to a better assessment of the role of diverse European schools of medical thought, in particular the British and French schools, in these fundamental transformations in medical knowledge in pathology and the clinic.

The aim of the present study is to further our understanding of the complex question of the relations of Great Britain and France in this domain. It will enable us to understand better the conditions present at the time that permitted the fundamental transformation of pathology and medicine. A thorough reading of this text will make it clear, first of all, that this great scientific innovation occurred very much before the Paris School and outside of it, and that the subsequent achievements of the Paris School in this area at the beginning of the nineteenth century owe much to a massive use of British works.

---

* The present study was made possible by a grant from the Social Sciences and Humanities Research Council of Canada. Unless otherwise indicated, all emphasis and translations of quotations from French are ours. We acknowledge the help of Alicia Sliwinski, Maryann Farkas and Geneviève Bazin, chef du Service des Collections Spéciales, Service des Bibliothèques, Université de Montréal.

Secondly, after examining the Paris School's reception of British anatomical-tissue pathology, we will demonstrate that this research tradition continued to develop in Great Britain in a relatively autonomous manner in the first three decades of the nineteenth century, even while it incorporated certain other developments from the Paris School which themselves rested on foundations the French had already borrowed from the British.

There were thus three important initial phases in the history of anatomical-tissue pathology. The first was its inception in Great Britain in the second half of the eighteenth century, and the formation of an important current of research in this area. The second was the reception of this pathology in France at the turn of the century and its appropriation by the Paris School, specifically by authors and practitioners like Pinel, Bichat, and Broussais, among others.

A key point about this phase should be made at the outset, because it has created confusion, contributing to a distorted vision of the history of tissue pathology: a certain number of British practitioners of the nineteenth century were unaware that clinicians of the Paris School (such as Pinel and Bichat) very liberally appropriated British achievements in this area. In some cases, British practitioners were not aware that what they assumed were new discoveries from France were, though clothed in a different rhetoric, in fact ideas and achievements which, in large part, had emerged from their own soil. As we shall see, this 'blindness' on the part of some British practitioners was not accidental. Often it can be explained by a kind of reformist vision in professional circles that tended to hold a selective and idealized view of Parisian medicine while at the same time deprecating or ignoring local achievements. By contrast, other British and, we might add, some French practitioners had seen this very clearly.

The third phase was a parallel development in the first three decades of the nineteenth century by which the two schools were mutually fertilized and refertilized by numerous exchanges and by contributions from both sides.

The present essay is not a study of precursors.[1] Its objective is quite different:

> 1) to delineate more clearly the theoretical and institutional context that permitted the development of anatomical-tissue pathology, and of Great Britain's research tradition in this domain,

2) to analyze the reception of this tradition in France, and

3) to provide a comparative analysis of new developments in this tradition in Great Britain and in the Paris School starting in 1800, demonstrating that there was continued interaction and cross-fertilization of these two traditions. This cross-fertilization was decisive for new developments in anatomical-tissue pathology in both countries, and each of the two schools was without doubt enriched by the other.

Historians have neglected to examine the creation of a tradition of works in anatomical-tissue pathology in Great Britain and their reception in France. Similarly, we have no comparative analysis of the development of this tradition in the two countries from the nineteenth century on, with the result that the contribution of the Paris School has been overestimated.

There can be no doubt that the contribution of the Paris School remains very important, in particular in the years 1810–1820. However, we can only make a more accurate evaluation of the French contribution by first situating it within a broader context, one which includes both earlier innovations and parallel developments in Great Britain, in order then to make a fair assessment of the impact of British contributions on French medicine.

This essay is also a contribution to a reinterpretation of classic theses, expounded in particular by Michel Foucault and E. H. Ackerknecht, on the birth of the clinic and on the development of anatomical-tissue pathology.[2] For these authors, Bichat's tissue pathology constituted a decisive and, for Foucault, a fundamental turning-point in the birth of the clinic. According to both, it was only at the Paris School that tissue pathology developed in the beginning of the nineteenth century.[3]

For some time now, a reinterpretation of the history of the Paris School, long considered a medical 'Mecca' of the early nineteenth century, has been underway. We have already contributed to this reinterpretation by showing that certain innovations in the institutions and concepts of the clinic, attributed to the Paris School and to the socio-institutional, politico-ideological and intellectual-scientific contexts of the French Revolution, were due in reality to foreign medical schools which in fact served as models for the Paris clinic from the end of the eighteenth century.[4] Moreover, these innovations were produced in the specific socio-political and intellectual contexts of each country which were very different from those of Revolutionary France.[5]

A Product of the Paris Clinical School?

I

We have shown this particularly in the case of anatomical-tissue pathology, by demonstrating that it is totally erroneous to think that no developments occurred in pathological and clinical anatomy between the work of Morgagni (1682–1771) and that of Bichat (1771–1802), and that there was a forty-year blockage or period of latency in this area due to the prevailing philosophy of clinical medicine, which was only interested in external symptoms and their classification.[6] We have shown, on the contrary, that during this period an important school of pathological anatomy and of clinical anatomy developed around the Hunters,[7] the Monros, and Matthew Baillie (1761–1823), etc. The works of the school of William and John Hunter[8] and Matthew Baillie (like those of the Monros at Edinburgh) in pathological anatomy and anatomico-clinical medicine were well known and considered as models in France, as elsewhere in Europe, at the turn of the century. When Baillie's *The Morbid Anatomy of Some of the Most Important Parts of the Human Body* was published in 1793, not one treatise with the term 'pathological anatomy' in its title had yet been published in France. As Baillie's biographer, A. E. Rodin, notes,[9] we can judge the success of this work by the number of editions: eight English editions from 1793 to 1838, three American editions from 1795 to 1820, and translations: one German translation (1793), two French translations (1803, 1815), one Italian translation (1807) and one Russian (1826). One can also assess the impact of the anatomico-pathological works of Hunter and Baillie by using an informal citation analysis; British physicians and surgeons, as well as foreigners, cited them frequently in publications as well as in their works on clinical subjects and on pathology. Of course, the works of the British school did not mark the beginning of a tradition of research and education in pathological anatomy; they contributed to the continuation of the Morgagnian tradition. Nonetheless, the British school in pathological anatomy (Hunter, Baillie, *et al.*) was innovative in comparison with the Morgagnian tradition in three ways:

> 1) Instead of presenting a large number of successive cases of anatomical lesions of different organic parts with the corresponding symptoms, as Morgagnians did, the Hunter–Baillie school, by abstracting and generalizing from a great number of cases, produced precise descriptions of diseased entities, with the goal of distinguishing the defining types of distinct morbid states. As

A Product of the Paris Clinical School?

Krumbhaar says of Baillie's treatise on pathological anatomy, 'it described in simple, clear language the lesions that the several organs and systems were prone to, much as in the special pathology sections of modern textbooks ... pathology was now treated as an independent science. The success of the book was prompt.'[10]

2) Morgagni linked pathological anatomy and clinical anatomy with physiology, in studying how lesions of organs give rise to functional impairments that produce disharmony in the economy of the organism, their clinical manifestations being proportionate to their location and nature.[11] The Hunterian school restructured the Morgagnian relationship between pathological anatomy and physiology by emphasizing knowledge of the dysfunction producing the lesion, as much as the lesion itself, and its disruptive effects on physiological equilibrium. One must, therefore, work back from an examination of altered structures to their causes in the disruption of functions (or 'physiopathology': that which Baillie, following John Hunter, calls 'morbid actions').[12] As J.-E. Dezeimeris (1799–1852) emphasized, the school of John Hunter proposed 'to investigate the laws of growth of irregular states of our parts, and to lay the foundations for a completely new pathological physiology'.[13] Dezeimeris opposed this *problématique* in pathological anatomy put forward by the Hunterian school with that descriptive or static approach, which, 'following Bayle, Dupuytren and Laennec, draws from the autopsy alone the history of the human body's abnormal modifications'.[14] Dezeimeris notes that 'the school that Hunter heads has, one must admit, the most philosophical approach, and *the compatriots of this famous surgeon left contemporary French writers quite far behind them*'.[15]

3) The British school of pathological anatomy did more than deepen and renew the Morgagnian tradition of 'gross pathological anatomy', or organ pathology; it also developed a pathological anatomy and a pathology that took into account tissues, and no longer just organs. This was a capital innovation, a development of the greatest importance that has been wrongly attributed to Pinel (1755–1826), to Bichat and to the Paris Clinical School.[16]

The thesis that there was, between Morgagni and Bichat, a void or stasis of nearly a half-century in the practice of and research in pathological anatomy and in anatomico-clinical medicine is therefore doubly false. First, because 'gross pathological anatomy', or organ pathology, was developed and renewed in an important way during this period, notably – but not uniquely – by the British school; and, secondly, because a sustained practice of autopsy and research on the location and the causes of diseases in the advanced sectors of clinical practice (medical and surgical) had allowed not only a continuation and renewal of Morgagnian anatomy, but also a displacement of the location of disease from the organ to the tissue.[17]

New ideas, techniques and accomplishments in pathology and clinical medicine did not appear miraculously or by intellectual spontaneous generation. One can develop notions of anatomical and tissue pathology only if one is already in a material and socio-institutional framework that permits anatomical and clinical research: i.e., in hospitals or other institutions where one may actively observe the sick and/or perform autopsies and thus acquire, through practice, anatomico-clinical experience. Such places and practices did exist in Britain (and elsewhere in Europe) at the end of the eighteenth century, thus allowing the formation of a body of knowledge in anatomical and tissue pathology. Indeed we have demonstrated in previous works the need to revise conventional history, supported by Foucault and Ackerknecht, which situates the beginning of clinical education and research at the Paris School. In particular, we must take into account the London clinic that preceded it.[18]

It is the existence of this institutional context that allows us to understand the progress of British pathological anatomy and the pathology of the Hunter–Baillie school and its successors; one finds there, as later in the Paris Clinical School, a combination of pathological anatomy of the organs and pathology of tissues.[19] In fact, in addition to demonstrating that the anatomical, physiological and pathological concept of tissues was already present in certain currents of the British clinic in the last decades of the eighteenth century – which compels recognition that British works in pathological anatomy were quite advanced for the era – we have shown that the leaders of the Paris School such as Pinel, Bichat, and Broussais (1772–1838) appropriated directly or indirectly a good part of these innovations into their own works – most notably in tissue pathology.[20] The pathological and clinical anatomy of the Hunter–Baillie school was, with the Morgagnian current, one of the models and major reference-points of the new French anatomical pathology that affirmed itself at the turn of the century (from Corvisart and Bichat up to Laennec and Broussais,[21] even though some of these authors retained only certain components or dimensions of the Hunterian model).

A Product of the Paris Clinical School?

It is worth noting that, even after the publications of Bichat's works, Baillie's book had no equivalent in France in the domain of pathological anatomy; it was judged essential to render it more accessible to French practitioners and students through a first translation in 1803 and a second in 1815. In the first translation Ferrall noted in a 'translator's foreword' that 'the need for a work of this nature, as much for those who practise as for those who study medicine, is so generally recognized that it would be totally superfluous to emphasize its utility'.[22] And Guerbois, the surgeon who did the second translation, noted in his preface of 1815 that 'The fame of Baillie's work and the number of its editions *prove clearly the full value that the public attaches to the method this practitioner has followed.*'[23] Guerbois gave the following translation of the first lines of the preface that Baillie put in the first edition of his book:

> Quelques maladies sont le résultat d'un travail pathologique qui ne *produit aucune altération dans le tissu de nos organes* et n'exigent par conséquent aucune recherche après la mort, mais il est *d'autres affections qui altèrent plus ou moins ce tissu*, qui devient alors le sujet particulier de notre étude.[24]

It is therefore clear that for early nineteenth-century French practitioners, Baillie's pathological anatomy dealt with organs but also with tissues. In fact, Baillie describes tissue lesions in the majority of organs, notably lesions of the arachnoid membrane, of the dura-mater, of the pia-mater,[25] the pleura,[26] the pericardium,[27] the peritoneum[28] and of the diverse mucous or internal membranes.[29] His description also highlights the analogies between the pathological processes in tissues of the same system, like the serous membranes, the mucous membranes, etc.[30] It comes as no surprise then that Baillie's treatise on pathological anatomy was a model in France, even after the publication of Bichat's works, if one considers, as do some historians of medicine, that, in Bichat's works, pathological anatomy remained in a programmatic and prescriptive state. In effect, opposing Morgagni and Bichat, M. D. Grmek, for example, emphasizes that Morgagni had written and published the *De sedibus* at the end of his life, after having accumulated a great deal of experience. In contrast, Bichat's writings all appeared at the beginning of his scientific life, since he died very young (at age 31). It is not surprising then that Morgagni's work was replete with facts and concrete achievements, while that of Bichat remained a programme, without doubt impressive, but nonetheless unfulfilled.[31] Moreover, the displacement of the location of disease from organs to tissues was not an accomplishment of Pinel and Bichat, but of many eighteenth-century European practitioners, and particularly of the British, who brought about this change, not individually, but through a medical tendency or the Hunterian tradition. As Georges Canguilhem underlined, our emphasis on the precedence of the British school over the Paris Clinical School in the development of tissue pathology is not a search for precursors. The issue is rather to re-analyze the conceptual and institutional context that made possible a great revolution in medical knowledge.[32]

The fundamental importance of the Hunterian contribution to anatomical and tissue pathology was recognized and emphasized by numerous clinicians and pathologists of the Paris School. Thus towards the end of the 1830s E. F. Dubois d'Amiens, professor of pathology at the Faculty of Medicine of Paris, proposed to follow the Hunterian model in this area. More interesting still, he opposed the Hunterian model to the work done by clinicians such as Cayol and his students, who were working in the period of greatest influence of the Paris School. He writes:

> Thus when they (vitalists such as Cayol and his students) say that all inflammation is an accidental reaction of the organism, they repeat what they have said of disease ... Therefore, instead of living eternally on these ideas, the least fault of which is being too general and without practical application, they ought instead to follow in the footsteps of the renowned Hunter, and thoroughly investigate varied symptoms that produce inflammation in diverse tissues and organs. Indeed, what use would there be in continuously repeating, in general pathology, that in all inflammation nature reacts, if we don't know how it reacts, and if there are not as many modes of reactions as there are different tissues in the organism? ... *Thomson teaches us that the great Hunter devoted more than thirty years of his life, not in repeating three or four definitions, but in deepening our understanding of the diverse nature of symptoms of inflammation in the tissues of the economy. Also, as Thomson remarks, his work, in establishing pathology on a solid foundation of observation, experience and analysis, marks a new epoch in the history of the art.*[33]

In the same period, Hunter's model is omnipresent in other treatises of the Paris Clinical School such as *Traité de pathologie externe et de médecine opératoire* (Paris: J.-B. Baillière, 1839), in 5 volumes, by Auguste Vidal, surgeon of the hospitals of Paris, and *Professeur agrégé* at the Faculty of Medicine of Paris.[34] In particular Vidal insists that the classifications of 'suppurative', 'adhesive' and 'ulcerative' given by

A Product of the Paris Clinical School?

Hunter to the inflammations of the tissues were still paradigmatic towards the end of the 1830s.[35] They would, moreover, remain so for a long time in the Paris School and elsewhere.

Numerous remarks by Vidal show that for the Paris clinicians, Hunter represents a very sophisticated model of pathology of the tissues. For example, in the chapter on the diseases of cellular tissue: 'Purulent accumulations are produced in all tissues: they have even been found in somewhat old blood clots; we see them at all levels in the breasts of all parenchyma, in the bones, but less frequently in the deep layers than in the tissues that are closer to the periphery. This remark is attributable to J. Hunter.'[36]

Dubois and Vidal cited Hunter, and not Bichat and the Parisian clinicians, as the model of research on tissue pathology. Following in the footsteps of the Hunterian school, French medicine exploited British models of anatomical and tissue pathology. These models would be transformed by the French clinicians, to be reimported afterwards by the British, who then incorporated some of these French contributions into their own research. Strangely enough, a recent work by Russell Maulitz,[37] which purports to be a comparative history of pathological anatomy and tissue pathology in France and Great Britain, focuses solely on 'the genesis of this tradition' by Bichat in France at the end of the eighteenth century and its development there at the beginning of the nineteenth century, in order then to examine the later importation into Britain of this new pathology, which the author labels 'Bichatian'. This interpretation obscures the fact that the ideas and practices circulating in Britain in the nineteenth century were in fact a reimportation of discoveries, innovations, and achievements which had first been transmitted from Great Britain to France, where they underwent adaptation and reformulation and were used as a basis for important developments. Great Britain's 'reception' of 'Bichatian' ideas on anatomical and tissue pathology was all the more willing because initially these ideas had been elaborated in Britain where an important body of research in both these fields had been developing for three or four decades.[38]

Maulitz's analysis takes us back to the received view, expressed most brilliantly but also most dogmatically by Foucault and Ackerknecht, that this great change in medicine began only after the French Revolution with practitioners like Bichat at the Paris Clinical School. I would argue that Maulitz's analysis is one-sided: it does not thoroughly treat the question of relations between the two countries in this area of pathology, but focuses primarily on the 'reception' of French pathology in Great Britain. It ignores both the reception of British anatomical and tissue pathology in France at the end of the eighteenth century and the continuation of an indigenous British tradition in the nineteenth century, by which time the two countries were reciprocally influenced.[39] I would also argue that, in order to study the comparative reception of anatomical and tissue pathology in England and France, one must begin not by studying the reception of the Bichatian tradition in the two countries, but instead the respective reception of the Hunterian tradition on each side of the English Channel. There can be no doubt that the Hunterian tradition was well received in France at the Paris Clinical School, notably by Bichat. Its reception in Britain was less spectacular, but it was both earlier and equally productive. This reception was a factor in the very positive welcome Bichat's work received in Britain, not surprising when one considers that British physicians found, within a different rhetoric, the central elements of Hunterian tissue pathology.

Given the importance of these questions for the history of medicine and for a reinterpretation of the Paris Clinical School, it is imperative to provide a detailed analysis of Anglo-French medical relations in the area. This analysis will allow us to elucidate further our own theses concerning the context of the rise of anatomical and tissue pathology in Europe in the eighteenth century and into the early nineteenth century. It will also allow us to show that Maulitz's theses – that Bichat is responsible for the birth of anatomical and tissue pathology while the same tradition is not present in Great Britain before Carswell and Hodgkin – are not admissible.

II

Maulitz himself agrees that it is arbitrary to study Anglo-French relations in pathology solely from the perspective of the French influence in Britain. In an article in which he describes the object of his book, he notes that, since tissue pathology emerged first with the Hunterian school and in the 'previous English medical context', the reimportation of 'Bichatian' ideas into Britain essentially closed the circle, in effect saying that British concepts of tissue pathology were imported into France, later to be reimported into Great Britain.

The author writes, 'I do not advance any strong thesis as to the ultimate, antecedent *origin* of this new "language of the body", much of it based upon the tissue pathology of Xavier Bichat, Gaspard Laurent Bayle and Théophile Laennec. (Indeed some have argued that the ideas embedded within it may be traced back to *the*

Hunterian school and earlier in the English context – in which case *one might conceive of my analysis as the "closing of the circle".)*[40] With regard to this statement, one must note that the central question is not 'the ultimate, antecedent origin', but the fact that the essential foundation of the *problématique* of tissues in pathology was built up by the British school through a body of practices, techniques and concepts.

We must also insist that if British medicine in the first decades of the nineteenth century reimported certain French elaborations, themselves based on British concepts of tissue pathology, it was in order to integrate them into developments of these concepts originating in England itself, and therefore to supplement innovations developed by British practitioners in the same era. Hence the question is not the British reception of concepts and practices in pathology which would not, or would no longer, be in use in Britain, nor is it a question of a lack of innovation and developments. It is simply a question of the integration into local developments of important advances which had been made elsewhere, but on the basis of British practices and concepts.

It is surprising, therefore, that the author defines the objective of his book as follows: 'I have not intended to provide a symmetrical comparison of French and British pathology in the era before the microscope, but sought rather to look at the reception of a *suite of medical ideas* in one culture after examining how they unfolded in another. My intention was to study the development of pathological anatomy and, in particular, tissue pathology, in France and then scrutinize various attempts to implant it in England.'[41] If one admits that the ideas of anatomical and tissue pathology are present in the 'British context' starting from, but even before, the Hunterian school, it seems extremely arbitrary, for a book claiming to record the history of a 'suite of medical ideas' about anatomical pathology in early nineteenth-century France and England, to decide not to make a symmetrical study of the subject in both countries, but to restrict the study to France, and to then look at its implementation in England. The inevitable result is the thesis that anatomical and tissue pathology was developed uniquely in France, and that it was only through its importation from France – a late importation moreover – that it could be implanted in Great Britain.

Maulitz endeavours to show that while anatomical and tissue pathology furnished a common language or a synthesis of pathology to an organizationally unified community of physicians and surgeons in early nineteenth-century France, it could not have been favourably received in Great Britain at the same time, because, due to the persisting tripartite division into physicians, surgeons and apothecaries, the elite of the medical community would have resisted the adoption of this pathology.[42] 'French' pathological anatomy would therefore have found 'adherents' only in the fringes of the community, outside of the medical 'establishment', notably in Scotland, at the new University of London (1828), among Dissenters and reformers like Thomas Hodgkin, or among the new generation of 'surgeon-apothecaries' who, working as 'general practitioners', questioned the privileges of the established medical corporations. Of course, it is pertinent to study the socio-institutional and socio-professional context in which a foreign body of knowledge is received in a given country, but it is also essential to differentiate between a foreign body of knowledge that is truly new, and one that is already present in the country, as was the case for anatomical and tissue pathology in Great Britain at the juncture of the eighteenth and nineteenth centuries.

Maulitz's argument is built on an initial double postulate: that not only tissue pathology, but also 'true' pathological anatomy began with Bichat.[43] This is, in fact, the same as saying that pathological anatomy began with tissue pathology, which is unacceptable for two reasons. Firstly, pathological anatomy and the method of anatomico-clinical correlations began with the school of Valsalva (1666–1723) and with Morgagni. The latter gave it a paradigmatic form, as historians of medicine established long ago.[44] Pathological anatomy was then developed, enriched and renewed before Bichat's time through the research tradition of the Hunter–Baillie school, as well as of other European schools: the German school of Haller, Meckel (Sr.), Ludwig, Soemmering, etc.; the Viennese school of Auenbrugger, Stoll, Frank, Vetter, etc.; the school of Sandifort (1740–1819); the Italian school of Morgagni's successors, etc.[45] Secondly, tissue pathology itself was not established by Bichat in France, but, as we have shown, by the British schools, particularly in the Hunterian circle.[46]

It should be noted that Maulitz acknowledges this, affirming, as we have, that before Pinel and Bichat a British tradition of tissue pathology already existed: he writes, in fact, of 'the chief exponents of the *English tissue pathology tradition*, notably John Hunter and James Carmichael Smyth',[47] and of a 'Hunterian strain of tissue pathology'.[48] He seems, therefore, to have placed himself in the centre of a contradiction, affirming on the one hand that French ideas and practices in pathological anatomy and tissue pathology

A Product of the Paris Clinical School?

were introduced into England in the years 1820–30, yet recognizing, on the other hand, that Britain had an important tradition of pathological anatomy and tissue pathology starting with the Hunter–Baillie school. He even admits that, strictly speaking, 'Bichatian' tissue pathology was not at all a French innovation. Speaking of ideas and techniques in tissue pathology that one finds in Scotland in the years 1800–10, he writes that:

> *To identify this receptivity with 'French ideas and techniques' would be to oversimplify the position*. In the first place, the now-dominant Bichatian mode of tissue pathology *was not, strictly speaking, a French innovation at all*. It could have sprung equally well from the Hunter–Baillie tradition, had English medicine and surgery been in a position to foster it.

And he adds:

> But it was the French who seized on the *pathology of tissues and textures that had been generated in both countries in the 1790s* and it was elaborated most completely by Xavier Bichat in 1799–1801; and it was the French who put this knowledge to work in the clinic. *On the availability of the tissue model in both medical cultures*, see Keel, 'La généalogie'. *The Scottish knew all this*.[49]

This passage contains several of Maulitz's theses which should be carefully examined. In fact, can the contradiction in his argument be explained by the fact that he contends that the British tradition of anatomical pathology had been interrupted, that it could only develop in France? Let us examine this thesis more closely. Maulitz rightly affirms that 'to identify this receptivity [of anatomical and tissue pathology in Britain] with "French ideas and techniques" would be to oversimplify the position'. But is this not precisely what he does throughout his book? He goes on to say that the 'Bichatian' model of tissue pathology was not a French innovation, that it could also have developed from the English Hunter–Baillie tradition, had the English been in a position to foster it, but that, in practice, it was the French who seized on the pathology of tissues and textures. Then, however, he immediately asserts that the tissue model was accessible in both medical cultures and that the Scottish already knew all this from their own medical tradition in the years 1800–10.[50] We are thus confronted with two incompatible theses. These two assertions are contradictory, and it is obvious that the second one is right.[51]

Maulitz also acknowledges explicitly in the passage cited above[52] that there had been a Hunter–Baillie tradition in tissue pathology preceding and independent of Bichat and the Paris School: 'It could have sprung equally from the Hunter–Baillie tradition had English Medicine and Surgery been in a position to foster it.' In fact, pathological anatomy and tissue pathology had continued to develop in Great Britain after Baillie, although in a form or in a style different from Paris medicine. As we have shown above, the qualitative and quantitative importance of the works of Hunter, Baillie and their partners or successors in pathological anatomy and anatomico-clinical pathology in fact fuelled the indigenous tradition in tissue pathology and certainly did not interrupt it.[53] It is impossible to cite all the works published in Great Britain by physicians and surgeons (or surgeon-apothecaries) on pathological anatomy or clinical anatomy (comprising tissue as well as organ pathology) between 1790 and 1830. However, as we will see, there were many.[54] In 1819, Gilbert Breschet (1784–1845) judged it useful to translate the *Treatise on the Diseases of the Arteries and Veins* by the British surgeon, J. Hodgson (1809; translated, Paris, 1819). In his preface to this translation Breschet, who, as demonstrator (*chef des travaux anatomiques*, successor of P. Béclard) in anatomy at the Paris Faculty of Medicine (later [1836] Professor of anatomy, successor of J. Cruveilhier) was in a good position to judge, made an eloquent comparison of French and British works (and those of other countries) in clinical and pathological anatomy:

> In France we possess a certain number of general treatises on medicine or surgery, and *not enough collections of observations or monographs* which contribute the most strongly to the advancement of the art... Too few surgical monographs have been written. There is an important branch of medicine for which *we have no general treatises*: this is pathological anatomy and, by this account, *the English, the Germans and the Italians* appear more advanced than us.[55]

To clearly define the relations in anatomical-tissue pathology between the British school and the Paris Clinical School, we must get rid of the false idea that the English were only the 'precursors' of Parisian clinicians. A close examination of the connections between Hunter and Bichat's works, and of the links between the two traditions, allows us to see that things were very different: what we see is a clear case first of appropriation and then later of parallel development.

One must understand once and for all that John Hunter did more than furnish some embryonic ideas on tissue pathology, and that Bichat appropriated much more than this from the works of the Scottish practitioner.[56]

A Product of the Paris Clinical School?

Within the framework of his considerable works in pathological anatomy, comparative anatomy and physiology, as well as in experimental pathology and surgery and in human physiology, John Hunter elaborated a very detailed and structured tissue-anatomical *problématique* which, on several counts, is even more complex than that of Bichat. This is particularly true with regard to the process of inflammation.[57] Bichat's understanding of the pathological state of tissues relied above all on dissection. Surgical-clinical experience contributed to his understanding, but surgery and experimental pathology played a smaller role than in Hunter's works in the development of histopathological knowledge. In contrast, physiological experimentation intervened systematically in Bichat's work to enhance understanding of normal histology. In addition, an important part of Bichat's understanding of tissues was derived from analytical techniques such as dissection, maceration, putrefaction, boiling, etc. These techniques for analyzing organs and tissues had already been used by Morgagni, Haller, and many others. Although Hunter, for his part, made use of reagents for the analysis of tissues and organic fluids, he did not limit himself to a study of solid parts using these methods. Like Bichat, but before him, Hunter drew an important part of his knowledge on tissue pathology from the systematic practice of dissection (Hunter opened thousands of cadavers); but it is important to emphasize that in his work the leading ideas of the tissue *problématique* were elaborated as much within the framework of experimental pathology and surgery (and of comparative anatomy and physiology) as within that of pathological anatomy. To put it another way, to form a tissue *problématique* it did not suffice to 'open a few corpses':[58] it was also necessary to have practical experience in pathological experimentation on animals, and considerable knowledge of histogenesis and pathology drawn from comparative anatomy and physiology.

For Bichat – who agrees with Hunter on this point – since the vital properties of each tissue make it different from others, each tissue also differs in diseases which are nothing other than alterations of these vital properties. Therapeutics must aim solely to restore their normal state. For Hunter diseases are localized at the level of tissues and they reveal themselves through alterations in the tissues' vital forces, but they are more complex than that. What determines an illness, and, in consequence, adequate treatment, is also the nature of the pathogenic cause that induces these tissue reactions and the state of the body's constitution (or the general state of reactivity of the body) or of the global physiological dynamic of the organism inside of which the pathological process takes place. Thus tissue reactions, or the alterations of vital properties of tissues, vary according to the state of the constitution, but, at the same time, the pathological processes that modify the vital properties of tissues react on the constitution. The form of these reactions depends on the affected part. The originality of Hunter's pathology was that, like Bichat's, it focused on the tissue, and furthermore, and to a greater extent than Bichat's, it was centred on a dynamic and experimental *problématique* of the evolution of lesions in tissues.[59]

We have shown in previous works that Hunter, rather than Bichat, was responsible for the revolution of 'decentralization of life' (Claude Bernard) in assigning a distinct life, not to each organ, as Bordeu did, but to each tissue. Physiological and, above all, pathological study – most often experimental – of most of the twenty-one tissues distinguished by Bichat are already well developed in Hunter's work. In comparing the writings of Hunter and Bichat on these points, we find substantial agreement between them.[60] This agreement is not due to fortuitous coincidence, but to Bichat's use of Hunter's work.[61] This is why, if we wish to compare the work of these two authors in tissue pathology, we must take into account the fact that Bichat made substantial use of Hunter's work on pathology, and even physiology, of tissues.[62] We must recall that Hunter broadly disseminated the concepts of this *problématique*, from the 1770s onwards, in his publications and through his teaching.[63]

In a recent essay, Christopher Lawrence, building on the work of Foucault, tries to establish the thesis that there was a fundamental epistemological rupture between the pathological localism of the eighteenth century, represented by Morgagni, and that of nineteenth-century pathology, represented by Bichat:

> It is the gulf that separates Morgagni from Bichat, not their proximity, that is striking. For Morgagni, according to Foucault, 'morbid kinship rested on a principle of organic proximity'. Thus 'asthma, pleuropneumonia, and haemoptysis formed related species in that they were all localized in the chest'. For Bichat, famously, 'Since every organized tissue has everywhere a general arrangement, and whatever its situation may be, retains the same structure and properties etc. its disease must unquestionably be the same.'[64]

The difference between these two local pathologies is therefore that one, that of the eighteenth century, is based on proximity of organs, while the other, that of the nineteenth century, is based on the analogy of tissues. But even if there was a certain distance between Morgagni's pathology and Bichat's, this does not refute the fact that already in the eighteenth century an important current of pathology existed for which the principle of analogy of the disease according to analogy of the structure and function of the affected tissue was already taken for granted.[65] This current is Hunterian pathology, and thus credit goes to Hunter and his students, Smyth and Baillie, for example, for having elaborated and implanted this *problématique*.[66] In fact, it was these authors who first demonstrated that, since each tissue is endowed with particular properties in the healthy state, it must be affected in a specific way by the cause of disease, and therefore that the same modes of lesion must always produce similar effects on all analogous tissues, whatever their place in the organism. Thus Hunter very clearly demonstrated that the process of inflammation always affects cellular tissue and serous membranes in the same way, and mucous membranes in another, whatever their position in the body. He also showed that the advance of inflammation is quite different, in fact inverse, in cellular tissue and the serous membranes on the one hand, and in mucous membranes on the other.[67] Furthermore, all of Hunter's work shows that in his *problématique*, the morbid or lesional process does not spread according to a principle of organic proximity, but according to the paths of a tissue geography.[68] This is true to such a degree that the absorption process in an ulcerative inflammation differs significantly depending on which tissue is affected in a given part of the organism, and one sees the abscesses spread following the paths specific to a given tissue, bypassing, so to speak, other proximate tissues or organs.[69]

The other point raised above, also problematic, is Maulitz's thesis of a genesis of tissue pathology in France independent of the British clinic. We have already argued that tissue pathology was not generated in France independently of British innovations between 1750 and 1800, and, in fact, that there had been direct and indirect appropriation by practitioners like Pinel and Bichat of the British *problématique*, concepts and innovations.[70] The first works of the French school are essentially transpositions and/or extensions of British and certain other non-French innovations. Yet, it must be acknowledged, it is also true that the Paris Clinical School built on these advances to develop its own style of tissue pathology and make extremely important advances that the British, and others, would in turn use. But, as for the beginnings of tissue pathology in France, it is still inadequate to speak of a 'derivation' from foreign developments; what we are really speaking about is a veritable appropriation by French clinicians of an entire body of knowledge produced by the English and others.[71] That is why it seems exaggerated to say that French clinicians *created* the new anatomico-clinical and tissue landscape of disease. We would rather suggest that they extended and enriched this new landscape in their own way and, if it is just to recognize the considerable importance of the contributions of the Paris Clinical School in the first decades of the nineteenth century, we must not forget that other European schools, notably the British, continued to furnish substantial contributions during this same period.

The exact relationship between British and French medicine regarding the question of the genesis and development of tissue pathology is a question that leaves the reader of Maulitz's book rather perplexed. Indeed, the author acknowledges that we have 'traced the notion of tissue specificity to James Carmichael Smyth', and that Pinel had prior knowledge of Smyth's work, which, after it was taken up by Pinel, 'stimulated' Bichat's work.[72] Bichat himself admitted that he had taken the basic concepts of the tissue *problématique* from Pinel. All historians of medicine have noted Bichat's debt towards Pinel, since, before our work on the question, it was not known that Pinel was only an intermediary: Bichat's debt for these concepts was to Smyth.[73] Maulitz also acknowledges that other Parisian clinicians were aware of British work on tissue pathology. Hence he admits, for example, that Laennec was aware of the works of Hunter, Johnstone, Baillie, and, more generally, that 'the medical community on both sides of the English Channel at the end of the eighteenth century was a well-knit one'.[74] Thus, it is difficult to understand how the author can acknowledge, on the one hand, that the French clinicians knew about prior British work on tissue pathology, and affirm, on the other, that tissue pathology in France was, perhaps, 'derived' from 'native French elements'.[75] Moreover, since the author admits that the late eighteenth-century French and British medical communities were closely linked (that concepts and techniques circulated easily between them),[76] it is difficult to understand how he can ignore the fact that Bichat was well acquainted with Hunter's works, to the point of appropriating a considerable part of his ideas, albeit without direct plagiarism as is the case of Pinel towards Smyth.[77] Bichat thus combined Hunter and (via Pinel) Smyth's contributions in order to formulate his own version of the *problématique* of tissue pathology.[78] As Elizabeth Haigh clearly showed, a great number of Bichat's ideas were borrowed from various medical authors.[79] In this regard Haigh observes that while no one works in isolation, the problem with Bichat was that he rarely acknowledged his intellectual debts.[80] She acknowledges our demonstration that the concept of tissues was not elaborated by Bichat, that the tissue *problématique* was present in the works of Hunter and his students, and that Bichat was well acquainted with Hunter's ideas,[81] even though he did not admit that he was in Hunter's debt for much of the tissue *problématique* in his own work.[82] Haigh also notes that we have shown that the concept of tissues as basic elements of the organism was present in the research of many other non-French (mostly English) clinicians before Pinel.[83] As we see it, Maulitz's thesis that tissue pathology developed in France towards the end of the 1790s could have been independent of tissue pathology developing and circulating in Great Britain since the 1750s cannot be sustained. Clearly, at the time this tissue pathology did not constitute a separate 'discipline'; rather it had emerged and developed as a new field of observation and research in the larger context of inter-related work in clinic, pathological anatomy, experimental pathology and surgery, obstetrics and physiology.[84]

III

Having established these points, we will now demonstrate that the British research tradition of anatomico-tissue pathology, generated in the 1750s, grew during the rest of the eighteenth century and continued to grow in Great Britain in a relatively autonomous manner during the first three decades of the nineteenth century. We will also show that it is precisely for this reason that, as early as 1800, British medicine was able to assimilate and incorporate new discoveries being developed in France on the basis of the pre-existing British model. Hence, it was unnecessary to wait for Carswell and Hodgkin in the 1830s and 1840s for those findings to be integrated into British practice. Finally, we will show that, while certain French results were imported into Britain during this period, conversely, English research continued to have an impact on the Paris School. Thus, from the beginning of the nineteenth century, a process of mutual cross-fertilization of ideas occurred.

Indeed, since the end of the eighteenth century and the beginning of the nineteenth century, the teachings of John Hunter and of Smyth were continued and further developed by renowned British practitioners and teachers such as Baillie and Cruikshank in London and John Thomson, Alexander Monro (tertius)[85] and

A Product of the Paris Clinical School?

Andrew Duncan (Jr) in Edinburgh. Through their teaching they reached a considerable number of students, and through medical societies a large number of colleagues. It is clear that Hunter's and Smyth's ideas did not go unrecognized unlike, for instance, those of Mendel in biology, which remained long isolated and unacknowledged. Many British authors of the time emphasized that Hunter's and Smyth's ideas were widely adopted as soon as they were circulated in Britain, and at times even nuanced, enriched or rectified on certain points, proving that work was being done in Britain on the notions of anatomico-tissue pathology. Thus, Andrew Duncan (Jr) (1773–1832), professor at the medical faculty in Edinburgh and president of the College of Physicians of the same city, affirmed explicitly in 1824:

> On the other hand, the effect of the difference of texture of the part inflamed is also so great, that since it was *particularly* pointed out by Dr C. Smyth, *it has perhaps been overrated*; and as phlegmon was stated to be the peculiar form of inflammation when seated in the cellular membrane, *the general adoption of his classification appears to have been the main reason why* the diffuse inflammation of the same texture has not hitherto been the subject of special consideration.[86]

It is clear that Duncan considered that Smyth's tissue classification was, from the start, of the utmost importance for the British and foreign medical communities. According to Duncan, this classification imposed a kind of 'paradigm' in tissue pathology which would eventually be overemphasized and would engender an epistemological obstacle to the consideration of other forms of tissue lesions. Thus we can say that even at the beginning of the third decade of the nineteenth century, the ideas relating to the tissue paradigm that Duncan supplemented and amplified with his own observations and research are not those of Bichat but those of Smyth.

Smyth's approach was largely disseminated at the Edinburgh medical school from the last decade of the eighteenth century; A. Monro (secundus) explained it to his students in the first lecture of his surgery course which was on inflammation.[87] Monro agrees with Smyth that inflammation takes on different characteristics according to the structure of the affected tissue. He observes, however, that the same kind of 'irritating matter' can attack and inflame very different tissues; and that very different kinds of 'infectious matter' can provoke inflammation in the same tissue, but that the appearance of the inflammation will vary according to the nature of the infection.[88] This does not in fact contradict Smyth's ideas[89] and is essentially convergent with Hunter's tissue theory.[90] To this effect, Monro (tertius) writes: 'In the following lecture, the first of his course of Surgery, my father has fully developed his views of the different inflammations of different tissues; and it will be observed, that these views are, in many respects, in the most perfect accordance with the opinion of the modern authors.'[91] Monro (tertius), professor of medicine, anatomy and surgery at the University of Edinburgh Faculty of Medicine in the early nineteenth century, himself published works following a histological approach that he presented as being in direct continuity with his father's (Monro secundus) and, above all, with Smyth's tissue theory.[92]

Further confirmation that Hunter and Smyth's theory of tissues was already well rooted in British medical circles at the beginning of the nineteenth century is given to us by George Gregory (1790–1853).[93] In a work entitled *Elements of the theory and practice of physic designed for the use of students* (1820), Gregory writes:

> The second, and by far the most important of all the sources of distinction among inflammations, is to be found in the structure of the part inflamed. Every part of an animal body, ..., is subject to inflammation, and according to its structure, is inflammation occurring in it, modified both in symptoms and in termination. It is an important and well ascertained fact, that inflammation, in by far the larger proportion of cases, is confined to one texture; that it spreads along that one without affecting other contiguous structures; and that almost all extensions of it from one structure to another are to be viewed as casual exceptions to a general law. For a long time this subject was either all together overlooked, or *but slightly attended* to by pathologists. Dr. Carmichael Smyth has unquestionably the merit of being the first who thought deeply and wrote expressly about it. *The views which he took of this great question are highly ingenious, extensive and accurate. Subsequent observations, indeed, have corrected some and enlarged others: but upon the whole, they may be considered as constituting the basis of all reasonings concerning the varieties of inflammation. John Hunter and Bichat pursued the same track of inquiry.* It was the fault of the latter author that he perhaps *refined* rather too much upon it. Physiologists reduce the fundamental textures of the body to five: viz. cellular membrane, serous membrane, mucous membrane, skin, and fibrous membrane; and accordingly, there are five varieties of inflammation founded on peculiarity of structure: viz. phlegmonous, serous, mucous, erysipelatous, and rheumatic.[94]

This passage, present in the first edition (1820), was part of the lectures he had been giving at the Windmill Street School, and a few years later, around 1815, at the St Thomas's Hospital school.[95] Thus we see that the elements of anatomico-tissue pathology were being taught in major medical schools in London long before Carswell's and Hodgkin's time.[96] It is interesting to note that even after Bichat's publications, it was Smyth's concepts of tissue pathology that Gregory resumed point by point (the typology of five kinds of inflammation for five types of membrane).[97] It is clear then that Smyth's (and Hunter's) teachings and works were being used and developed in London at the beginning of the nineteenth century. Nonetheless, we should mention that Gregory is in error when he places Smyth's work on tissue pathology before Hunter's, whereas the reverse is true. In fact John Hunter began his research on tissue pathology in the 1750s, continuing the work of his brother William. Smyth himself had been a student at the Windmill Street School, thus benefiting from the Hunters' research.[98]

We must also stress the fact that Gregory criticized Bichat for excess of subtlety in rendering the tissue *problématique* in pathology and physiology. As he pointed out, the physiologists of his time limited the number of the organism's principal tissues to five (as did Smyth).[99] Indeed, as we have previously noted, a kind of taxonomic mania in pathology appeared in France after Pinel and Bichat. This mania for classification, or pathological 'scholasticism', developed at the Paris School was, moreover, denounced by members of the school. Thus in 1820, René-Louis Villermé (1782–1863) wrote:

> That the inflammations of one kind of membrane show strikingly similar traits; that inflammations of the serous tissue never have the appearance of mucous inflammations, that from this point of view, the classification of membranes provided an immense service to observational medicine, this is undeniable. But it seems to me that we were much less happy when we identified as many different inflammations as there are tissues in the composition of an organ. In all conscience, can we suppose a membrane's severe inflammation does not affect in any way another membrane to which it is linked most intimately? Have the inflammations of the dura-mater, of the pia-mater, of the internal, external and rachidian arachnoid ever been distinguished aside from in books? To define the inflammation of each of these parts as a different disease and to acknowledge varieties for each of these inflammations, is this not an unnecessary multiplication of types? ['n'est-ce pas multiplier les

A Product of the Paris Clinical School?

êtres sans nécessité?'] Must we absolutely differentiate a metritis *per se*, a uterine peritonitis and a uterine catarrh? Haven't we multiplied the varieties of peritonitis to the extreme? ... Seven or eight varieties of pharyngitis have been discerned, always dependent on the location of the inflammation; the types of ophthalmia have been multiplied *ad infinitum*. We should finally recognize these excesses and above all dare to point them out.[100]

Now, as we have shown,[101] if clinicians at the Paris School had not exceeded Smyth's *problématique*, distorting it through a morphological-classificatory system still based on natural history's taxonomic model, they could have avoided such harsh criticisms. Furthermore, had they better assimilated the Hunterian tissue *problématique*, they would have found ways to correct these exaggerations. In fact it was precisely by going back to the Hunterian *problématique* that some Parisian clinicians would be able to criticize the hyper-classificatory course their school was taking in tissue pathology. This deviation towards a histological classification with scholastic overtones no doubt corresponds to a rigid and dogmatic application of the analytical method cherished by the Ideologues, and to an attachment to natural history's epistemological model of classification, deviations found in the first generation of clinicians at the Paris School (Pinel, etc.).

For Hunter, pathology and anatomical pathology were not based on a model taken from natural history; instead, both are dialectically related to physiology.[102] Indeed, as Palmer observes, the whole Hunterian *problématique* is characterized by 'that alliance between Pathology and Physiology which forms the characteristic feature of his doctrines'.[103]

Moreover, as Dezeimeris emphasized, anatomico-pathologists were divided into two schools at the beginning of the nineteenth century, 'the first, following John Hunter, investigates the laws of development of the irregular states of our bodily parts and lays the foundation for a completely new pathological physiology; the second, following Bayle, Dupuytren and Laennec, draws from autopsy alone the history of abnormal modifications of the human body'. Thus, Dezeimeris contrasts an anatomical pathology linked to physiology to an essentially morphological pathological anatomy typical of a great part of the Paris Clinical School. This cleavage between a Hunterian 'physiological' school and a morphological school is encountered in the field of pathological anatomy of tissues. It was almost certainly the classificatory and morphological model

A Product of the Paris Clinical School?

of natural history that induced a significant part of the Paris School to adopt an essentially descriptive and morphological anatomico-tissue pathology. And without a doubt, it is precisely because many British practitioners, following the Hunterian tradition in the clinic and in pathological anatomy, conceded an important role to the physiological dimension of pathogenesis in their works that the fundamental concepts of tissue pathology were not easily discerned, even though they were already instrumental in their pathology. Indeed, for the Hunterians, the concepts of tissue pathology are not simply anatomical; they are also 'physiopathological'. Of course, by giving considerable weight, in the study of organic lesions, to cause and constitution, next to tissue structure, and by giving equal weight to the pathological process as to its static product (the anatomical alteration), a false impression may arise: the histopathological *problématique* would appear less elaborated in a physiological framework than in a morphological construct, while, in fact, the opposite is true.[104]

We should stress that Laennec himself rectified Bichat's hyper-classificatory casuistry from the point of view of descriptive pathological anatomy.[105] In Britain, the development of the tissue *problématique* was not marked by these types of taxonomic exaggerations; it should be noted that this did not prevent the further consolidation of observation and research in early nineteenth-century Britain. In fact the opposite is true.

To this effect, it is quite surprising that Maulitz did not mention those British practitioners of the period who produced treatises on normal general and pathological anatomy (e.g., Craigie),[106] and that he ignored very important works in tissue pathology, such as Bright's work. These practitioners combined British contributions in tissue pathology with those of the French (and with the German tradition and that of other European schools). Reading Maulitz, one would be led to believe that, except for Farre and the group of practitioners at the Academy of Minute Anatomy (1825) and the London Ophthalmic Infirmary (founded in 1804–5),[107] there was no tissue pathology in Britain during the entire period between Hunter and Baillie's generation and that of Carswell and Hodgkin.

An examination of Hodgkin's work, taken here as one example among many, demonstrates that his research on tissue pathology (and his teaching) was not merely based on French work, but also on British studies (Baillie, Bright, Craigie, Abercrombie, Baron, Knox, Carswell, etc.). In fact, Hodgkin draws attention to the works of the preceding generation (Hunter, Smyth, the Monros, Home, Cline, etc.).[108] Indeed, he emphasizes the importance of Baillie's works (and therefore of the Hunterian tradition) for the development of pathological anatomy throughout Europe in the late eighteenth century, and situates his own work within the scope of the British tradition (and within the earlier Morgagnian tradition), as well as within the French one.[109] It is worth noting that Hodgkin also refers to the studies in tissue pathology of the Vienna school (De Haen, Stoll, etc.) and the achievements of the German school (notably Meckel junior), as well as the Italian school.[110] The preface to Hodgkin's work clearly shows that he considers that Great Britain, France, Germany and Italy all hold an important position in the development of pathological anatomy and tissue pathology, and that this discipline grew through contributions from the different schools and through reciprocal exchanges and use of information.[111]

It is therefore inaccurate to state that ideas about tissue and anatomical pathology were not further developed in Britain in the early nineteenth century. In an important chapter of his book,[112] Maulitz himself shows that the Hunter–Smyth tradition of tissue pathology evolved quite independently from the 'Bichatian' tradition: he is referring to the studies in tissue pathology completed at the Academy of Minute Anatomy and at the London Ophthalmic Infirmary by practitioners such as Saunders, Farre, Lawrence or John Dalrymple, as well as to other practitioners who collaborated with the *Journal of Morbid Anatomy*, founded by Farre in the late 1820s. Maulitz also names Scottish practitioners such as Duncan (junior) and Thomson (1765–1846) who, in his view, combined both British and French traditions of tissue pathology. However, the author should have taken account of the essential fact that, in addition to this group of physicians and surgeons, many other British practitioners carried on the British tradition of tissue pathology, integrating the concept of tissues into their pathological anatomy and their anatomico-clinical practice. These practitioners often declared themselves solely within the Hunter–Smyth tradition, but sometimes simultaneously mentioned Bichat and/or the French studies in the field, and combined the two traditions in their own research.

Amongst those practitioners, we can begin with Baillie, and continue with many others: R. Willan (1757–1812),[113] Ch. Bell (1774–1842),[114] J. Baron,[115] J. Cheyne (1777–1836),[116] A. Cooper (1768–1841),[117] A. Monro (tertius), J. Abernethy (1764–1831),[118] W. Lawrence (1783–1867),[119] B. C. Brodie (1783–1862),[120] George Gregory, J. H. James (1789–1869),[121] J. Yelloly (1774–1842),[122] J.

Abercrombie (1780–1844), J. Hodgson (1788–1869),[123] B. Travers (1783–1858),[124] C. Hastings,[125] J. Armstrong,[126] J. Wardrop (1782–1869),[127] C. Badham,[128] R. Bright (1789–1858),[129] D. Craigie, etc.

We might consider John Abercrombie, M.D., as an example. A member of the College of Physicians of Edinburgh, Abercrombie is the author of *Pathological and Practical Researches on the Diseases of the Stomach, the Intestinal Canal, the Liver and other Viscera of the Abdomen* (Edinburgh, 1828) and *Pathological and Practical Researches on Diseases of the Brain and the Spinal Chord* (Edinburgh, 1828). These works clearly demonstrate that research in tissue pathology was occurring in Britain before Carswell's and Hodgkin's publications. For example, in the first treatise the pathology is organized uniquely around tissue structures: see 'View of the structures concerned in this inquiry, and the principal morbid conditions to which they are liable: I) Peritoneum, II) Muscular Coat, III) Mucous Membrane' (pp. 27–35).

The second part of the essay, entitled 'Of the inflammatory affections of the more external parts of the intestinal canal, including peritonitis and enteritis' (pp. 151–93) reviews all forms of peritonitis and enteritis based on the author's case studies beginning in 1810. The same is true for the next part: 'Of the inflammatory affections of the mucous membrane of the intestinal canal' (pp. 194–265). This chapter is divided into three sections: I) Active inflammation of the mucous membrane of the intestinal canal, II) Of the chronic diseases of the mucous membrane, III) Ulcers of the mucous membrane without prominent symptoms. In this study we find a very detailed analysis, largely based on the author's observations during his practice, of pathology of tissues of the organs of the abdominal region. Of course, the author also cites a certain number of his colleagues' observations on the subject, but they essentially complement his own inquiries. Abercrombie gives equal if not more consideration to British practitioners' observations on tissue pathology (Smyth, Hunter, Monro (tertius), Alison, Annesley, Travers, Hamilton, Knox, Cheyne, Marshall Hall) as to observations made by French practitioners such as Pinel, Bretonneau and Louis. Furthermore, in his works, Abercrombie rectifies certain points of the analyses made by practitioners like Bretonneau and Rostan. Other British practitioners similarly revised the works of French authors in the field.

In 1820, C. Hastings of the Hunterian school wrote on the very first page of the preface to his treatise on the inflammation of

A Product of the Paris Clinical School?

mucous membranes:

> *It will be admitted, that the effects of inflammation vary considerably in the different textures of the human body, and that it is of the first importance accurately to distinguish the morbid changes which occur in these several textures when inflamed* ... Until the appearance of Dr. Badham's essay on bronchitis, in which he has given an excellent outline of this genus of diseases, there was no separate work, in our own language at least, on the inflammation of the mucous membrane of the lungs. The author of the following treatise has, *for some years, had frequent opportunities of witnessing cases of this description, and of ascertaining the state of the lungs after death*; so that he has gradually accumulated many facts which appear to him calculated to throw additional light on this interesting though still obscure disease.[130]

Hastings then embarked on a detailed analysis of all the varieties of bronchitis and their different effects on tissues, citing a large number of anatomico-clinical observations. He did cite with approval the works of Bichat in physiology, but he mainly used British studies on tissue pathology of mucous membranes and corresponding anatomico-clinical observations. Indeed he constantly referred to the works of Badham, Armstrong, John Cheyne,[131] Baron, Duncan (Jr), Chevalier, Warren, Wilson Philip, etc.

These examples, chosen amongst many others, show that during the 1820s anatomico-tissue pathology was developing in Britain in a relatively autonomous manner. It was not a question of British medicine passively assimilating French tissue pathology.

Having said this, we should not forget that there were also important interactions between France and Britain in this field. Thus Gendrin considered Abercrombie's work on diseases of the brain, which analyses in detail the pathology of membranes and the inflammation of tissues, important enough to translate it into French in 1832. However, in the footnotes, Gendrin incorporated many observations of his own which were later included by Abercrombie in the third edition of his work in 1834. There was thus a relationship of mutual enrichment between English and French medicine in the field of tissue pathology.

R. Carswell (1793–1857) made note of British contributions in tissue pathology, mainly those of Hunter and Thomson.[132] In turn, in his treatise of general and pathological anatomy, Craigie explicitly recognized the British tradition of tissue pathology, extending from Hunter and Smyth to Thomson (1765–1846),[133] to be independent of and prior to the French movement (from Bichat to Béclard). In his work he made use of both these traditions, as well as the German one (Meckel, etc.). His aim was to complete the French and English trends of tissue pathology because, in his view, notwithstanding these achievements, no comprehensive system of tissue-based pathological anatomy existed at the time (1826).[134] Hence Craigie defined the objective of his treatise as follows:

> In the arrangement of the materials in which it consists, I found it impossible to adopt the methods in ordinary use. Without pretending to determine the comparative merits of the methods of Baillie, Conradi, Meckel, and Cruveilhier, each of which has peculiar advantages, I may be permitted to observe, that the first object in tracing the progress and effects of pathological processes is to fix the boundary between what is sound and what is morbid, and that every morbid process always bears some relation to the proper characters of the texture in a sound state. For these reasons, I have chosen as the basis of the arrangement, the distinction of the component tissues of the animal body, as derived from the similitude and difference of their anatomical characters; and, *though the advantages of this method have been recognized by John Hunter, Carmichael Smyth, Bichat, Dr. Thompson and Béclard*, I am not aware that any complete system of pathological anatomy has been hitherto constructed according to its principles. The present attempt is, I believe, *the first instance in which it has been carried to the length of a full though elementary treatise.*[135]

It would therefore be in Britain in the late 1820s that the project of a complete pathological anatomy based on the distinction of the human body's tissues would be fully achieved. Does this mean that anatomico-tissue pathology did not exist before Craigie? Of course not, no more than it started with Bichat. In fact, as Craigie himself pointed out, tissue pathology (or the application of the principles of general anatomy to pathology) began at the Edinburgh school and the William Hunter school, and it was through the works of John Hunter and Smyth that the first major achievements were made in this field.[136] As we can see, if anatomical and tissue pathology grew in a somewhat uneven way in Britain, nonetheless it did continuously develop from the time of Hunter to Thomson and Craigie and later during Carswell and Hodgkin's period. Furthermore, Maulitz himself recognizes that for Scottish clinicians in the early nineteenth century, Bichatian tissue pathology was not new since, to be precise, it was not really Bichatian and these

A Product of the Paris Clinical School?

clinicians already had their own British tradition. The author admits in fact, in agreement with our thesis, that the Scottish knew all this.[137] But we should add that the Scottish practitioners were not the only ones who knew all this: this was equally true for many other British practitioners, particularly the Hunterians in London.

IV

Within the limits of this essay it is impossible to offer an exhaustive analysis of the socio-institutional context of the development of anatomical and tissue pathology in Britain in the eighteenth and nineteenth centuries. We have dealt with some of these questions in earlier works.[138] Our intention is to complement those works, showing that this field was first constituted in Great Britain in a conceptual and institutional context of research and educational practices that was receptive despite obstacles,[139] and that a relatively autonomous tradition could have developed in these circumstances in the first decades of the nineteenth century in the advanced sectors of British medicine.

As we have seen, Maulitz would have us believe that the institutional and socio-professional context in Great Britain was not favourable to the development of anatomical and tissue pathology, thus explaining its apparent eclipse after Hunter and Baillie. In our earlier works we proposed a different analysis. We should add that one must not confuse the formal frameworks of the profession and of medical institutions with the actual practices that in fact further medical knowledge. At that time, indeed, it was often outside the sphere of official medical institutions that knowledge progressed. We should also note that in Paris, as elsewhere, formal official structures hindered the advancement of knowledge. In fact, at the beginning of his book, Maulitz himself stresses that professional and institutional pressures and traditions in pathology of the Paris School kept Bichat in a marginal position with regards to the academic and professional centres of the Faculty of Medicine. Bichat never held an academic post at the Faculty, and even Bayle and Laennec accomplished most of their work outside the walls of this institution – Bayle was never a professor there and Laennec was only appointed in 1823, three years before his death. According to the author, during the entire Napoleonic era, 'Bichatian' tissue pathology was unable to gain a foothold at the *École pratique de dissection* or in lectures on pathology at the Faculty of Medicine. Bichat's pathology could only slowly infiltrate the dominant school of anatomical pathology, which remained Morgagnian and centred on the organ, not the tissue. It

A Product of the Paris Clinical School?

was only during the 1820s that it began to be present in the official educational system.[140] According to Maulitz, therefore, during this period the Faculty of Medicine does not appear as a centre for creation of new medical knowledge, but subsequently becomes the authority that legitimizes it.[141] We could even say that the Faculty incorporates the work produced outside its walls.[142] In Britain, as in France, the development of anatomico-tissue pathology during the nineteenth century often occurred outside the confines of corporations and academic educational institutions (such as London's Royal College of Physicians and the medical faculties at Oxford and Cambridge) and in an official socio-institutional context which was, in many respects and for reasons different from those in France, far from favourable. Nevertheless, a favourable informal socio-institutional context did exist.

Why Maulitz does not apply the same standard for England as he does for France remains puzzling. According to him the tripartite division of the medical profession into physicians, surgeons and surgeon-apothecaries in nineteenth-century Great Britain constituted the principal obstacle to the continuation of the Hunter–Baillie tradition of anatomical and tissue pathology. It prevented the anatomico-localist approach in surgery from being applied in medicine, as it was in France, where the two professions, medicine and surgery, were united after the Revolution. Yet for some time now, a number of works have emphasized the fact that in England these divisions were strictly formal, that in practice the great surgeons also had medical training (and practised in both fields), and that many surgeon-apothecaries, who were half-way between medicine and surgery, were educated in and practised in both branches. Long before the Apothecaries Act of 1815, surgeon-apothecaries were *de facto* general practitioners working simultaneously in medicine and surgery. A considerable number of surgeon-apothecaries identified themselves as surgeons and/or physicians, often joining the respective professional corporations.[143] Furthermore, a significant number of physicians also were initiated into surgery and pathological anatomy (for instance in the schools of William and John Hunter and their successors, in hospitals and hospital schools, in Edinburgh, etc.).[144] British surgeons and surgeon-apothecaries without a doubt contributed as much, if not more, than physicians to the field of anatomical and tissue pathology in the early nineteenth century. But this does not imply that this pathology did not evolve at the time: in fact, a number of British physicians did indeed contribute substantially to this field.

A Product of the Paris Clinical School?

These physicians often had surgical training in the same way that surgeons and surgeon-apothecaries also received fairly significant training in medicine.[145]

It has often been said that the physicians of the Paris School were able to develop the anatomico-clinical approach because they had adopted the anatomico-localist point of view of eighteenth-century surgeons or of the surgical clinic. If this is indeed one of the essential conditions for the development of the anatomico-clinical approach, it is then quite logical that it made significant advances in England – before the Paris School. The anatomico-localist point of view was widespread in the clinical practice of advanced medical circles, given that many practitioners who also worked in 'internal' clinical medicine – surgeons and surgeon-apothecaries employed in hospitals and institutions in particular – had a background primarily in clinical surgery; hence they would necessarily apply the anatomico-localist approach. Moreover, as we have seen, physicians engaged in clinical practice in institutions often acquired significant training in anatomy and surgery. They were thus also inclined to incorporate the anatomical point of view into medicine. The *de facto* decompartmentalization in England between the different practitioners in the realms of education, practice and research – despite rivalries and power conflicts between the different professional corporations – is a characteristic of the British medical milieu of the time and a very positive factor in the affirmation of an anatomico-surgical point of view in the internal clinic. Moreover, it also led to a genuine interpenetration of medicine and surgery, allowing the affirmation of a medico-physiological point of view in surgery, giving this craft a more scientific basis. This interaction between and interpenetration of different medical branches was also favoured by close collaboration between physicians, surgeons, surgeon-apothecaries and apothecaries in clinical practice (in hospitals, infirmaries and dispensaries), in clinical research (again in institutions: for diagnosis, treatment, dissection, etc.) and in the medical societies, despite the different professional allegiances of the practitioners.[146]

Thus, with regards to the affirmation of an anatomical point of view in medicine, the socio-professional context of medical practice was as favourable for the rapid development of clinical practice in Britain in the late eighteenth and early nineteenth centuries as in France, where, in 1794, medicine and surgery were officially united. We know that interaction between medicine and surgery already existed in clinical practice in France before the laws of 1794, which led, *de facto*, to an increasing link between the two branches in the avant-garde of these professions. But it is quite certain that in Britain, as early as the last decades of the eighteenth century, the interaction and collaboration between practitioners in the various branches and the polyvalence of some elite practitioners promoted the adoption of an anatomical approach in the clinic (which in the Hunterian school combined with the 'physiopathological' approach to morbid processes in medical and surgical clinic). Despite the inertia of corporations like the Royal College of Physicians of London, a considerable number of practitioners or clinicians from diverse professional backgrounds were able to consolidate the anatomical and localist approach to disease that was characteristic of the Hunter–Baillie tradition.

It is also important to emphasize that the concepts of anatomical and tissue pathology obviously did not fall from the English heavens. They emerged within a framework of institutional structures and medical practices that made their development possible. Indeed, these concepts could only be generated through clinical experience based on the observation of a significant number of medical and surgical cases in diverse institutional settings. These settings, in which one acquired practical knowledge of organic lesions of organs and tissues through dissection, surgical operations, treatment of wounds, and so on, ranged from hospitals to infirmaries, from dispensaries to military hospitals (standard and in the field) and to private practice. The schools and museums of anatomy were also places where one could obtain medico-surgical and anatomico-clinical knowledge. Research in clinical medicine, pathological anatomy, experimental pathology, etc., was conducted in formal, semi-formal or informal ways in these diverse institutional settings. Clearly it is in such a material field of clinical experience and practice that important concepts of lesions of organs and tissues took shape as early as the 1750s.[147]

Of course the development of this knowledge was uneven and encountered various obstacles, in England as elsewhere, and sometimes more than elsewhere. Nonetheless it was sufficient to allow the development and growth of an anatomical and tissue pathology. True, legal, economic (high cost of cadavers), and socio-cultural impediments that complicated dissection in Great Britain should in principle have hindered the advancement of pathological anatomy and the anatomical clinic. Yet, remarkably, despite these obstacles it was in Britain that pathological anatomy made the most significant progress in the last decades of the eighteenth century and

A Product of the Paris Clinical School?

British practitioners continued to produce very important results in the first decades of the nineteenth century. The fact is that, despite these hindrances, dissection was practised on a large scale by a significant number of practitioners and it was part of the system of practical training.[148]

Maulitz writes that the concern of his book pertains less to a genealogy of ideas than to the unravelling of the story of a tradition. According to him, the emergence of a tradition 'depends upon a great deal more than the enunciation of key ideas. It depends upon even more than the sharing of those ideas among members of an elite, educated community given to reading memoirs of their peers.'[149] The author asserts that by this definition the medical community on both sides of the English Channel shared close ties. He also admits that this is a very important factor which explains how a 'line of intellectual ideas', like that of anatomical and tissue pathology, develops. But he goes on to say that 'minds thus drawn together do not in themselves form a tradition. Something very different, something in the nature of a conjunction of institutions, professional groups *and ideas* is needed to effect such a change.'[150]

The problem is that there was indeed an indigenous tradition of pathological anatomy and tissue pathology in Britain between 1750 and 1800 (as Maulitz himself avers), independent of the French tradition. This understanding logically leads to trying to determine what could have made this tradition possible: how did it come into existence and how was it transmitted, that is, in what kind of scientific and socio-institutional context? Is it not extreme idealism to assume that key concepts of tissue pathology appeared spontaneously in the realm of pure ideas? It is obvious that the emergence of new ideas in pathological anatomy and the anatomical clinic in Great Britain depended as much on material conditions as Maulitz claims they did in France. But these material conditions are as much of a scientific and technical nature as of a socio-institutional and professional nature. The key ideas or basic concepts (the *problématique*) of tissue pathology did not appear miraculously or by chance in Britain. These ideas or concepts could not have appeared and developed without a structure of scientific medical practice (and of its socio-institutional context) providing a context for their development.[151] For Maulitz, one of the essential conditions for the development of a tradition in pathological anatomy was the existence of an 'institutional context for the reinforcement and dissemination of theoretical notions about tissue pathology'.[152] We have demonstrated that a favourable institutional context – although mostly informal or semi-formal – did exist in Great Britain, as it later did in France. In addition, we cannot agree with the division the author establishes between the theoretical notions miraculously appearing outside of a necessary institutional context, and the dissemination and reinforcement of ideas which require this appropriate context. In our view, a favourable – formal or informal – institutional context is necessary both for the production of ideas or concepts and for their dissemination. Indeed, the concepts of anatomico-tissue pathology of Hunter, the Monros, Baillie and their students could never have been produced without a favourable institutional (as well as technical and scientific) context (anatomico-clinical practices, the interpenetration between medicine and surgery, etc.). Moreover, an institutional context which promotes the creation and elaboration of new theoretical notions in a given field will usually also favour their further development and diffusion.

It seems to us, therefore, that Maulitz clearly betrays an idealistic stance when he writes: 'Theoretical notions [about anatomico-tissue pathology] were as nothing without the milieux within which they might be put into practice.'[153] In reading this one might think that the British concepts in anatomico-tissue pathology were generated in a purely intellectual or theoretical space and pre-existed all anatomico-clinical, surgical and experimental practices. In fact, practice itself (and the institutional structures which sustained it) was the means by which these concepts could be constituted. Within the framework of this practice, these concepts would develop and spread. It is undeniable that a significant practice of dissection and of clinico-pathological correlation must have already existed in British medicine at that time for it to be able to 1) renew the gross pathological anatomy of the Morgagnian school, and 2) move beyond the pathology of organs to a pathology of tissues.

It is evident, nevertheless, that ideas that were first conceived and elaborated in a given country (in this case Great Britain) can, when transferred to another country (France), undergo new parallel developments which can even surpass in some areas those of the country of origin. (If France surpassed Great Britain in some areas of internal medicine from the 1820s onwards, for example, it did not in anatomico-clinical surgery.) It is also clear that the greater facilities available in Paris for experience in the anatomico-clinical field made the French capital a 'magnet' for British and foreign students, as Maulitz and others rightly point out.[154] This certainly enabled students to acquaint themselves with new local developments in anatomico-clinical medicine through direct experience, and not merely through the writings of French clinicians. However, this does not mean that the British did not develop their own local anatomico-clinical tradition and make contributions to this field. True, British medical students arrived in great numbers in Paris after Waterloo; but this does not invalidate our thesis: that anatomico-tissue pathology was first constituted and developed in England in the eighteenth century and that a significant body of research continued to develop in the early nineteenth century, as several French clinicians who travelled to Great Britain at the time discovered. For this reason many British practitioners and researchers, already working on anatomico-clinical research, did not feel the need to go to Paris in order to acknowledge the value of French innovations (for example, mediate auscultation). In the same way, many Parisian clinicians felt no need to cross the English Channel in order to assimilate the anatomico-tissue pathology of Hunter, Smyth, Baillie and their peers and successors.[155] If leading British clinicians read about, understood and assimilated French innovations without difficulty, it is because they already had considerable anatomico-clinical experience, just as French clinicians were able to easily understand and assimilate the innovations of the British tradition because of their own substantial anatomico-clinical practice.

In another context, Warner has shown that the transfer of knowledge between countries is a complicated and selective process. For instance, what British practitioners and students retained from France and Paris medicine during the first decades of the nineteenth century differs greatly from what their American counterparts borrowed.[156] Each tended to focus on the characteristics of Paris medicine which had the greatest implications or consequences for their own country's medical profession. Through this process of selection, the English and the Americans constructed very different images of the Paris Clinical School. The British tended to stress above all the model of medical polity or professional organization, while the Americans mainly focused on the Paris School's epistemological model of sceptical empiricism.[157]

In a similar vein, Jacyna, in describing Carswell's and Thomson's stay in France, and in particular at the Hôtel-Dieu in Lyons, observes that it was not a mere passive process of assimilation but a genuine interaction between 'medical cultures'. The visitors' background and orientation influenced their perceptions of French medicine and guided what they selected from it. It is quite significant that the two Scots did not find what they were looking for in Paris, and therefore proceeded to Lyons in order to complete their clinical experience, mainly in the field of surgery.[158] While cognizant that they found in France a rich terrain of experience for themselves, given their earlier training, they were nonetheless often critical towards French clinical practices. They noticed various inadequacies in comparison to what they had learned and seen in their own country, in the field of pathological anatomy, for example.

In 1815, John G. Crosse, another British practitioner visiting France, pointed out this paradox: although France offered more opportunities than England for practising dissection, pathological anatomy and clinical surgery were more advanced in England than in France.[159]

The transfer of knowledge is not a process of passive assimilation even when it is acquired through the reading and study of foreign medical writings and not through the medium of visiting practitioners or students. Thus, as we have shown, the Paris School was quite selective in its assimilation of British anatomico-tissue pathology. Pinel and Bichat integrated it into a highly systematic classificatory paradigm, derived from the analytic philosophy of *Idéologie* as applied to the natural history of diseases. This paradigm was not included in Hunter's, Smyth's or Baillie's *problématique*. On the other hand, Pinel and Bichat neglected – or perhaps were unable to assimilate and develop – some core elements of the anatomico-tissue pathology *problématique*, elements one could find in the works of Hunter and the Hunterians. Only later were these elements taken into account by the Paris School, first by Broussais and afterwards by medical writers like Andral.

For example, in determining the nature of a lesion, the proponents of the British School attached considerable importance to the cause and to the constitution, in addition to the tissue structure. They were more interested in the physiopathological dynamics of morbid processes (including the tissue level) than in their static product. What was paramount for Pinel, however, was the classification of diseases in relation to tissues, while for Bichat it was the classification of tissues *per se*, but essentially from the perspective of normal anatomy and physiology.[160]

Moreover, Hunter's histopathological *problématique* allowed the conception of both organic solids and fluids as tissues. This original concept of tissues allowed the integration of a solidistic and neo-humoral pathology into a localist approach to disease, which simultaneously gave considerable weight to both the constitution and general state of the organism. Now Bichat, who was entrenched in Pinel's solidistic paradigm, focused on solids as tissues and was less interested in the place of organic fluids in pathology, with the exception of a few general declarations of principle mentioning their important role in disease.[161] Another innovation in Hunter's study of tissues, also to be found in the works of his followers, is the common use of the microscope for the analysis of tissues in normal as well as pathological states.[162] As we know, Bichat and many later members of the Paris School refused, due to their sensualist purism, to use the microscope in pathological anatomy and, consequently, they were not in a position to integrate this important component of the Hunterian anatomical/tissue pathology.[163] One can see how the particular intellectual tradition or epistemological orientation of a medical school can guide it in many ways in the selection and appropriation of elements from another school's body of knowledge. This selection can have positive results: Pinel's and Bichat's contributions to the creation of the great Parisian tradition of 'descriptive' or 'empiricist' clinic, for example.[164] However, this selection also had a negative aspect, for it left aside, for a time at least, research in anatomico-tissue pathology, of a different, more experimental and physiopathological, orientation. This other trend in research had already brought fruitful results in Great Britain and elsewhere and would continue to do so. Bichat did not exploit other elements of the Hunterian research *problématique* in his selective assimilation. These include the experiences in transplantation of tissues in order to determine their physiological properties and understand their reactions in the pathological state,[165] and Hunter's studies in comparative histogenesis.[166]

When dealing with the transfer between countries of elements extracted from a specific body of knowledge (as is the case of anatomico-tissue pathology), the political aims and strategies of the medical circles into which these innovations are imported are not the sole factors determining the kind of selection, assimilation and reconstruction of those elements that will be made. It also often depends on requirements of the scientific tradition and on the established orientation of research in the recipient country. Thus, it would appear that Pinel's and Bichat's incorporation of British anatomico-tissue pathology into a classificatory framework that was central to their approach is the result of their intellectual habits, based on the philosophical model of *Idéologie* prevailing in Parisian medicine, rather than the requirements of the politics of the profession. In addition, research trends in Paris (prior to the works of Magendie), when compared to the Hunterian tradition, appear less oriented towards physiological and experimental pathology, the use of the microscope for the analysis of tissues, the histological approach to organic fluids and the correlation of all these studies with comparative anatomy, comparative physiology and pathology.[167]

On the other hand, it seems that the requirements of professional politics of a country's medical community explain substantially the overall manner in which the selection/assimilation of elements of foreign medicine is made, as well as the way in which the resultant model is constructed for implementation at home. This explains why, in some cases, foreign scientific models are favoured over earlier native ones, even though the latter are older and sometimes are more sophisticated in some aspects.

A case in point is Hunterian pathology. Indeed it is likely that one reason why some British practitioners did not fully acknowledge the importance of the Hunterian school in pathological anatomy and tissue pathology (and more generally in clinical anatomy) was the tension existing between the various groups of reform-minded medical practitioners, with surgeon-apothecaries at their head, and the conservative professional corporations. Maulitz claims that surgeon-apothecaries were advocating a reform of the medical profession in their own interests and were thus highly critical of London's medical establishment. (Their principal target was the Royal College of Physicians, of course, but perhaps even more so the Royal College of Surgeons.)[168] Generally, it can be said that the majority of practitioners who did not belong to these traditional professional associations were reformers opposed to the London medical establishment, which came from both Royal Colleges.

We know that at the beginning of the nineteenth century, John Hunter was already a dominant symbol for the surgical profession, and in particular for the Royal College of Surgeons.[169] Hunter was acclaimed as the man who had raised surgery from the status of a craft to that of a science. But at the same time he was also the most important symbol of London's medico-surgical establishment and medical elite, of which the Royal College of Surgeons was the institutional pillar for surgeons. All members of the College, and in particular its successive presidents, loudly proclaimed their Hunterian heritage (including pathological and clinical anatomy) and considered themselves as its disciples. Likewise, Baillie was a pillar of both the Hunterian establishment (composed of physicians and surgeons having key positions in London's hospitals) and the Royal College of Physicians, where he obtained the highest rank of Fellow in 1789.[170] After Hunter's death, Baillie took his place as

A Product of the Paris Clinical School?

dominant symbol of the London medical elite.

It is thus clear why surgeon-apothecaries and other reformers from various medical fields were unwilling to give Hunter and Hunterians like Baillie full credit, refusing to acknowledge the breadth of their achievements in pathological anatomy, tissue pathology and, more generally, in anatomico-clinical medicine. They preferred to praise Bichat and the French School since, as Warner has shown, the 'anti-elitist' and 'meritocratic' Paris School was the model of professional politics for many reform-minded British medical circles in which surgeon-apothecaries played an important role.[171]

Conclusion

In conclusion, we would say that the present study demonstrates that anatomico-tissue pathology was constituted in Great Britain – and not in France – during the last decades of the eighteenth century. We have shown that it continued to grow in British medicine in the early nineteenth century – not only at the Paris Clinical School – after which time there was an important and mutually enriching interaction between the two medical milieux during the first three decades of the nineteenth century. Until now the emphasis historians have put on the contributions of the Paris Clinical School has resulted in the neglect of those of British medicine and others. Possibly the overvaluation given to the Paris Clinical School during the first half of the nineteenth century by some British and American practitioners (who constructed highly idealized models of the Paris School for their own profession's political ends) is to a large extent the cause of the underestimation by historians of medicine of British contributions to anatomical and tissue pathology and of the importance of the interaction of British medicine and the Paris Clinical School. It should be noted that while contributions of the Paris School have been overvalued, the study of important developments in laboratory medicine (the use of the microscope, for example; see contribution of Ann La Berge in this volume) or of developments after 1848 (see contribution by Joy Harvey) has been neglected as a result of acceptance of Ackerknecht's famous thesis of the 'dead end'. It was not only the British and Americans who elaborated idealized images of the Paris School, each based on their own particular professional aspirations. It seems that another idealized vision of the School, where we find certain aspects from the two others, was also constructed by some members of the Paris School themselves, as well as by some of their successors. This was how the legend of Pinel and Bichat as founders of tissue pathology was forged in part by the Paris School itself as one of its founding myths. The act of creating founding heroes, of proclaiming that Parisian medicine had made a radical break with medicine of the Ancien Régime or of other countries corresponded with the need to affirm the superiority of the system and the professional organization – which formed the basis for medical science – put in place since the Revolution. The more that French medical science was deemed original, the less it seemed to owe to the past or to other countries, the more the new socio-institutional and professional system that underpinned this medical science could be seen as positive and worthy of consolidation.

Thus we see that, by accepting on face value the thesis of the Paris School's radical break with the medical past in France and in other countries, of absolute and/or unique innovation, as well as total autonomy of the scientific developments of this School with regard to other schools, some historians of medicine, including Foucault, have only strengthened a highly idealized image that was initially constructed in great part to promote the socio-professional strategies of the French – in particular the Parisian – medical corps in the early decades of the nineteenth century.[172]

Notes

1. See here, 124.
2. See M. Foucault, *La Naissance de la Clinique* (Paris: Presses Universitaires de France, 1963), and E. Ackerknecht, *Medicine at the Paris Hospital, 1794–1848* (Baltimore: Johns Hopkins Press, 1967).
3. For Foucault, the Bichat tissue *problématique* made possible a conceptual mastery of death (or a decomposition into partial, successive, and plural death of tissues) which constituted the fundamental revolution of pathology by which it was the knowledge of death that made possible knowledge of life. See *The Birth of the Clinic: An Archeology of Medical Perception*, trans. A. M. Sheridan (London: Tavistock Publications, 1973), 144–5. But this conceptual mastery of death was already part of the Hunterian *problématique*, which Foucault half-recognized: *ibid*. See O. Keel, 'Les conditions de la décomposition analytique de l'organisme: Haller, Hunter, Bichat', *Etudes philosophiques*, 1 (1982), 37–62. See also on this point S. J. Cross, 'John Hunter, the animal economy and late eighteenth-century physiological discourse', in W. Coleman and C. Limoges, (eds), *Studies in History of Biology*, 5 (1981), 1–110. Cross, comparing the works of Hunter and Bichat, shows that it was the

A Product of the Paris Clinical School?

former who elaborated this *problématique* in the area of anatomical pathology, but he failed to take into account the tissue basis of Hunterian anatomical pathology, which would in fact reinforce his thesis. Cross writes: 'Death became conceptualized and entered the field of positive knowledge in various forms with Hunter, in addition to that of morbid nosology.' *Ibid.*, 33.

4. See O. Keel, 'Cabanis et la généalogie de la médecine clinique' (Ph.D. dissertation, McGill University, 1977); *idem*, *La généalogie de l'histopathologie* (Paris: Vrin, 1979); *idem*, 'La pathologie tissulaire de John Hunter', *Gesnerus*, 37 (1980), 47–61; *idem*, 'John Hunter et Xavier Bichat. Les rapports de leurs travaux en pathologie tissulaire', *Actes du XXVIIe Congrès International d'Histoire de la Médecine* (Barcelona: Delfos, 1981), vol. 2, 535–49; *idem*, 'La constitution de la *problématique* de l'anatomie des systèmes selon Laennec', in *Commémoration du Bicentenaire de la Naissance de Laennec, 1786–1826 : Colloque organisé au Collège de France les 18 et 19 février 1981. Paris : Revue du Palais de la Découverte*, no. spécial 22 (1981), 189–207; *idem*, 'Haller, Hunter, Bichat'; *idem*, 'La place et la fonction des modèles étrangers dans la constitution de la problématique hospitalière de l'École de Paris', *History and Philosophy of the Life Sciences*, 6 (1984), 41–73; *idem* , 'The Politics of Health and the Institutionalisation of Clinical Practices in Europe in the Second Half of the Eighteenth Century', in W. Bynum and R. Porter (eds), *William Hunter and the Eighteenth Century Medical World* (Cambridge: Cambridge University Press, 1985), 207–256; *idem*, 'La problématique institutionnelle de la clinique de la fin du XVIIIe siècle aux années de la Restauration', *Canadian Bulletin of Medical History*, 2 (1985), 183–206 and 3 (1986), 1–30; *idem*, 'L'Ecole Clinique de Paris et la naissance de l'histologie', *Gesnerus*, 44 (1987), 209–20; *idem*, 'Les rapports entre médecine et chirurgie dans la grande école anglaise de William et John Hunter', *Gesnerus*, 54 (1988), 323–43; *idem*, 'Percussion et diagnostic physique en Grande-Bretagne au 18e siècle: l'exemple d'Alexander Monro Secundus', in R. Bernabeo (ed.), *Actes du XXXIe Congrès International d'Histoire de la Médecine* (Bologna: Monduzzi, 1988), 868–75. We have also emphasized that certain innovations were already initiated in French medicine and surgery at the end of the Ancien Régime and that they were combined with foreign innovations to serve as models at the Paris School. See Keel, 'Cabanis'; *idem*, 'Modèles étrangers de la problématique hospitalière de l'École de Paris'; *idem*, 'The Politics of Health'. For the role of Parisian surgery as model, see also the works of Temkin, Entralgo, Huard, Imbault-Huart, Gelfand, etc. cited in

Keel, 'The Politics of Health', 208, note 1. On the situation of medical instruction in France before the Revolution, see also L. Brockliss, 'L'enseignement médical et la Révolution. Éssai de réévaluation', *Histoire de l'éducation*, 42 (1989), 79–110; and his contribution in this volume. For the importance, in France as elsewhere, of military medicine in the emergence of a new practice of clinical medicine and pathology before the Paris School, see O. Keel and Ph. Hudon, 'L'essor de la pratique clinique dans les armées européennes (1750–1800)' *Gesnerus*, 54 (1997), 37-58.

5. See on this point our works cited in the preceding note.
6. This is the thesis of Foucault, among others: 'Morgagni published his *De sedibus* in 1760 ... Yet forty years later, Bichat and his contemporaries felt that they were rediscovering pathological anatomy from beyond a shadowy zone. ... The clinic, a neutral gaze directed upon manifestations, frequencies, and chronologies, concerned with linking up symptoms and grasping their language, was, by its structure, foreign to the investigation of mute, intemporal bodies; causes and locales did not interest it: it was interested in history, not geography. Anatomy and the clinic were not of the same mind: strange as it may seem to us now that anatomy and the clinic are inseparably linked, and seem to us always to have been, it was clinical thought that for forty years prevented medicine from hearing the lesson of Morgagni.' *Birth of the Clinic*, 126.
7. For convenience, we will refer to the Hunterian school or the school of John Hunter, but in fact, in using this term, we are also including, as is often done, the achievements of William Hunter and those of his students. See Keel, 'The Politics of Health'; *idem*, 'Médecine et chirurgie dans l'école de William et John Hunter'. On the collaboration between John and William Hunter, see also C.H. Brock (ed.), *William Hunter, 1718–1783: A Memoir by Samuel Foart Simmons and John Hunter* (Glasgow: Thomson Litho Ltd, 1983).
8. John Hunter (1728–1793) has been considered by historians of medicine as the founder of pathological anatomy in England. See e.g. A. Castiglioni, *Histoire de la médecine* (Paris: Payot, 1930), 497. This statement is correct, but one must not forget the very important contributions of anatomists and practitioners like Douglas, Nichols, Pott, William Hunter, the Monros, W. Stark, etc. See Keel, *La généalogie*; *idem*, 'Médecine et chirurgie dans l'école de William et John Hunter'. On the importance of the contribution of John Hunter and of the Hunterians to pathological anatomy and anatomical clinic, see also Cross, 'John Hunter', and G. Quist, *John Hunter, 1728–1793* (London: Heinemann, 1981).

A Product of the Paris Clinical School?

9. See A. E. Rodin, *The Influence of Matthew Baillie's Morbid Anatomy. Biography, Evaluation and Reprint* (Springfield, Illinois: Ch. C. Thomas, 1973),10.
10. See E. B. Krumbhaar, *Pathology* (New York: Hoeber, 1937), 66.
11. We must emphasize that Morgagni's *problématique* is not a descriptive presentation, in the natural history style, of organic lesions, and that physiology of the Hallerian type occupies a central place in his theoretical framework. See L. Belloni 'Morgagni', in Ch. Gillespie (ed.), *Dict. Scient.Biogr.* See also V. Cappelletti and F. Di Trocchio (eds), *De sedibus, et causis. Morgagni nel centenario* (Rome: Instituto della Enciclopedia Italiana, 1986).
12. See Baillie, in Rodin, *Matthew Baillie*, 67.
13. J. -E. Dezeimeris, 'Aperçu des découvertes faites en anatomie pathologique durant les trente dernières années qui viennent de s'écouler et de leur influence sur les progrès de la connaissance et du traitement des maladies', *Archives de médecine* (June 1829), 161. Note that Dezeimeris himself belonged to the Paris School and that he was its official historian.
14. *Ibid.*
15. *Ibid.* Our emphasis. Note that the statement of Dezeimeris on the superiority of the British school in pathological anatomy holds, according to him, for all the period 1800–1830.
16. In fact, even Morgagni, like the other Italian anatomo-clinicians of his era, though primarily interested in the pathology of organs, nonetheless took account, at least in certain cases, of lesions of membranes. See further in this essay.
17. See Keel, *La généalogie.*
18. See our works cited in note 4. See also H. de Almeida, *Romantic Medicine and John Keats* (Oxford: Oxford University Press, 1991), 5 ff and ch. 1: 'The London medical circle', 22–33, where the author summarizes our thesis (pp. 26–27) and confirms it for the situation in London at the beginning of the nineteenth century. On the transformation and 'modernization' of the London medical scene and practices in the second half of the eighteenth and early nineteenth century, see also S. Lawrence, *Charitable Knowledge: Hospital Pupils and Practitioners in Eighteenth-Century London* (Cambridge: Cambridge University Press, 1996), see *inter alia* 164 ff. For similar trends more generally in Britain, see I. Loudon, *Medical Care and the General Practitioner, 1750–1850* (Oxford: Clarendon Press, 1986); *idem*, 'Medical Education and Medical Reform', in V. Nutton and R. Porter (eds), *The History of Medical Education in Britain* (Amsterdam: Rodopi, 1995), 229–49; C. Lawrence, 'The Edinburgh Medical

A Product of the Paris Clinical School?

School and the End of the "Old Thing" 1790–1830', *History of Universities*, vii (1988), 259–86; L. Rosner, *Medical Education in the Age of Improvement* (Edinburgh: Edinburgh University Press, 1991); M. Fissell 'The Disappearance of the Patient's Narrative and the Invention of Hospital Medicine', in R. French and A. Wear (eds), *British Medicine in an Age of Reformation* (London, New York: Routledge, 1991), 92–109.

19. For the analysis of this socio-institutional framework in Great Britain, see Keel, 'The Politics of Health'; *idem*, 'Médecine et chirurgie dans l'école de William et John Hunter'; see also other articles in W. Bynum and R. Porter (eds), *William Hunter*; and references in note 18 here.

20. See Keel, *La généalogie*; *idem*, 'La pathologie tissulaire de John Hunter'; *idem*, 'John Hunter et Xavier Bichat'; *idem*, 'Haller, Hunter, Bichat'; *idem*, 'L'École Clinique de Paris'.

21. We have already insisted on the fact that a relatively important current of pathology and the clinic based on pathological anatomy (and the Morgagnian tradition) existed in medicine – and not only in French surgery (Desault, etc.) – before the Paris School and before Bichat's period (e.g., Sénac, Lieutaud, Pujol, Portal, the work done by Corvisart before the time of his professorship at the Paris School, doctors interested in surgical diseases, etc.). See Keel, 'Modèles étrangers de la *problématique* hospitalière de l'École de Paris'; *idem*, 'The Politics of Health'; and M.-J. Imbault-Huart, 'L'école pratique de dissection de Paris de 1750 à 1822, ou l'influence du concept de médecine pratique et de médecine d'observation dans l'enseignement médico-chirurgical au XVIIIe siècle et au début du XIXème siècle' (Ph.D. dissertation, Université de Paris I, 1973). However, up to 1800, there were not in France developments in the area of pathological anatomy on the scale of those of the Hunter–Baillie school.

22. See *Traité d'anatomie pathologique du corps humain par M. Baillie*, trans. M. Ferrall, M.D. (Paris: Samson, 1803), viii.

23. See *Anatomie pathologique des organes les plus importants du corps humain par M. Baillie*, trans. M. Guerbois (Paris: Crochard, 1815), xv, our emphasis.

24. *Ibid.*, 1. Baillie's original text is: 'Some diseases consist only in morbid actions, but do not produce any change in the structure of parts; these do not admit of anatomical inquiry after death. There are other diseases, however, where alterations in the structure take place, and these become the proper subjects of anatomical examination.' See Rodin, *Matthew Baillie*, 67.

25. *Ibid.*, 266–77.

26. *Ibid.*, 96–101.
27. *Ibid.*, 75–83.
28. *Ibid.*, 130–8.
29. Baillie had observed that the lesion is often confined to one of the constituent tissues of an organ without affecting the others. See Rodin, *Matthew Baillie*, 170–1.
30. See the descriptions in Baillie's treatise republished in Rodin, *Matthew Baillie*. See more generally on the serous and mucous membranes 131 ff. and 146 ff. On tissue pathology in Baillie's works and the recognition of these works by clinicians like Laennec, see Keel, 'La constitution de l'anatomie des systèmes selon Laennec', 202 ff. It should be noted that Baillie's activities as anatomist and anatomo-pathologist lasted more than twenty years. See Rodin, *Matthew Baillie*, 10. Moreover, Baillie, far from being a naturalist, was an excellent anatomo-clinician who, in the wake of Hunter, gave what became the standard descriptions of many entities, notably cirrhosis and emphysema, the formation of peritoneal and pleural adhesions by inflammation, etc. *Ibid.*, 28 ff.
31. See M. D. Grmek, 'Morgagni e la scuola anatomo-clinica di Parigi', in V. Cappelletti and F. di Trocchio (eds), *De sedibus*, 180. This even-handed comparison of Morgagni and Bichat also applies to Hunter and Bichat at a subsequent stage of pathological anatomy. Hunter, with his students, pursued research in pathological anatomy of organs and tissues for forty years. See Keel, 'John Hunter et Xavier Bichat'; *idem*, 'Haller, Hunter, Bichat'.
32. See G. Canguilhem, Preface to Keel, *La généalogie*. Most historians of medicine have presented tissue pathology as a result of the application by Pinel and Bichat of Condillac's analytical method to pathology (see e.g. Foucault, *The Birth of the Clinic*, 133 ff.). The earlier development of the British school obliges us to reconsider the conditions that made possible this fundamental scientific innovation.
33. See E. F. Dubois, *Traité de pathologie générale*, 2 vols (Paris: J.-B. Baillière, 1837), vol. 1, 282–3. Our emphasis. In 1847, Dubois was elected *secrétaire perpétuel* of the Académie de médecine.
34. See in particular in the first section entitled 'Surgical diseases in which the tissues could be affected' and the constant references to Hunter and 'his genius'. See, for example, vol. 1, 2, 4, 8, 12, 21, 25, 58, etc.
35. *Traité de pathologie externe*, 2 ff.
36. See *Traité de pathologie externe*, vol.1, 226.
37. See Russell C. Maulitz, *Morbid Appearances: The Anatomy of Pathology in the Early Nineteenth Century* (Cambridge: Cambridge University Press, 1987).

38. Two members of the Paris School, A.-J.-L.Jourdan and F.-G. Boisseau, emphasized, in their preface to their French translation of *Lectures on Inflammation, Exhibiting a View of the General Doctrines, Pathological and Practical of Medical Surgery* (Edinburgh: William Blackwood, 1813) by Hunter's disciple, J. Thomson, that Bichat's writings could only have been well received in the British Hunterian medical environment: 'England sees the dawn of a new, more rational medicine. Hunter, a man of genius, so attentive in his observations, so fertile in his deductions, so ingenious in his experiments, gave an example, in his treatise on inflammation, of what the *well-reasoned marriage of anatomy and physiology to pathology* can bear. When the *writings of Bichat were published, they could only be embraced by Hunter's readers*: the perceptive minds recognized that *the truth began to emerge from all over Europe*.' See *Traité médico-chirurgical de l'inflammation* (Paris: J.-B. Baillière, 1827), 2, our emphasis. Of course, Jourdan and Boisseau indicate that there were also readers of Hunter in France and that Hunter's work had prepared the ground for a good welcome to Bichat's writings there as well. Therefore before turning to the study of how Bichat's work was received in Great Britain, one has to study how the works of Hunter and his school helped promote the favourable reception of Bichat's writings in France.
39. See Keel, *La généalogie*; *idem*, 'La pathologie tissulaire de John Hunter'; *idem*, 'John Hunter et Xavier Bichat'; *idem*, 'Haller, Hunter, Bichat'; *idem*, 'L'École Clinique de Paris'.
40. See Maulitz, 'Intellectual migration: the case of pathological anatomy', in R. Numbers and J. Pickstone (eds), *British Society for the History of Science and the History of Science Program, papers and abstracts for the joint conference* (Madison: Omnipress, 1988), 197. 'Origin' emphasized by author, other emphasis is ours.
41. Maulitz, *Morbid Appearances*, vii, our emphasis.
42. The author writes that in England, 'theoretical pathological anatomy, though adumbrated by John Hunter, was not, in fact, enrooted by his later followers'. Maulitz, *Morbid Appearances*, 247–8, note 22. We show in the present text that this assertion is not at all founded. On this point, see also our works cited in note 4.
43. After having admitted that pathological anatomy had already begun its growth with Morgagni and Hunter (see following note), Maulitz writes nevertheless: 'In this discussion however, I am *by choice [?] and convention [?]* using the phrase "pathological anatomy" to mean *something more specific*. By that phrase I wish to denote an approach to the theory and practice of pathology that, while not resorting to the microscope, relied nonetheless on emerging notions of

histopathology. This approach, also known sometimes as tissue pathology, was first clearly systematized by Xavier Bichat.' See *Morbid Appearances*, 3 (our emphasis and question marks). But we must then ask: in this case where does the arbitrariness of the personal choice and of convention stop when compared to what has already been established by the whole history of medicine? One could also well decide that the 'true' pathological anatomy or the 'true' anatomical pathology only begins after Laennec, or Cruveilhier, or Rokitansky, etc. Yet, in each case, it is only a question of a new stage in the tradition of pathological anatomy and not the birth of this branch of knowledge.

44. See *inter alia* R.E. McGrew, 'Pathology', in *Encyclopaedia of Medical History* (New York: McGraw-Hill, 1985), 238; L. S. King, *The Medical World of the Eighteenth Century* (Chicago: University of Chicago Press, 1958), ch. 9: 'The Rise of Modern Pathology': 'Giovanni-Battista Morgagni is generally considered the *founder of truly* modern pathology', 271. King also emphasizes the progress from the Morgagnian approach to the Hunterian approach: 'In pathology, attention had generally been *directed to the organs as the seats of disease, but the traditional past was no longer satisfactory.* Hunter, we have seen, had studied general pathologic reactions rather than specific organs changes', 290, our emphasis. King also notes, but only in passing, that the Hunterian physiopathological approach was combined with a tissue approach in pathology: 'We should point out parenthetically that Hunter anticipated Bichat in distinguishing certain general tissue types and their reactions', 288. Note that Maulitz admits from the outset that his point of departure is arbitrary: 'My account of the growth of anatomical pathology begins with Bichat's career. But the tale *need not* begin here. *The history of pathology in the century before him teems with major figures in the field of morbid anatomy, men like John Hunter and Giovanni Battista Morgagni*' (and Baillie whom the author forgot to mention here). See *Morbid Appearances*, 3. Our emphasis. We wonder why, then, the author who proposes to write the history of the development of anatomical pathology does not begin with the first stages, i.e. the Morgagnian tradition and the Hunter–Baillie tradition.

45. On the importance of pathological anatomy in the works of many clinicians in Europe during the second half of the eighteenth century and on the fact that these works served as models for the Paris Clinical School, see Keel, 'Cabanis'; *idem*, *La généalogie*; *idem*, 'Modèles étrangers de la problématique hospitalière de l'École de Paris', and the references in these works.

46. We must emphasize that there were also important elements of tissue pathology in many schools or medical (and surgical) currents of the eighteenth century based on anatomical pathology (for example, in the Italian school: Morgagni himself, Cotugno, etc.; in the Vienna school: De Haen, Stoll, etc.; in the German school: Walter, etc.). In the British, mainly Hunterian, clinic, the tissue *problématique* had undergone decisive developments in the last decades of the eighteenth century. On these points, see Keel, 'Cabanis'; idem, *La généalogie*; idem, 'Haller, Hunter, Bichat'; idem, 'L'Ecole Clinique de Paris'.
47. Maulitz, *Morbid Appearances*, 144, our emphasis.
48. *Ibid.*
49. *Ibid.*, 252, note 26, our emphasis.
50. *Morbid Appearances*, 252, note 26. See also *ibid.*, 143–5.
51. Maulitz also acknowledges that an English current of tissue pathology at the beginning of the nineteenth century, such as the one represented by Farre and his group of the Academy of Minute Anatomy, for example, situates itself directly in the wake of the Hunterian tradition and that it owes very little, if anything, to the 'Bichatian' school. See *Morbid Appearances*, ch. 8, 175–97. This chapter is very interesting, but it introduces implications which, in fact, contradict the thesis of the book.
52. *Ibid.*, 252, note 26.
53. See Keel, *La généalogie*; idem, 'La constitution de l'anatomie des systèmes selon Laennec'; idem, 'Modèles étrangers de la *problématique* hospitalière de l'École de Paris'; idem, 'Médecine et chirurgie dans l'école de William et John Hunter'. See further in the text.
54. See further in the text.
55. *Traité des maladies des artères et des veines* (Paris: Gabon, 1819), ix. Our emphasis.
56. See Keel, *La généalogie*; idem, 'La pathologie tissulaire de John Hunter'; idem, 'John Hunter et Xavier Bichat'; idem, 'Haller, Hunter, Bichat'; idem, 'L'Ecole Clinique de Paris'. Maulitz agrees with us that the works of Hunter embrace the pathology of tissues as well as that of organs in his global system of pathological anatomy, and that we find in Hunter 'a sophisticated analysis of the "surfaces taking on inflammation", i.e. the membranes and the tissues'. See *Morbid Appearances*, 178. He even acknowledges that as of 1780 '*he [Hunter] explicitly used the language of tissues and textures …*', *Morbid Appearances*, 114 ff. He also underlines, as we have, that Hunter took not only pathological lesions into consideration, but also the general effects of tissues, both solid and fluid, on the body. *Ibid.*, 114. All

this represents much more than 'first insights'.

57. On these points see Keel, La généalogie; *idem*, 'John Hunter et Xavier Bichat'; *idem*, 'Haller, Hunter, Bichat'. Maulitz affirms, without demonstrating it, that Hunter had not insisted as much on 'tissue inflammation' in his *Treatise on the Blood, Inflammation and Gunshot Wounds* (1794) as Bichat later did in his *Traité des membranes* (1800) and in his *Anatomie générale* (1801). We are in total disagreement with this assertion. See further in this text.

58. 'Open a few corpses' is, as we know, the title of ch. 8 (which deals with Bichat) of *The Birth of the Clinic*. Contrary to Foucault's assertions, what rendered the anatomico-tissue *problématique* possible was neither the application of Condillac's analytical method to pathology by Pinel, Bichat and the Paris School, nor the sole act of 'opening a few corpses' in Paris hospitals after the Revolution, nor is it simply the combination of these two factors. The conditions which made possible the development of tissue pathology were present during the second half of the eighteenth century in Great Britain through the collaboration in the hospital of physicians and surgeons of the Hunterian school on the one hand, and, on the other, by the intertwining of research in pathological and clinical anatomy with research in physiopathology, experimental surgery and pathology, obstetrics, comparative anatomy and physiology.

59. We have developed this analysis in Keel, 'John Hunter et Xavier Bichat'; *idem*, 'Haller, Hunter, Bichat'.

60. It is significant that this 'resemblance' or 'isomorphism' between Hunter's tissue-centred approach and Bichat's had been underlined by a student of Hunter, J. Adams (1756–1818), who thought that Bichat had no cognizance of Hunter's works and had arrived by himself to the same results. After having recalled Hunter's theses according to which the inflammatory process follows a reverse course depending on the type of tissue affected (starting with the adhesive stage in the serous membranes and with the suppurative stage in the mucous membranes, albeit with some exceptions), Adams writes: 'Such is the different order of inflammation according to the texture and office of the part inflamed ... M. Bichat, without knowing what was done by Mr. Hunter, has made an ingenious work on the different forms of inflammation, according to the texture of the membranes inflamed. Abstracted from the French verbiage, the whole is reducible to those laws of inflammation which Mr. Hunter has so long taught, and of which, in two instances, an epitome is here offered' (i.e. in the treatise on venereal disease). J. Hunter, *A Treatise on The Venereal Disease, with an Introduction and Commentary by*

Joseph Adams, M.D. (London: Sherwood, 1810), 17. Note that Bichat certainly knew of this work by Hunter (first edition in 1786) which had been translated into French by Audiberti M.D. as early as 1787 (Paris: Méquignon) and which had great repercussions.

61. On these points see Keel, *La généalogie*; *idem*, 'La pathologie tissulaire de John Hunter'; *idem*, 'John Hunter et Xavier Bichat'; *idem*, 'Haller, Hunter, Bichat'; *idem*, 'L'Ecole Clinique de Paris'.

62. We have presented in another essay the references to some of the principal passages in Hunter which deal with the questions of the different tissues and of the processes of adherence, suppuration, ulceration, absorption, of gangrene and tumours. In comparing these texts with those of Bichat, we find a surprising number of similarities for each system. See Keel, 'John Hunter et Xavier Bichat', 537, note 6. On the modifications of lesions according to the different tissues as exposed in Hunter's works; see also Keel, *La généalogie*, and *idem*, 'La pathologie tissulaire de John Hunter'; *idem*, 'Haller, Hunter, Bichat'.

63. *The Treatise on the Blood, Inflammation and Gunshot Wounds* (which gives an account of this *problématique*) was published in 1794 but had been completed as of 1762. It constituted the subject matter of the author's teachings since at least 1770, and, as of this date, we find Hunter's anatomical and tissue concepts in his works. See Keel, *La généalogie*. Hunter's treatise was first translated into French by J. Dubar, *officier de santé* at the Ostende military hospital, under the title: *Traité sur le sang, l'inflammation et les playes d'armes à feu* (Ostende: Schedelwaert) in the year VII (1799). Bichat knew at least this work by Hunter, since he mentions him and various elements of the Hunterian doctrine in his *Traité des membranes* (1799, edited by F. Magendie, Paris: Gabon, 1827, 211, *passim*) and in his *Anatomie générale, appliquée à la physiologie et à la médecine, 1801*, edited by E. Serres M.D., P.-N. Gerdy M.D. and P.-Ch. Hughier, M.D. (Paris: L'Encyclopédie; Béthune, 1834), 626 (*Encyclopédie des sciences médicales*, 1re division, t. 3) where there is explicit reference to Hunter's theses on blood and to other results of the latter's research; 153. See also *ibid.*, 232, 238, 394, 395 and *passim*.

64. See C. Lawrence, 'Democratic, Divine and Heroic: the History and Historiography of Surgery', in C. Lawrence (ed.), *Medical Theory, Surgical Practice: Studies in the History of Surgery* (London & New York: Routledge, 1992), 21.

65. We must emphasize that Morgagni himself had noted, in observations dating from the first half of the eighteenth century, the analogy of diseases (as inflammation) of certain membranes that were located in different areas of the body, but were similar in their

structure (such as the pleura, the pericardium, the peritoneum, etc. or such as the mucous membranes). Moreover, Morgagni, when opening corpses, did not limit himself to the observation of organs, he also carefully examined the lesions of membranes. See for example in the XXXIV anatomico-medical Letter of *De Sedibus* the examination of the peritoneum, the pleura and the pericardium. On pathology at tissue level in eighteenth-century European civilian and military medicine before Bichat and the Paris School, see Keel, 'Cabanis'; *idem*, *La généalogie*; Keel and Hudon, 'L'essor de la pratique clinique dans les armées'.

66. A similar *problématique* is also found in the works of the professors of Edinburgh's School of Medicine such as A. Monro (secundus) and A. Monro (tertius). See Keel, *La généalogie*, 71 ff. and 110; *idem*, 'La constitution de l'anatomie des systèmes selon Laennec'; *idem*, 'Percussion et diagnostic physique en Grande-Bretagne au 18e siècle'. See also in text.

67. See *inter alia* 'The Blood, Inflammation and Gunshot Wounds', in J. F. Palmer (ed.), *The Complete Works of John Hunter*, 5 vols (American edition, Philadelphia: Haswel & Barrington, 1841), vol. 3, 276–7. Our references are from this American edition. The first edition is: J. F. Palmer (ed.), *The Works of John Hunter ... with Notes*, 5 vols (London: Longman, 1835–7), including one vol. of plates, 1837.

68. One of the more explicit passages on this point is in the same treatise. See *ibid.*, vol. 3, 281–2.

69. See *ibid.*, vol. 3, 440.

70. Cf. Keel, *La généalogie*; *idem*, 'John Hunter et Xavier Bichat'; *idem*, 'Haller, Hunter, Bichat'; *idem*, 'L'Ecole Clinique de Paris'; *idem*, 'La constitution de l'anatomie des systèmes selon Laennec'.

71. In his text, Maulitz says 'The French clinicians created a new landscape of disease. It was a landscape derived, perhaps from native French elements, or perhaps from elements found elsewhere.' See *Morbid Appearances*, 225. Bichat's appropriation of Hunter's ideas had been underlined by many British and French practitioners at the time. See *inter alia*, John Thomson, *Lectures on Inflammation, Exhibiting a View of the General Doctrines, Pathological and Practical of Medical Surgery* (Philadelphia, 1817); we use the American reprint of the first edition (Edinburgh, 1813), 127–28: 'To this enumeration of textures I shall only add, that I am inclined to believe it will be found, that as there are no two parts of the human body precisely the same in structure, or which possess vital properties in the same degree, so there is no texture or organ in which *inflammation follows exactly the same progress, and produce the same local and constitutional*

effects. But for a fuller account of these textures, *particularly in the sound state*, I must refer you to the "Anatomie Générale" of the late most ingenious Professor Bichat of Paris. *It is to be regretted that Professor Bichat should nowhere in that work have acknowledged the obligations which he lay under to Mr. Hunter, of whose facts and reasonings he has made a liberal use. How familiar the effect of structure in modifying the phenomena of inflammation was to the mind of Mr. Hunter must appear to any one who will take the trouble to read what he has said with regard to it in various parts of his Treatise on Inflammation*', our emphasis. Note that Thomson underlines that Bichat's tissue *problématique* in the *Anatomie générale* is applied essentially to *normal anatomy* – and less so to pathology.

72. See *Morbid Appearances*, 4.
73. See *inter alia* the review of our work, *La généalogie de l'histopathologie* by W.R. Albury, in *Bull. Hist. Med.*, 55 (1981), 290.
74. See *Morbid Appearances*, 4.
75. See note 71.
76. At that time, the circulation of concepts and techniques does not operate abstractly in the realm of the ideas: it is a material process which operates through various concrete channels or vehicles such as medical journals, monographs, translated works or extracts of foreign medical journals or books published by local presses. Maulitz underlines the importance of English medical journals at the beginning of the nineteenth century for the reception and dissemination of 'Bichatian' ideas in British medicine. We must say that the medical journals played the same role, but in the opposite direction, during the eighteenth century, for the reception and dissemination in France of British ideas on anatomical and tissue pathology. During the nineteenth century, these exchanges go both ways.
77. However, Bichat was accused by Richerand of having plagiarized Andreas Bonn in his *Traité des membranes*. A great number of other authors of the time insisted that Bichat had been credited the concepts of membrane and the decomposition of the organism into tissues while, in fact, this credit belonged to Haller and Bonn and others for the normal state; and to Hunter and Smyth and others for the pathological state. See our analysis on this issue in Keel, *La généalogie*; *idem*, 'Haller, Hunter, Bichat'; *idem*, 'L'Ecole Clinique de Paris'. See also Palmer: 'To *Haller* is *undoubtedly* due *the merit of having first analytically divided the animal body into its component tissues*, and *ascertained their distinctive physiological properties*; while *to Hunter we must accord the merit of applying this mode of inquiry to pathological investigations, conceiving that as each texture was endowed*

A Product of the Paris Clinical School?

with peculiar properties in a state of health, it would likewise in the same manner be affected in a special manner by the causes of disease, and consequently, that the same modes of lesions would always produce similar effects on the analogous structures of the body. Bichat still further extended this system in his *Anatomie générale*, which appeared in 1801, *but without acknowledging to Hunter; and it is undoubtedly to this source that we must ascribe the great and rapid advance which have been made in pathological knowledge during the present century*.' See *The Blood, Inflammation and Gunshot Wounds, with Notes by James F. Palmer*, in J. F. Palmer (ed.), *The Complete Works of John Hunter*, vol. 3, 493–4, our emphasis. This passage by Palmer clearly establishes that Bichat neither founded the analytical division of tissues composing the human body (this is due to Haller), nor did he found this division from the pathological point of view (this is due to Hunter).

78. In the *Examen des doctrines médicales et des systèmes de nosologie*, third edition (Paris: J.-B. Baillière, 1829–34), Broussais clearly stated that Bichat had 'taken ideas from Hunter and Pinel, giving credit to Pinel': 'Bichat *s'étant aussitôt emparé des idées de Hunter* et de Pinel, dont *il fit honneur à ce dernier*', vol. 3, 514, our emphasis.
79. See E. Haigh, 'Xavier Bichat and the Medical Theory of the Eighteenth Century', *Medical History* Supplement, no 4 (London: Wellcome Institute, 1984), 10 ff.
80. *Ibid.*
81. Bichat obviously also knew of Smyth's ideas through the intermediary of Pinel's writings.
82. *Ibid.*, 93, note 8 and 120, note 7.
83. *Ibid.* Monro (tertius), who was well acquainted with the contributions of the British school to the development of the tissue *problématique*, explicitly claimed the pre-eminence of Smyth in relation to Bichat. See A. Monro, *Outlines of the Anatomy of the Human Body in Its Sound and Diseased State*, 4 vols (Edinburgh: A. Constable, 1813), vol. 1, 4. Many years later, Monro (tertius) would not hesitate to restate the pre-eminence of the British school, recalling that the 'modern system of general anatomy' was 'based' on the works of the British school (Hunter, Monro (secundus), Smyth). See Monro (tertius), *Essays and Heads of Lectures on Anatomy, Physiology and Surgery by the late Alexander Monro secundus* (Edinburgh: Maclachlan, Stewart and Co., 1840), lviii. See also Keel, 'Haller, Hunter, Bichat', 56 for the entire passage.
84. See Keel, *La généalogie*; *idem*, 'John Hunter et Xavier Bichat'; *idem*, 'Haller, Hunter, Bichat'.

85. On the development of Smyth's concepts in the works and teachings of Monro (tertius) in Edinburgh, see Keel, *La généalogie*, 76 ff. For a re-examination of 'the mythology of the inadequacy' of Monro (tertius) as an anatomist, see C. Lawrence, 'Edinburgh Medical School', 265 ff.
86. 'Cases of diffuse inflammation of the cellular texture; with the appearance on dissection and observations', *Transactions of the Medico-Chirurgical Society of Edinburgh*, 1 (1824), 473–650, see 9, our emphasis. This text of nearly 180 pages presents a great number of cases, showing that Duncan's research in this field was very systematic. At no point does Duncan make any reference to Bichat. For numerous other positions of practitioners of the era showing the very positive reception in Great Britain to Hunter's and Smyth's tissue *problématique*, see Keel, *La généalogie*.
87. See Monro (secundus), 'Of the characters, causes, consequences, and mode of treatment of inflammation', in A. Monro (tertius) (ed.), *Essays*, 36 ff. One has to bear in mind that this *problématique* in pathology was conveyed to a large audience: 'The core of medical education for all groups of students was Monro's course on anatomy and surgery', L. Rosner, 'Students and Apprentices: Medical Education at Edinburgh University, 1760–1810' (Ph.D. dissertation, Johns Hopkins University, 1986), 386.
88. *Ibid.*
89. For Smyth's conceptions on the issues brought up by Monro, see Keel, *La généalogie*, 54 ff.
90. See Keel, *La généalogie, ibid.*
91. See *Essays*, 26. On Monro's (secundus) tissue pathology, see Keel, *La généalogie*; *idem*, 'Percussion et diagnostic physique en Grande-Bretagne au 18e siècle'.
92. On this point, see Keel, *La généalogie*, 76 ff. Curiously, Monro's role in the dissemination and development of the tissue *problématique* in Great Britain has always been neglected. Nevertheless, as early as 1813, Monro (tertius) published a treatise on normal and pathological anatomy based on the study of tissues that we can consider as a treatise of general anatomy. See A. Monro (tertius), *Outlines of the Anatomy of the Human Body in its Sound and Diseased State* (Edinburgh: A. Constable, 1813). This treatise is the transcription of the lectures he gave for many years at Edinburgh's Medical School. See also Keel, *La généalogie*, 78–83.
93. George Gregory, M.D. (Edinburgh, 1811) had also previously studied at the Windmill Street School founded by W. Hunter. He also acquired training in surgery as he qualified as a surgeon (member of

A Product of the Paris Clinical School?

the Royal College of Surgeons of England in 1812 and assistant-surgeon during the Napoleonic Wars). Like a certain number of British practitioners, particularly those who had been through the Hunters' schools, Gregory acquired training and practice in both medicine and surgery which obviously predisposed him to an anatomo-localist approach to disease. (For other similar cases, see Keel, 'Médecine et chirurgie dans l'école de William et John Hunter'.) In 1824 Gregory became physician at the Smallpox and Vaccination Hospital and at the General Dispensary. He was accepted as 'licentiate' at the Royal College of Physicians of England in 1816 and as fellow in 1839. See 'George Gregory', *Dict. Nat. Biogr.*

94. *Elements of the Theory*, third edn (London: Burgess & Hill, 1828), 159; refined is emphasized by Gregory. Other emphasis is ours. Like most of the books published in London, this monograph was published simultaneously in Edinburgh and the reverse holds true, e.g., Thomson and Monro (tertius), Craigie, etc. Usually they were also simultaneously – or just a short while after – published in other medical centres in Great Britain and in the United States. Consequently, works dealing with tissue pathology reached a large medical audience and received wide coverage in medical journals.

95. *Dict. Nat. Biogr.*

96. All of Gregory's work is based on pathological anatomy and on a tissue approach in pathology. Gregory mentions and uses numerous British contributions in this field: Smyth, Hunter, Baillie, Monro (tertius), Farre, Arnold, Hooper, Duncan (junior), Thomson, Clutterbuck, Cheyne, Pemberton, Noble, Jeffrey, etc. as well as those of Frenchmen such as Bichat, Laennec, etc.

97. On this point see Keel, *La généalogie*.

98. On these points see Keel, *ibid.*

99. On the reduction of Bichat's twenty-one tissues into three principal tissues according to Haller's model in Béclard's general anatomy and in other anatomists and physiologists, see Keel, 'Haller, Hunter, Bichat'; *idem*, 'L'Ecole Clinique de Paris'.

100. Article entitled 'Membrane', in Alard, Alibert, Barbier *et al.* (eds), *Dictionnaire des sciences médicales* (Paris: J.-B. Baillière, 1812–22), vol. 32, 208.

101. See Keel, *La généalogie*, 34 ff.

102. As Klemperer notes with pertinence, Hunter clearly broke away from the descriptive model of natural history: 'His [Hunter's] appreciation of morbid anatomy as a key to the comprehension of clinical symptoms is frequently illustrated by the detailed clinical abstracts accompanying the pathological specimens of his museum. Yet, he did

not limit his inquiry to the seats and proximate causes of diseases but extended its scope to a search for the hidden causes and the mechanisms by which they act. The morphologic alteration of organs was for him the *product* of disease and the disclosure of the *morbid process* the aim of his investigations. He was convinced that knowledge of pathogenesis was the foundation for an understanding and ultimate alleviation of disease. ... It can be affirmed that his dynamic concept ushered in a new era of pathology', 'John Hunter's contribution to pathology', *Bull. N.Y. Acad. Med.* 37 (1961), 283, our emphasis.

103. See Palmer, *The Complete Works of John Hunter*, vol. 3, 7. See also Klemperer, 'John Hunter's contribution', in *Bull. N.Y. Acad. Med.*; Cross, 'John Hunter', in *Studies in the History of Biology*; G. Quist, *John Hunter 1728–1793*; L. S. Jacyna, 'Physiological principles in the surgical writings of John Hunter', in C. Lawrence (ed.), *Medical Theory*, 135–52.

104. As C. Fr. Heusinger forcefully states in the preface of his *Histologie* (Eisenach: J. Fr. Bärecke, 1822): 'We know what powerful influence Pinel and Bichat exerted on the course of pathological anatomy: but this influence was quite different from that of Hunter. While the latter spread the seeds of the most fecund ideas, the example of Pinel and Bichat only promoted thorough observation and comparison. To my eyes, the merit of the two schools is equally great' (p. 36). Heusinger ignored the fact that the histological *problématique* in the pathology of Pinel and Bichat was itself derived from Hunter and Smyth's school. Otherwise, he would have had an even more positive appreciation of the British school.

105. See 'Anatomie pathologique', in Alard *et al.* (eds), *Dictionnaire des sciences médicales* (Paris: J.-B. Baillière, 1812–22), vol. 1 (1812), 49.

106. See D. Craigie, *Elements of General and Pathological Anatomy* (Edinburgh: Adam Black, 1828). For the dissemination of the *problématique* of general anatomy in the courses in London, see R. D. Grainger's manual, *Elements of General Anatomy Containing an Outline of the Organisation of the Human Body* (London: S. Hyghley, 1829). Grainger had the most important private school of anatomy (with many students) in London where he taught general anatomy starting in 1825. See Mazumdar, 'Anatomy, physiology and surgery: physiology teaching in early nineteenth-century London', *Canadian Bulletin of Medical History*, 4 (1987), 136.

107. See *Morbid Appearances*, ch. 8.

108. See T. Hodgkin, *Lectures on the Anatomy of the Serous and Mucous Membranes* (London: Sherwood, 1836–40), vols 1 and 2.

A Product of the Paris Clinical School?

109. See *Lectures on the Anatomy*, vol. 1, 11. Hodgkin's text clearly shows that, contrary to what Maulitz writes, Baillie's work had a considerable impact on the British medical milieu where it stimulated the tradition of works in pathological anatomy, and it also had a considerable impact abroad: 'The *Morbid Anatomy* of Dr. Baillie – for years confessed, even by our rivals, to be the most complete treatise of the kind which had ever appeared – soon received the hommage of translation in France, Germany and Italy', *ibid*. And he adds: 'I am ready to subscribe to the remark of Rothe, that *no physician should be without this book*, and, *from my own experience*, do not hesitate to state, that *even now, we are acquainted with, comparatively, few morbid appearances which have not been seen and described by Dr. Baillie ...*', *ibid.*, vol. 1, 12. Our emphasis.
110. *Ibid.*, vol. 1, 27, 41, 49, 168.
111. *Ibid.*, vol. 1, iii.
112. See *Morbid Appearances*, ch. 8: 'Pathology and the Specialist: The London Academy of Minute Anatomy', 75–197.
113. See R. Willan, *Description and Treatment of Cutaneous Diseases*, 4 vols (London: Longman, 1798–1805). See also T. Bateman (1778–1821), *A Practical Synopsis of Cutaneous Diseases According to the Arrangement of Dr. Willan*, 8 vols (London: Longman, 1808). In these works we find a great number of observations on tissue pathology.
114. See C. Bell, *A System of Dissections, Explaining the Anatomy of the Human Body, the Manner of Displaying the Parts and their Varieties in Diseases*, 2 vols in one (Edinburgh: Mundell, 1798).
115. John Baron, physician at the 'General Infirmary at Gloucester', is the author of *An Inquiry Illustrating the Nature of Tuberculated Accretions of Serous Membranes and the Origin of Tubercles and Tumors in Different Textures of the Body* (London: Longman, 1819). He cites as model the histopathological approach and the description of the inflammation of serous membranes by James Carmichael Smyth (72–4) and he criticizes and rectifies Bichat who identified tubercles as the product of chronic inflammations of serous membranes, considering them as affections exclusive to this tissue, while 'tubercles exist in almost every texture, and their origin and essential character will probably be found to be the same wherever they are discovered' (75).
116. Dr John Cheyne published, in 1809, *The Pathology of the Membrane of the Larynx and Bronchia* (Edinburgh: Mundell).
117. See, for example, A. Cooper, *Surgical Essays* (London: Cox and Son, 1818) written with B. Travers, surgeon at St Thomas's Hospital, which contains numerous observations on tissues. See also Cooper, *Lectures on the Principles and Practice of Surgery as Delivered in the*

A Product of the Paris Clinical School?

Theatre of St. Thomas's Hospital (London: F. C. Westley, 1829).

118. See, for example, J. Abernethy, *Lectures on Anatomy, Surgery and Pathology, Including Observations on the Nature and Treatment of Local Diseases Delivered at St Bartholomew's Hospital* (London: J. Bulcock, 1828), also in *Lancet*, no. 26. Abernethy was responsible for setting up the Museum of Anatomy and Pathological Anatomy at St Bartholomew's Hospital where he had founded the medical school in 1791. See 'John Abernethy', *Dict. Nat. Biogr.* and see H. Haeser, *Lehrbuch der Geschichte der Medicin und der Epidemischen Krankheiten*, 3 vols (Iena, 1875–82, reprint Hidelsheim & New York: Georg Holms, 1971), vol. 3, 952.

119. See, for example, W. Lawrence, *Lectures on Surgery, Medical and Operative Delivered at St. Bartholomew's* (London: F. C. Westley, 1832). In 1802 Lawrence was named prosector at St. Bartholomew's Hospital. *Dict. Nat. Biogr.* and Haeser, *Lehrbuch der Geschichte*, vol. 3, 955.

120. See, for example, *Pathological and Surgical Observations on Diseases of the Joints* (London: Longman, 1818); *Lectures on Various Subjects in Pathology and Surgery* (London: Longman, 1837)'.

121. See *Observations on some of the general principles and of the particular nature and treatment of the different species of inflammation* (London: Thomas & Underwood, 1821). On James and tissue pathology, see Keel, *La généalogie*, 61–8.

122. Yelloly was a physician at London Hospital from 1807 to 1818 and the founder, with A. Marcet in 1805, of the Royal Medical and Chirurgical Society. He presented many observations of anatomico-tissue pathology to the Society. See, for example, 'Observations on the vascular appearances in the human stomach, which is frequently mistaken for inflammation of that organ', *Transactions of the Medico-Chirurgical Society*, 4 (1813), 371–424.

123. See *A Treatise on the Diseases of Arteries and Veins* (London: T. Underwood, 1815).

124. See, for example, *Inquiry into the Process of Nature in Repairing Injuries of the Intestines Illustrating the Treatment of Penetrating Wounds and Strangulated Hernias* (London: Longman, 1812).

125. Charles Hastings, M.D. (1794–1866), physician at the Worcester Infirmary, published among other things *A Treatise on Inflammation of the Mucous Membrane of the Lungs, to which is Prefixed an Experimental Inquiry Respecting the Contractile Power of the Blood Vessels and the Nature of Inflammation* (London: Thomas & Underwood, 1820). He had training first in surgery, then in medicine, which was typical of a certain number of British physicians of the time. See Keel, 'Médecine et chirurgie dans l'école de William

A Product of the Paris Clinical School?

et John Hunter'. Moreover, from 1832 on, he was the principal force in the Provincial Medical and Surgical Association (which united the two branches of the profession). This organization became the British Medical Association in 1856 and he was named permanent president. See 'Charles Hastings', *Dict. Nat. Biogr.*

126. John Armstrong (1784–1829) was a physician at the Fever Institution of London. He was a most appreciated private teacher, and had a major influence on medical practice in Great Britain. After his death, his lectures on pathological anatomy and on the clinic were published under the title: *Lectures on the Morbid Anatomy, Nature and Treatment of Acute and Chronic Diseases*, (ed. Joseph Rix) (London, 1834). First American edition by J. Bell, M.D., 2 vols (Philadelphia: Desilver, Thomas & Co., 1837). We can see from this work that Armstrong gave a significant place to tissue pathology in his lectures. On Armstrong, see H. Haeser, *Lehrbuch der Geschichte*, vol. 3, 901. See also 'John Armstrong', *Dict. Nat. Biogr.*

127. See, for example, *Essays on the Morbid Anatomy of the Human Eye*, 2 vols (Edinburgh: Ramsay & Co., 1808–18). Wardrop was the first to classify the various inflammations of the eye according to the structures attacked.

128. Charles Badham (1780–1845), physician at the Westminster General Dispensary, published in 1808, *Observations on the Inflammatory Affections of the Mucous Membrane of the Bronchiae* (London: J. Callow). A second edition, revised and augmented, was published in 1814 under the title *An Essay on Bronchitis, with a Supplement Containing Remarks on Simple Pulmonary Abscess*. In this treatise, chronic and acute bronchitis were for the first time separated from peripneumonia and pleurisy and from other diseases for which they were mistaken, and their differential history and diagnosis were established. See 'Charles Badham', *Dict. Nat. Biogr.*

129. See, for example, *Reports of Medical Cases Selected with a View of Illustrating the Symptoms and Cure of Diseases with Reference to Morbid Anatomy*, 2 vols (London: Longman, 1827–31).

130. *A Treatise on Inflammation of the Mucous Membrane of the Lungs, to which is Prefixed an Experimental Inquiry Respecting the Contractile Power of the Blood Vessels and the Nature of Inflammation* (London: Thomas & Underwood, 1820), vii–viii. Our emphasis.

131. *The Pathology of the Membrane of the Larynx and Bronchia* (Edinburgh: Mundell, Doig and Stevensen, 1809).

132. See *Illustrations of the Elementary Forms of Disease* (London: Longman, 1838). See *inter alia* 21–35. It is normal that Carswell makes reference to 'professor Thomson of Edinburgh' (21) since he had been his student and had been responsible for supplying colour

illustrations of the different morbid appearances of the different parts of the body for William Thomson and David Craigie's course on pathology. See W. Thomson and D. Craigie, 'Notice of Some Leading Events in the Life of the Late Dr. John Thomson', *Edinburgh Medical-Surgical Journal*, 67 (1847), 131–93 (p. 178). The authors of this biographical note emphasize that Thomson appears as an essential link in the British anatomo-pathological tradition which continues with Carswell and others. See 179. On the influence of Thomson in Edinburgh, see L. S. Jacyna, 'Robert Carswell and William Thomson at the Hôtel-Dieu of Lyon: Scottish views of French medicine', in R. French and A. Wear (eds), *British Medicine in an Age of Reformation* (London, 1991), 111 ff. He attracted 250–280 students to his military surgery course in 1815, in which he was arguing 'that pathological knowledge showed there should be no distinction between physicians and surgeons'. See C. Lawrence, 'Edinburgh Medical School', 271; Thomson and Craigie, 'Notice', 163 ff. More generally, on his influence on medicine in Britain, see here following notes 133 and 135.

133. Thomson was named surgeon at the Royal Infirmary in 1800 and from then on taught surgery. He mainly gave lectures on the clinic in this institution. In 1805 he was named to the chair of surgery which had just been established by the College of Surgeons of Edinburgh and, in 1806, was named professor to the newly created chair of military surgery at the University of Edinburgh. He left his appointment at the Royal Infirmary in 1810, but continued to teach. He would finally be named professor of general pathology in 1832. Thomson tells us in his preface to his *Lectures on Inflammation* (Edinburgh, 1813) that this work (which gives a lengthy account of the tissue *problématique*) is the introduction for a series of lectures he had given since 1805 at the Royal College of Surgeons of Edinburgh (see III). From this date, if not before, Thomson had thus greatly diffused tissue pathology through his teachings and his research. These works by Thomson had a profound influence in Great Britain: 'This important series of lectures was founded on the Hunterian theory of inflammation and moulded the opinion of the profession for many years.' See 'Thomson', *Dict. Nat. Biogr.* We must also note that Thomson, who was first trained as a surgeon, received a diploma of M.D. from the University of Aberdeen in 1808, and in 1815 was accepted as 'licentiate' in the Royal College of Physicians of Edinburgh because he became a consultant physician as well as a consultant surgeon. Thus Thomson represents another incarnation of the double training and/or double practice (medicine and surgery)

that we find in numerous British practitioners of the era. See Keel, 'Médecine et chirurgie dans l'école de William et John Hunter' and *supra*. Moreover, J. Thomson gave a series of lectures on practical (clinical) medicine starting in about 1822. From 1829 to 1831 he gave this course with his son William who also had double training. See Thomson and Craigie, 'Notice', 131 ff.

134. See D. Craigie, *Elements*.
135. See Craigie, *Elements*, Preface, vii, our emphasis. We must emphasize that according to W. Thomson (1802–52) and D. Craigie, the authors of the 'Notice of Some Leading Events in the Life of the Late Dr. John Thomson', Thomson was the author who further developed Smyth's tissue *problématique* in pathology: 'One of the most important parts of Dr. Thomson's *Lectures on inflammation*, was the examination of the influence of different textures on this process, and on its effects. Though Dr. Carmichael Smyth had given a short view of this subject in 1790, yet Dr. Thomson had the undisputed merit of giving the first clear and comprehensive exposition of it, elucidated by the lights of morbid anatomy and pathology, and enriched with much new information', 158. According to William Thomson, who is the son of John, and to Craigie, these British developments in tissue pathology are independent of Bichat and the Paris School.
136. 'The distinction of the animal body into separate kinds of texture thus introduced and recognized (by Haller) was confined principally to anatomy and physiology. *The merit of applying them to pathology is divided between William Hunter, William Cullen, and John Hunter ... In the Nosology, Physiology and First Lines of Dr. Cullen, we find the author making frequent allusion to the organic properties of the various substances which enter into the composition of the animal body, and employing these distinctions as the foundation of his Pathology ... In the hands of John Hunter this system was carried to still greater perfection; and his work on Inflammation contains the rudiment of many of the improvements which pathology has derived from this source. General anatomy was thus beginning to attain insensibly the form of a science, and to be cultivated with assiduity as the surest basis of pathological knowledge ... I have already alluded to the application of the distinctions of general anatomy to pathology in the writings of Cullen and John Hunter. A more complete specimen of this was given in 1790 by Dr Carmichael Smyth*'. Craigie, *Elements*, 9-12, our emphasis.
137. 'To identify this receptivity with "French ideas and techniques" would be to oversimplify the position'. On the availability of the tissue model in both cultures, see Keel, *La généalogie*. The Scottish knew all this, *Morbid Appearances*, 252, note 26.

138. See Keel, *La généalogie*; *idem*, 'Modèles étrangers de la problématique hospitalière de l'École de Paris'; *idem*, 'The Politics of Health'; *idem*, 'Médecine et chirurgie dans l'école de William et John Hunter'.

139. For complementary analyses on these points in Great Britain and elsewhere in Europe, see Keel, works cited in note 4. See also for Great Britain the works cited hereinafter.

140. See *Morbid Appearances*, chaps 1, 2, 3 and 4.

141. See *Morbid Appearances*, 35, 58, 64, 103.

142. We have sustained the thesis that it is often on the fringe of the university establishment that discoveries were made and that medical knowledge in the field of the clinic progressed during the eighteenth and early nineteenth centuries. This holds true for both Paris and London medicine. See Keel, 'Modèles étrangers de la problématique hospitalière de l'École de Paris'; *idem*, 'The Politics of Health'; *idem*, 'La problématique institutionnelle de la clinique'.

143. On these points, see for example Loudon, *Medical Care*, 51. See also I. Waddington, *The Medical Profession in the Industrial Revolution* (Dublin: Gill & Macmillan Ltd, 1984), who writes: 'However, this tripartite classification of practitioners can be very misleading if it is assumed that *this professional division corresponded to what practitioners actually did in the day-to-day practice of their profession*, rather than simply to their formal or legal status. Indeed, it may be argued that the key to understanding many important aspects of the development of the medical profession in the early nineteenth century lies precisely in a recognition of the fact that *this tripartite classification no longer bore any clear relationship to the everyday structure of medical practice*', 9. Our emphasis. We already find this argument in S. W. Holloway, 'The Apothecaries Act of 1815: A Reinterpretation', 2 parts, *Medical History*, 10, no. 2 (1966), 107–29; and 10, no. 3 (1966), 221–36; and 'Medical Education in England, 1830–1858: A Sociological Analysis', *History*, XLIX (1964), 299–324. Thus, we must ask how Maulitz can assert that the separation between medicine and surgery is the major socio-institutional factor acting as an obstacle to the development of the Hunterian tradition in pathological anatomy in Great Britain, while, as Holloway puts it so well: 'the practice of physicians, surgeons and apothecaries was inextricably intermingled' *ibid*. We have already stated in previous works that the increasing approximation of medicine and surgery in Great Britain was one of the conditions for the rise of anatomico-clinical pathology. See Keel, *La généalogie*, *idem*, 'The Politics of Health', *idem*, 'Médecine et chirurgie dans l'école de William et John Hunter'.

144. See Keel, 'Médecine et chirurgie dans l'école de William et John Hunter'; *idem*, 'The Politics of Health'. See also Loudon, *Medical Care*, and R. Porter, 'Medical education in England before the teaching hospital: some recent revisions', in J. Wilkins (ed.), *The Professional Teacher* (London: History of Education Society, 1986). Porter justly remarks on the informal education system in Great Britain at the time: 'in any case, pupils commonly combined several modes of instruction: apprenticeship, a spell at Edinburgh, visits abroad, pupilage in London, etc.'. And, as he notes further: 'Above all, this story offers a further warning against confusing educational forms, or shells, with realities. Here as so often in the history of education, informal, personal private, temporary agencies of instruction prove to have been far more alive and influential than the carcass of the medical education represented by the English universities and the London corporations.' 'Medical Education', 39.

145. See examples in preceding section on the double medical and surgical training of a significant number of British practitioners. On this point see also L. S. Jacyna, '"Mr Scott's Case": A View of London Medicine in 1825", in R. Porter (ed.), *The Popularization of Medicine 1650–1850* (London & New York: Routledge, 1992), 252–86; C. Lawrence, 'Edinburgh Medical School'.

146. Surprisingly, Maulitz acknowledges that in the English medical community, the 'medicosurgical *raprochement* [sic] was more primitive' than in the Paris School. See *Morbid Appearances*, 105.

147. On these points see our works: Keel, *La généalogie*; *idem*, 'The Politics of Health'; *idem*, 'Médecine et chirurgie dans l'école de William et John Hunter'.

148. See Loudon, *Medical Care*, 172. On the practice of dissection in London since the eighteenth century, see also Keel, 'Médecine et chirurgie dans l'école de William et John Hunter' and the references in the notes of this article. See also R. Richardson, *Death, Dissection and the Destitute* (London; New York: Routledge & Kegan Paul, 1987); Porter, 'Medical Education'; De Almeida, *Romantic Medicine*, ch. 1; and S. Lawrence, 'Entrepreneurs and Private Enterprise: The Development of Medical Lecturing in London, 1775–1820', *Bull. Hist. Med.*, 62 (1988), 172 : 'By the late eighteenth century, London had become not only a center for surgery, anatomy, firsthand dissection, and hospital experience, but also a training ground in medicine, chemistry and midwifery. The evidence suggests that many London students pursued an education suitable for general practice without regard to the ostensible professional divisions embodied in the traditional London medical corporations.'

149. Maulitz, *Morbid Appearances*, 4.
150. Maulitz, *Morbid Appearances*, 4, our emphasis. The author adds: 'This sort of juncture appeared in France at the end of the eighteenth century', *ibid*. However, we find this kind of a "juncture" of institutions, of professional groups and of ideas which render possible the rise of pathological anatomy in many countries during the last decades of the eighteenth century. This is the case in Great Britain, Italy, Austria and Germany. See Keel, 'Cabanis'; *idem*, 'Modèles étrangers de la *problématique* hospitalière de l'École de Paris'; *idem*, 'The Politics of Health'.
151. On the technical, institutional and socio-professional conditions of the development of anatomical and tissue pathology and of the localist clinic in Great Britain during the eighteenth century, see also Keel, *La généalogie*, ch.VII: 'Les conditions de possibilité du Mémoire de Smyth: institutions et disciplines'. See also *idem*, 'Modèles étrangers de la *problématique* hospitalière de l'École de Paris'; *idem*, 'The Politics of Health'; *idem*, 'Médecine et chirurgie dans l'école de William et John Hunter'.
152. Maulitz, *Morbid Appearances*, 4.
153. Maulitz, *Morbid Appearances*, 4.
154. It should be noted, however, that the attraction of students and young practitioners towards a centre and the memoirs of these travellers are not necessarily accurate indicators of the scientific vitality of the centre. J. Warner very justifiably gives this warning with regard to the English and Americans studying in Paris in the early nineteenth century: 'the act of migration and the accounts of travellers may be doubtfully reliable indicators of the intellectual vibrancy of a center'. 'The Medical Migrant's Baggage Unpacked: Anglo-American Construction of the Paris Clinical School', in R. L. Numbers and J. V. Pickstone (eds), *British Society for the History of Science and the History of Science Society: Program, Papers, and Abstracts for the Joint Conference* (Madison: Omnipress, 1988), 217. In recent papers, Warner's criticism is more radical: 'Richard Shryock, for example, expressing a view historians have almost uniformly shared, attributed the migration to Paris to what he called "the scientific supremacy of the French metropolis" ... In fact, there is surprisingly little evidence that will support this interpretation. ... Instead, ..., what led Americans to choose Paris over London as a place of study was the social structure of Paris medical education more than the intellectual vibrancy of the Paris School, ... As portrayed in American accounts, ..., its facilities, talent and medical culture made London a serious rival of Paris.' See Warner, 'American

A Product of the Paris Clinical School?

Doctors in London during the Age of Paris Medicine', in V. Nutton and R. Porter (eds), *The History of Medical Education in Britain* (Amsterdam, Atlanta: Rodopi, 1995). See also Warner, this volume. See further in this text.

155. On this dynamic interaction between European medical schools of the era, where each one in turn occupied a dominant position, but not necessarily in all fields, and where exchanges continued to be reciprocal, see Keel, 'Modèles étrangers de la problématique hospitalière de l'École de Paris'.

156. See John Harley Warner, 'The Selective Transport of Medical Knowledge: Antebellum American physicians and Parisian Medical Therapeutics', *Bull. Hist. Med.*, 59 (1985), 213–31; *idem*, *The Therapeutic Perspective: Medical Knowledge, Practice and Identity in America, 1820–1885* (Cambridge, Massachusetts: Harvard University Press, 1986); *idem*, 'The Medical Migrant's Baggage Unpacked'; *idem*, 'The Idea of Science in English Medicine: The "Decline of Science" and the Rhetoric of Reform, 1815–45', in R. French and A. Wear (eds), *British Medicine in an Age of Reform* (London & New York: Routledge, 1991), 136–64. See also Warner's contribution in this volume.

157. See Warner, *The Medical Migrant's Baggage*, 214.

158. See L. S. Jacyna, 'Robert Carswell and William Thomson at the Hôtel-Dieu of Lyon: Scottish Views of French Medicine', in French and Wear (eds), *British Medicine*, 110–35. In a passage of his book, Maulitz recognizes that there was in fact a mutual impact or a relation of reciprocity between the (advanced) British students in Paris and the local medical milieu. The British did not passively absorb the Parisian experience: they came with their own stock of knowledge and experiences: 'The French setting affected their guests, while the English began in turn to make their impression on the French'. (*Morbid Appearances*, 151). But, if Maulitz shows that the English students were able to set up their own course of pathological anatomy in Paris, and if 'that impact, moreover seems to have been a mutual one' (*ibid.*), why does he defend the thesis throughout his entire book that anatomical and tissue pathology could only have been implanted in England through French influence (notably by the British students who had sojourned in Paris)? Why not also concede a mutual impact or a reciprocal influence, especially if one takes into account the fact that this pathology had initially developed in Great Britain?

159. See John Green Crosse, *Sketches of the Medical Schools of Paris* (London: J. Callow, 1815), 104.

160. On these points, see Keel, *La généalogie*; idem, 'Haller, Hunter, Bichat' and above in the text.
161. See Keel, 'La pathologie tissulaire de John Hunter'; *idem*, 'Haller, Hunter, Bichat'.
162. On this point see Keel, 'John Hunter et Xavier Bichat', 543 ff.
163. On the question of initial resistance to the use of the microscope at the Paris Clinical School, and on its subsequent use in pathology, which seems rather late in comparison with Great Britain, see the contribution of Ann La Berge in this volume; *idem*, 'Medical Microscopy in Paris, 1830–1855', in A. La Berge and M. Feingold (eds), *French Medical Culture in the Nineteenth Century* (Amsterdam & Atlanta: Rodopi, 1994), 296–326.
164. We have seen that Americans favoured this 'empiricist' or sensualist epistemology in their construction of an idealized image of the Paris Clinical School. However, this 'empiricism' could also constitute an impediment for various avenues of research. The glorification of the clinical 'empiricism' of the Paris School no doubt has also been an obstacle to the analysis of aspects of the history of the clinic and of pathology (and, notably, of anatomical and tissue pathology) since, as J. Warner pertinently suggests, the image of the Paris School propagated by historians like Ackerknecht probably derives from the idealized image of this school which Ackerknecht had found in the writings of American physicians who had studied in Paris (E. Bartlett, etc.). Ackernecht seems to have accepted this image at face value, instead of critically examining it as an idealized construction which was certainly related to some realities but filtered through a process of overvaluation answering the needs and interests of the American medical profession at the time.
165. See Keel, 'John Hunter et Xavier Bichat', 543 ff.
166. See Keel, 'Haller, Hunter, Bichat', 57 ff. In the *Anatomie générale*, Bichat takes into consideration only the genesis of tissue in the human species.
167. See Keel, 'John Hunter et Xavier Bichat'; *idem*, 'Haller, Hunter, Bichat' and above in text.
168. *Morbid Appearances*, ch. 7: 'After Waterloo: Medical journalism and the surgeon-apothecaries'. We would like to point out, however, that Maulitz paints too unilateral a portrait of many practitioners, notably the reformers of the surgeon-apothecaries group (Kerrison, Haden, Alcock, Clark, Johnson, etc.), who were also editors of various new medical journals. Maulitz implies that they 'discovered' tissue pathology solely through the works of Bichat and French clinicians, publicizing it to English medicine through the publication of extracts

or translations in their journals. Yet, on careful examination of the writings of these practitioners, we see that they mention British currents of anatomical and tissue pathology and that they are also based on these contributions.

169. L. S. Jacyna, 'Images of John Hunter in the Nineteenth Century', *History of Science*, 21 (1983), 85–108.

170. See Rodin, 'Matthew Baillie', 9. Baillie was an Oxford M.D. (1789) and had been appointed as Physician to St George's Hospital as early as 1787, probably through his uncle John Hunter's 'protection', who was the leading surgeon there; *ibid.* Hence, to reformers, Baillie should have appeared as a symbol of the hospital medico-surgical establishment as well as of the Royal College of Physicians' establishment. Note that James Carmichael Smyth, M.D. (Edinburgh, 1764) appointed as physician (as early as 1775) to the Middlesex Hospital, London – had also been a Fellow of the College of Physicians of London since 1788: admitted *speciali gracia* – in spite of the fact that he was an Edinburgh M.D. – to the Fellowship and thus member of the medical 'establishment'. He had been a Licentiate of the College since 1770. At the London College of Physicians, he was Censor in 1788, 1793, 1801; he delivered the Harveian oration in 1793; and was named an Elect 26 June 1802. See Keel, *La généalogie*, 102; and W. Munk, *The Roll of the Royal College of Physicians of London*, 2nd edn, 3 vols (London: Royal College of Physicians, 1878).

171. See Warner, *The Medical Migrant's Baggage*; idem, 'The Idea of Science'. On the reformists' medical politics and strategy and their construction of an idealized French – especially Parisian – model, see also A. Desmond, *The Politics of Evolution: Morphology, Medicine and Reform in Radical London* (Chicago: University of Chicago Press, 1990).

172. See also note 164. For discussion of the monolithic, idealized and simplistic image of the Paris Clinic still present in the history of medicine, see also the beginning of the contribution by L. S. Jacyna and the contributions of others (Warner, Brockliss, etc.) in this volume.

4

Pious Pathology:
J. L. Alibert's Iconography of Disease

L. S. Jacyna

Introduction

The protagonist of this paper is Jean Louis Alibert, a French physician who lived between 1768 and 1837 and who studied and practised medicine in Paris. He was among the most successful Parisian medical practitioners of the early decades of the nineteenth century, and acted as physician to both Louis XVIII and Charles X. Alibert is, however, chiefly remembered as an author, in particular, for publishing pioneering works dealing with diseases of the skin. Alibert was from 1802 physician to the Hôpital Saint-Louis which he transformed into an establishment devoted exclusively to the treatment of skin disorders. It was from this source that he derived most of the materials for his research.

The most immediately striking feature of Alibert's publications is the pictures they contain. Alibert employed the latest technologies to produce vivid coloured illustrations of the cases he discussed.[1] Contemporary commentators emphasized the importance of the media Alibert employed to the overall impact of his works: in the words of one reviewer, 'precious facts strike the eyes with all the sumptuousness of typography, with all the magnificence of the colours of the paintbrush and all the finesse of the processes of the engraver's needle ... It is, in short, an excellent work undertaken with an excellent method.'[2]

Alibert has attracted the attention of a number of historians. He has, for instance, served in the well-established role of the founding figure of a medical speciality: according to Mark Allen Everett, Alibert was 'The Father of French Dermatology'.[3] More recently, Elizabeth Williams has tried to insert him into a different genealogy;

she views the distinctive features of Alibert's work as exemplary of the discourse of 'anthropological medicine' in nineteenth-century France. The most salient feature of this discourse was the impulse to create a medically based 'Science of Man' which would be relevant not only to clinical but also to social and political practice.[4]

The pictorial aspect of Alibert's opus has been considered by some art historians. In her discussion of early nineteenth-century medical illustration, Susanne Dahm draws upon the explanatory strategies of traditional art history to proffer an interpretation of the lavish coloured prints that are the most immediately remarkable feature of Alibert's books. Medical illustrations, she argues, reflect more general trends in painting: they manifest shifts in 'Zeitgeist'. Thus the representations in Alibert's early works show a clear neo-classical influence; they depict individuals with 'classical beauty', whose clothes and coiffure recall the ancient world. Later illustrations, in contrast, take more care to depict individual characteristics and so carry the imprint of romanticism.[5]

Some of the paintings do appear to vindicate Dahm's argument. Not only the features but also the drapery of this figure, for instance (Fig. 1), have clear classical allusions. The lesion on the shoulder is incongruous and incidental to this scheme of reference. Others of the pictures do not, however, conform to Dahm's generalization, which, moreover, is hardly adequate as an overall account of these depictions.

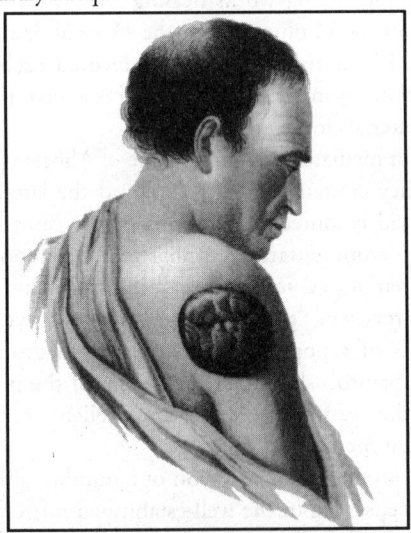

Figure 1
Alibert, *Nosologie naturelle*, facing page (f.p.) 336, plate (pl.) B.
Reproduced with the permission of the
Wellcome Institute for the History of Medicine Library.

Pious Pathology

In her book, *Body Criticism: Imaging the Unseen in Enlightenment Art and Medicine*, Barbara Maria Stafford has provided a different appreciation of the visualizations of disease found in Alibert's works. She seeks to provide a grand narrative which describes the rise of the visual image to its predominant place in contemporary culture. Alibert has a not inconsiderable part in this story. Stafford maintains that:

> Alibert ... should be inscribed in the annals of art history as the diagnostician of blighted, or modern, looks. It is impossible to imagine nineteenth-century French Realist portraiture without this trailblazing truth-sayer.[6]

Stafford's analysis of Alibert's depictions of skin disease contains valuable insights. But neither she nor Dahm address a crucial issue: the role that these pictures play in the totality of Alibert's literary project. They need to be understood as illustrations integral to a medical text rather than as self-sufficient works of art. Conversely, while Williams describes some of Alibert's text, she ignores these pictorial representations. It is with the relationship between the pictorial and the literary in Alibert's work that I will be chiefly concerned.

In approaching this task I have derived considerable assistance from an essay on ancien régime French painting by Norman Bryson. He draws a distinction between the 'discursive' and the 'figural' aspects of an image. The former term denotes 'those features which show the influence over the image of language'; while the latter refers to 'those features which belong to the image as a visual experience independent of language'.[7]

The text that informs an image may be immediate – taking the form of an inscription on a picture frame, for instance, or of the livret provided for visitors to a salon. It may be more remote as when a picture refers to some familiar historical, religious, or mythical narrative. Bryson maintains that in some cases the discursive element of a painting is so dominant that it exhausts the significance of the representation. But in other cases a surplus meaning resides in the figural aspects of the image. As well as its relation to an explicit text, a picture may allude to a variety of codes prevalent in a culture and intelligible to those who view it.

In the present case text and image coexist within the covers of the same volume. Because Alibert's paintings are presented as illustrations, they are – prima facie – subordinate to the verbal component of these works: the discursive element is predominant.

Pious Pathology

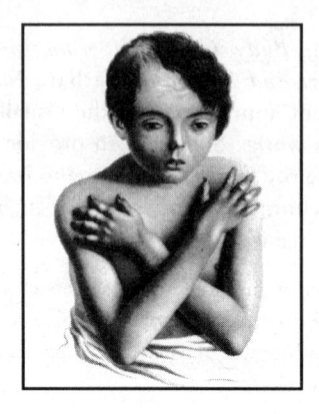

Figure 2
Alibert, *Nosologie naturelle*, f.p. 448, pl. B.
Reproduced with the permission of the
Wellcome Institute for the History of Medicine Library.
'[I]t was necessary to make him speak to know that a breath of life still animated him. He remained for a long time in the hôpital Saint-Louis where our nuns gave him the nickname of the Mummy, because he resembled a dessicated cadaver.'[8]

In some cases the priority of word over figure is quite clear. Take this picture from Alibert's *Nosologie naturelle* of 1817 (Fig. 2). The accompanying text relates to a patient who resembled a phantom. The plate accordingly shows a shrivelled child whose skin is drained of colour. The face shows little sign of life: the eyes stare blankly while the mouth hangs open with the tongue visible. The arms are folded across the chest. This serves to display the state of the fingers to which Alibert had alluded in the case history; but it is also the proper posture of a corpse. The drapery around the waist suggests a shroud.

In other cases, however, the signification of the picture is not so thoroughly determined by the text. Some of the images possess layers of meaning additional to their discursive function; in other words, they cease to be merely illustrations of a verbal text and become texts in themselves. The legibility of these pictorial texts depends upon familiarity with a range of iconic codes. An involved set of cultural cross-references needs to be recognized, therefore, before the full meaning of these signs can be retrieved.

The point may be illustrated by reference to a depiction taken from Alibert's *Description des maladies de la peau* (1806). It is of a woman suffering from what Alibert calls 'scrophule vulgaire' (Fig.

188

Pious Pathology

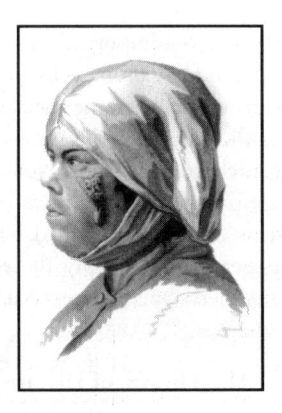

Figure 3
Alibert, *Descriptions des maladies de la peau*, pl. 46.
Reproduced with the permission of the
Wellcome Institute for the History of Medicine Library.

3). There is a wealth of seemingly otiose detail to this image: we are shown the woman's headscarf and enough of her clothing to see that she is wearing a drab functional garment. These details are not, however, superfluous and insignificant. They are signs that identify the patient as a woman of the people; she, like her disease, is vulgar. The message is reinforced by a more subtle system of signification within the portrait. The woman's head is presented in profile to display the lesion on her cheek. This point of view also draws attention, however, to the facial angle and to the prominent lower

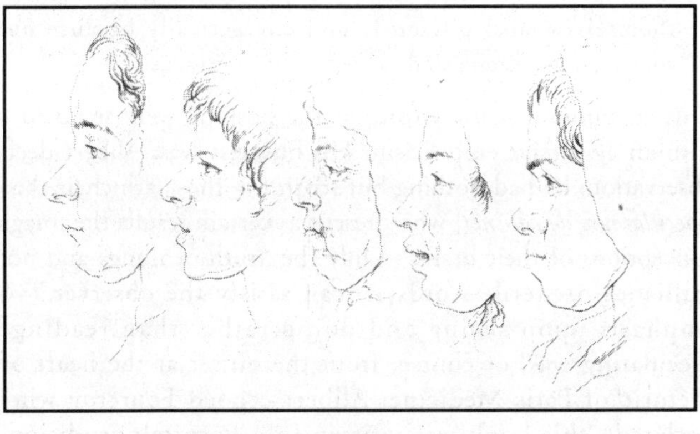

Figure 4
Lavater, *L'art de connaître les hommes par la physionomie*,
tome V, f.p. 381, pl. 245, women's faces.
Reproduced with the permission of the
Wellcome Institute for the History of Medicine Library.

lip. For the physiognomist the import of these signs was plain: they implied feebleness of mind.[9] (Compare Lavater's drawings, Fig. 4.) There is thus a consonance between the social station of this woman and the illness that afflicts her. The illustration also makes a coded statement about her intellectual capacity. None of this is hinted at in the history of the case; in this instance there is a figural meaning to the image far in excess of that determined by the verbal text. The remainder of this paper seeks to apply these methods of analysis more extensively to Alibert's medical texts and to the illustrations that accompany them.

The Theatre of Disease

Alibert's commitment to what Erwin Ackerknecht called Hospital Medicine[10] was unmistakable. On numerous occasions he insisted on the hospital's title as the premier site for the evolution and exposition of medical knowledge. The hospital's advantages in part derived from the sheer wealth of pathological material presenting there: the Hôpital Saint-Louis, Alibert declared, was 'the sewer of all the countries of the world'.

> Located in a place where these maladies incessantly present and renew themselves I have been better able than any other to unravel the confusion introduced into the works of the ancients; I have been able to follow the progress, the periods, the decline, the recrudescence, the metamorphoses of the various exanthemata. It is in hospitals that their various characteristic traits manifest themselves most obviously and energetically because one contemplates them in all the epochs of their existence.[11]

This encomium to the virtues of the hospital went hand in hand with an aggressive empiricism. His business was, Alibert declared, observation: he had nothing but scorn for 'those armchair theorists [*spéculateurs de cabinet*] who present as certain results the imaginary conceptions of their brains'. Only the 'truth of things and not the brilliance of sterile words ... can satisfy the observer.'[12] Such emphasis upon seeing and doing rather than reading and speculating was, of course, from the outset at the heart of the rhetoric of Paris Medicine. Alibert echoed Fourcroy when he declared: 'this book was written in a hospital; erudition was altogether superfluous'.[13]

The hospital was therefore the location where the senses of the clinician – and, above all, the medical gaze – could best be trained. In the hospital 'one acquires such practice in contemplating these hideous objects, that I have often been known to point out and to name a species of eruption even when scarcely the slightest trace of it remained on the skin: so true is it that vision is the sense with the most powerful memory'.[14]

Alibert drew comparisons between the enterprise of the nosographer and that of the naturalist; both were engaged in a classificatory exercise. On this analogy, the hospital was a collection of specimens, equivalent to the botanist's cabinet or the zoological museum, that offered opportunities for observation. But the hospital could serve also as a laboratory: Alibert detailed inoculation experiments undertaken in the Hôpital Saint-Louis to investigate the contagiousness of various diseases.[15]

Alibert's favoured metaphor for the hospital is, however, neither that of the museum nor the laboratory. Instead, he repeatedly speaks of the hospital as a theatre. Thus he asserted that it was only in the 'hôpital Saint-Louis that one can study [dartrous diseases] under all their different aspects; it is only in this theatre that all is displayed to the attentive eye of the observer'.[16] Associated with this image of the hospital as a theatre is a preoccupation with spectacle. The Hôpital Saint-Louis was a stage that offered the most novel objects to the view of those who wished to study skin diseases according to philosophic principles; moreover, 'What spectacle leaves stronger, more permanent impressions upon the spirit of the observer?'[17] Within this metaphor the patients of the Hôpital Saint-Louis figured as actors presenting certain striking appearances to the eye of the observer.[18]

It is the essence of spectacle that it impresses the observer in some way. Alibert takes pains to describe his own and others' reactions to the striking sights they encountered in the hospital: compassion, amazement, and horror are the most frequent responses elicited by the theatre of disease.

> The hospital presented a spectacle deserving pity ... when one sees walking in the courts of this vast building that multitude of individuals whose face is terribly disfigured, and who are bereft ... of the most important characteristics that compose the human physiognomy.[19]

Alibert is therefore also concerned with the audience for the spectacle he describes. This comprises in the first instance himself and his colleagues in the hospital; at its most extensive, however, the audience includes the readers who access these appearances at second hand through Alibert's text and pictures.

Alibert did not, therefore, maintain a purely objective,

Pious Pathology

dispassionate attitude to disease. On the contrary, he takes pains to describe his own affective responses to what he has witnessed and invites others to display a similar degree of sensibility. There is nothing 'clinical' – in the sense of cool and detached – about Alibert's version of the medical gaze.

Alibert's published works attempted to give a wider audience access to the theatre of disease that was the Hôpital Saint-Louis. The most obviously spectacular aspect of these books was the illustrations. The sheer size of these plates – especially those in the *Description des maladies de la peau* (1806) – their colours, as well as the details of their composition, all cooperate to make these illustrations imposing. Alibert made it clear that this was his intention:

> In order to imprint a seal of authenticity upon what I have written, to augment the energy and power of my discourses, to perpetuate and animate, as it were, all my descriptions [*tableaux*], I have felt it necessary to have recourse to the ingenious contrivances of the paintbrush and of the engraver's needle. I have wished to reinforce the impressions by the physical image of the objects that I want to offer to the contemplation of the pathologist; I have ... desired, by means of the terrifying colours of the painter, to instruct, so to speak, the vision by vision, to emphasize and to contrast more the characteristics of skin diseases, to fix their finest nuances, in a word, to strike the senses of my readers, and to reproduce vividly before

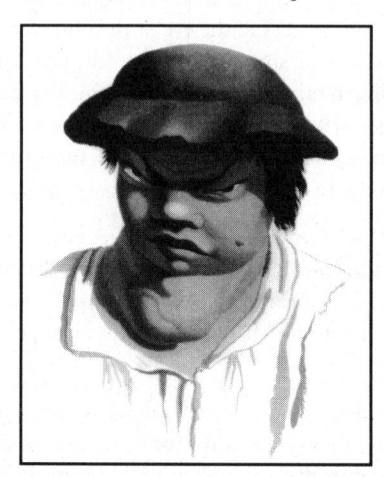

Figure 5
Alibert, *Descriptions des maladies de la peau*, pl. 49.
Reproduced with the permission of the
Wellcome Institute for the History of Medicine Library.

them the various phenomena that have amazed my gaze.[20]

Alibert provided a utilitarian justification for this stress upon the visual: illustrations would, he argued, give a new precision to clinical description and enable medicine to take its proper place among the natural and physical sciences. But it is clear that these spectacular devices were also designed to astonish the reader and to evoke in him or her an emotional reaction.

The textual portion of the book could serve the same end; in various passages Alibert strained his descriptive powers in an effort to compose a verbal tableau that would impress and move his readers. Here is his word picture of the 'scrofulous' inhabitants of the Lozère who sometimes made their way to the Hôpital Saint-Louis:

> They were almost all in a frightful state of emaciation ...; the thyroid appeared monstrous; the colour of their skin was dirty and muddy [*terreuse*]; the epidermis was hard and calloused on various parts of the body; their hands and forearms were dessicated like the limbs of an Egyptian mummy; their nails were curled; ... they had a dull and, so to speak, lifeless gaze; the voice [was] harsh and hollow, as if it came from a grave.[21] (Fig. 5)

Although it does contain a good deal of information about these patients' symptoms, this description goes well beyond the remit of a clinical picture.[22] There is, indeed, more of the gothic than of the clinic about it; the reader is meant to be appalled as well as informed. The repertoire of Alibert's theatre of disease did not, however, consist solely of spectacular pictorial or verbal tableaux. What made it true drama was its preoccupation with narrative.[23]

Storylines

A demotion or dismissal of the patient's subjective account of his or her condition is supposed to be a definitive aspect of the rise of Hospital Medicine.[24] It is something of a surprise, therefore, to find that Alibert, operating within the very citadel of Hospital Medicine, was much concerned with how his patients perceived and explained their illnesses.

He took pains, for instance, to explore the phenomenological aspects of the diseases that he encountered. He records that 'I questioned the patient about the kind of sensation that he experienced: he told me that at that time he felt a sort of tingling in the fingers, a species of pain [*travail*]: that was his expression'.[25] Alibert's anxiety to preserve the words and metaphoric resources used by patients to express their experience of disease is also evident in his discussion of psoriasis. Individuals afflicted with this condition, he reported, 'speak only of acridity, of hot blood, of scorching fire, etc.: I am on the grill that made a martyr of saint Lawrence, a wretched clergyman told me'.[26]

Still more striking is the care Alibert took to report his patients' own accounts of the aetiology of their condition and of its place in their total biography. He claimed that patients were anxious to tell their tale: 'they are not afraid to breathe their groans and to recount the story of their suffering'. Such narration might even have a therapeutic effect. Moreover, allowing patients to speak for themselves was, Alibert argued, the most instructive form of clinical teaching.[27]

Into these accounts Alibert introduced prevailing medical beliefs about the interaction of the moral and the physical; and, in particular, on the influence that disturbances of the passions could have upon the body.[28] In the case of one 23-year-old man, skin disease was perceived as the result of emotional excess coupled with intemperate personal habits:

> For nearly fifteen months he experienced violent sorrows, and was tormented by two equally strong passions, jealousy and love. In the winter of 1805 every morning on rising from bed he washed his head with cold water. One day several pimples appeared about the crown of the head which intermittently gave rise to quite acute itching.[29]

The case of Marguerite Ferrant gave a still more striking example of how external eruptions could follow internal crises. This woman, who suffered from tinea, was much ill-used by her husband and even by her children. When she was calm the affected parts of her skin suppurated, the scabs detached themselves, and she seemed cured; when, however, 'her sorrows were worst, the scabs were dry and she experienced severe headaches'.[30]

The effects of emotional distress could even be transmitted to others. A 20-month-old infant presented at the Hôpital Saint-Louis with the symptoms of a 'mucous tinea'. This affliction manifested itself at a time when his nurse experienced very serious distress. Her husband had been carried off in front of her to be conveyed to prison; she then fell very ill – indeed, she suffered a brief attack of insanity [*manie*]. Despite this lamentable incident, she continued to feed the child until her milk was entirely exhausted. Almost immediately, the child's head was covered with yellow scabs.[31]

Patients sometimes reached deep into their own and even their

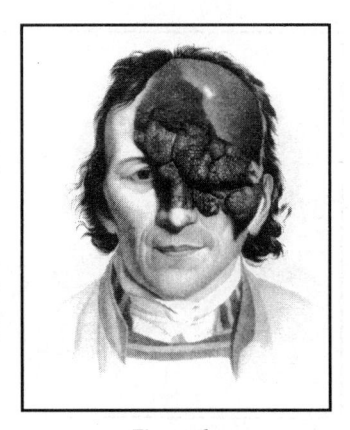

Figure 6
Alibert, *Monographie des dermatoses*, f.p. 803, 'spalaco-dermie frontale'.
Reproduced with the permission of the
Wellcome Institute for the History of Medicine Library.

parents' biographies to find events that might explain their condition. Thus Alibert recounts the tale of a gardener called Delaitre, also known as 'La Taupe' – or 'The Mole'. He had been born in 1756 of 'very healthy' parents.

> His mother has, he says, often recounted that early in her pregnancy three men had come into her garden, and had there come upon the body of a dead mole; his mother having returned to look at this animal, was so startled that she cried out, and placed her right hand on her eye and forehead on the same side.
>
> She gave birth after nine months, and her infant was marked by the excrescence known as mole which had the same situation, the same size, and the same appearance as it has today.[32] (Fig. 6).

Alibert added that, according to Delaitre, the colour and texture of his mole changed at the time of year 'when the mulberry bushes lose their flowers' – a good example, incidentally, of Alibert's scrupulous rendition of a patient's own words. Here, however, he added a caveat, noting that he had not been able to verify this claim himself.[33] Otherwise, Alibert presented the narratives given by this and by his other patients without any sceptical asides; he merely notes that this is Delaitre's story 'as told by himself'.

Alibert was not, however, merely a passive reporter of his patients' accounts. There is evidence that in some cases he edited and structured these narratives in accordance with his own views of what was relevant

Pious Pathology

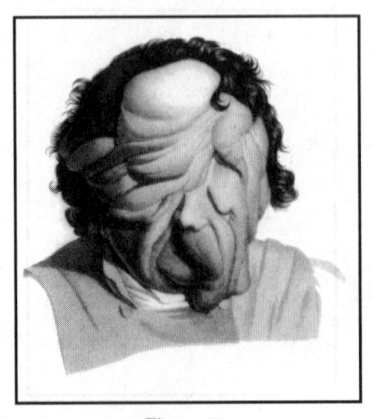

Figure 7.
Alibert, *Monographie des dermatoses*, f.p. 796, 'dermatose faciale'.
Reproduced with the permission of the
Wellcome Institute for the History of Medicine Library.

and important. In deciding which narratives to recount he exercised a further form of editorial control. By studying the ways in which Alibert employed this discretion it is possible to discern something of the criteria with which he operated and of the effects he was trying to achieve.

Among the most extensive of these narratives is the tale of J.-B. Lemoine, a shepherd who was afflicted with what Alibert called 'dermatose hétéromorphe' (Fig. 7).

> This unfortunate man had lost the sight of one eye at the age of six months; when he was twenty years old, he lost the remaining eye, after having suffered violent head aches. He despaired at being no longer able to work; boredom overtook him until he tried to go out for walks, guiding himself with a stick. He made his way to a wood close to the village and, wishing to make his excursion useful, he began by cutting birchwood to make brooms. So encouraged was he by his initial success that he thought himself capable of watching the cows; true he could only be trusted with one. Lemoine was besides familiar with all the places where he walked .... During the period of nearly twenty years that he did this job, he had never lost his way; if he ever strayed for an instant, he soon found his path again by orientating himself by the sun glimmering through his eyelids.
>
> He enjoyed all his intellectual faculties. One of the greatest sorrows his deformity caused him was that he was unable to marry. He loved his parents dearly. Sometimes he was seen to laugh when

Pious Pathology

someone told him a joke ....

To this point the story is sad yet uplifting. The reader is invited to sympathize with Lemoine for his early loss of sight and consequent feelings of uselessness; but he is also asked to admire the resourcefulness with which he overcame these handicaps. Lemoine's capacity, despite his bizarre appearance, for the normal human emotions of filial love, joy, and sadness is emphasized. The narrative belongs to the genre of sentimental drama with a pastoral setting.

Then matters take a tragic turn. The reader is informed that Lemoine now

> sleeps in a barn to which is brought all that he needs; for this wretch had been excluded from the paternal home because of a vow taken by his sister when she married never again to look on his face, afraid that a child of hers might one day bear the imprint of the same deformity.[34]

Because of his affliction Lemoine was thus cut off from the familial links that were so dear to him.

There is little in this lengthy account to instruct readers in the nature of Lemoine's condition. There is, however, much to reveal to persons of sensibility the personal tragedy that may result from such deformity. Pathology is displaced by pathos.

Central to the pathetic effect of this tale is the incongruity between Lemoine's spiritual potential and the hideous bodily garb he is forced to wear. Elsewhere, however, Alibert insisted upon the validity of the physiognomic axiom that the outer envelope faithfully represented the individual's inner essence. The transformations of the body in disease served only to emphasize this correspondence.

Alibert ventured beyond the confines of the Hôpital Saint-Louis to find cases that illustrated these principles. He had observed in the streets of Paris one Thomas Quart whose nickname was the 'Rogue' [*gueux*]. Quart made a living by collecting rags from the street and by begging. He thus belonged to the bohemian demi-monde of the city and was one of the dangerous classes. He was, moreover, a wastrel who soon spent on drink whatever money he obtained; on one occasion he was so drunk that he mistook a window for a door and fell two storeys onto a paved courtyard. Quart displayed, moreover, 'an invincible aversion for work'.

Quart's origins were exotic: he was born in Poland of a native woman and a French father. Because of political disturbances in Poland, at the age of eighteen he came to live in France; he thus conformed to the stereotype of a rootless 'nomad'. According to Alibert, Quart possessed

> a sinister air and always seemed famished. His long, bushy beard; his thick, arched eyebrows, endowed him with a sombre and farouche aspect. Almost his entire person was covered in hair. To this truly picturesque body was joined a revolting dirtiness, in which he appeared to take pleasure, and which made him hideous to contemplate.[35]

What justified Quart's presence in a work devoted to diseases of the

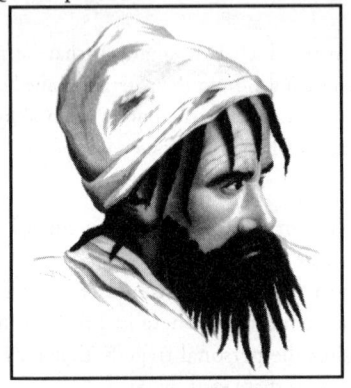

Figure 8
Alibert, *Descriptions des maladies de la peau*, pl. 6.
Reproduced with the permission of the
Wellcome Institute for the History of Medicine Library.

skin was the fact that he suffered from a rare condition called 'plica' in which the strands of the hair grow together in one or several masses. In Quart's case the hair is shown to have formed a series of spikes in keeping with his ferocious and farouche nature (Fig. 8). There is also a strong hint that this affliction was a punishment for Quart's vicious lifestyle: Alibert does not hide his disgust for the man's dirty and drunken habits.

In other cases too Alibert suggests that plica is a chastisement for those who breach the canons of acceptable behaviour. He notes that another beggar, who was on good terms with Quart, suffered from the same disease. There is no hint that the second man may have contracted the condition through his acquaintance with Quart; instead, Alibert stresses the similarities in the 'manner of existence' of the two. The second beggar also 'drank immoderately; and was revoltingly filthy, [he was] continually devoured by vermin'. There is a suitably moral ending to the tale: this man died from burns incurred after falling into a drunken sleep in front of a fire.[36]

Plica was not confined to the lowest reaches of society; it could afflict even formerly respectable individuals if they strayed from the paths of propriety. Thus Élénore Gaudray had for long been in the service of a well-known Paris actress. At the age of seventeen, however, she became infatuated with a drunken soldier with whom she cohabited; soon Élénore herself began to manifest an excessive taste for brandy and other spirits. She underwent 'a sort of degradation'. This moral decline was reflected in her health and in her bodily figure. She fell ill, coughing and spitting blood. Her face

> became rubicund, and her complexion inflamed like that of persons who habitually take alcohol in excess. A viscous humour, the smell of which was as peculiar as it was stale, soon poured out over all parts of the head. The poor woman made futile efforts to clean and to untangle her hair; from day to day it agglutinated to form a large, thick crest [*calotte*] ... [37]

Alibert noted that when this mass of hair was humid the woman's pulmonary symptoms were relieved; when it was dry, they were aggravated. The scalp seemed to serve therefore as a conduit for the vicious humours generated within her body. Despite the lessons of disease, Gaudray continued to abuse alcohol.

Some of Alibert's stories about disease therefore conform to the conventions of the cautionary tale: those who fail to observe the laws of bourgeois morality will suffer bodily afflictions as well as social stigma. The case of Quart and his fellow beggar reveals a particular concern to articulate the connections between dirt, depravity, and disease among the urban poor which was not peculiar to Alibert.[38] Indeed, aspects of his work can be related to the endeavour to figure the menacing 'Other' within the nineteenth-century city; in particular, his depiction of Thomas Quart served to make that Other safely visible to respectable eyes.[39]

The individual was, to some extent, answerable for his or her fall from health; illness was the natural consequence of vice. But Alibert's text also shows an awareness that individuals were not altogether masters of their own destiny; the biographies of even the humblest might be shaped by the great events of history.

Bodily Revolutions

A recognition of the fact that the drama of individual life is played out on a stage set by history is apparent in Alibert's tale of Thomas

Quart. Soon after he came to France, Quart's plica gave him much pain. But he then found his way to the forest of Senart where he entered a monastery. The religious order that he joined required its members to shave their hair and beard. Quart remained in this situation until the age of thirty – 'occupying himself with rural labours'. The implication is that during this period of his life he enjoyed a remission from his affliction. This idyllic existence was, however, to be brutally terminated: 'His monastery having been destroyed in the revolutionary disturbances that agitated France, he fell into the most frightful destitution'. To survive he had to labour in public works funded by the republican government. From this time he took little care of his person and his condition soon recurred.[40]

Two themes in particular should be abstracted from this narrative. The first is the deleterious effect of the disasters of the French Revolution upon individual health. The second is the wholesome character and curative potential ascribed to religion.

The baleful influence of the Revolution is a motif that runs through Alibert's case histories. This topos in Alibert's writing can be viewed as an extended footnote on Rousseau's axiom that 'everything depends on politics'.[41] In Alibert's gloss, this principle applied especially to the health of the individual member of a polity. In an essay written under the Directory, when the influence on his work of *Idéologie* was still most apparent, Alibert had held that the 'philosophic physician' should pay special attention to the effect that 'legislation' exerted upon populations.[42] He was at this period in his career especially concerned to demonstrate the baleful effects of despotism upon national health; people forced to live under regimes that failed to respect the rights of the individual were, in particular, prone to endemic diseases of the skin.[43]

Conversely, Alibert maintained that the Revolution in France had at first exercised a beneficial influence on the nation's health. Certain diatheses, such as hysteria and hypochondriasis, had disappeared thanks to the salutary reformations that occurred after 1789. But this wholesome tendency was reversed after the Revolution entered its radical phase: during the period when 'Robespierre covered the land with scaffolds, blood, and mourning, the famous Desault had remarked that aneurisms became infinitely more common at the Hôtel-Dieu of Paris'.[44]

In his later work Alibert's previous critique of the despotic governments of the ancien régime is quietly dropped. He continued to insist, however, on the ways in which social conditions and political events could impinge upon the health of populations.[45] By

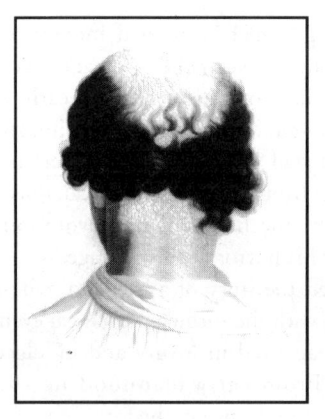

Figure 9
Alibert, *Descriptions des maladies de la peau*, pl. 11.
Reproduced with the permission of the
Wellcome Institute for the History of Medicine Library.

causing famine and forcing people to eat vitiated food, for example, social disturbances did much to spread disease. Thus during the 'awful times of the Terror' all kinds of skin disease became more prevalent because of bad diet.[46]

The pathogenic effects of the Revolution sometimes worked through the more occult channels of the passions. Such was the case with a patient at the Hôpital Saint-Louis named Le Tellier. Before the Revolution he had been valet to a member of the Paris Parlement; 'We believe', Alibert explained,

> it useful to report this detail of his biography because of its influence upon the development of the skin disease of which he was subsequently the victim. Here is the fact, as it occurred in the stormy period we have just recalled. One day as he crossed one of the bridges over the Seine, he saw his former master shamefully dragged towards the frightful punishment of the guillotine. At this spectacle, he was struck with such terror, that a furfuraceous eruption suddenly occurred all over the surface of his body.[47] (Fig. 9)

This narrative serves to draw attention to the atrocities committed during the Terror; but it also conveys more subtle meanings. Threats to the proper relationship between master and servant had been a common cultural concern even before the Revolution; the rebellious valet was, for instance, a stock figure of eighteenth-century French drama.[48] By openly attacking traditional hierarchies and patterns of deference, the Revolution greatly heightened these concerns.[49]

Alibert's story assuaged such fears: it demonstrated the strength of the natural sympathy between the valet and his former employer. The narrative can therefore be seen as an early contribution to a nineteenth-century genre of nostalgia for an imagined past in which master and servant had been bound together in a relationship of mutual loyalty.[50] Far from rejoicing in the calamity that had befallen his former master at the hands of the revolutionaries, Le Tellier's skin made manifest his horror at this outrage.

Alibert recounted the story of a 'vieillard' whose medical history had also intersected with the turbulent political events of the time. As a youth this man had lived in luxury and indulged an immoderate taste for spirits. From early manhood he suffered from the consequences of this indulgence in the form of violent attacks of gout. His symptoms included insomnia, nervous spasms, nausea, retention of the urine, and constipation; all forms of treatment failed to relieve the condition. Then there occurred an 'astonishing metamorphosis':

> all the misfortunes which had succeeded one another and which had, so to speak, been interconnected, suddenly vanished at the famous epoch when political troubles began to agitate France. This man was doubly unfortunate: he lost his fortune and his titles [*dignités*], and the acute sorrow that he suffered produced an incomprehensible change in his physical condition. His sufferings ceased; but his whole body became covered by a flaky eruption which had a horrible and repulsive appearance .... From that time the internal pains ceased: the functions of the viscera regained the calm and vigour of health; his appetite was voracious, and digestion was effected with unfailing regularity.[51]

The synergy between revolutions in the physical and political bodies is more complex in this than in Le Tellier's case. The Revolution appears to act as a cathartic, curative event – or, to be more precise, as an agent which effects a metamorphosis in the nature of the ailment afflicting the body. This transformation was brought about by displacing an internal visceral pathology to the surface of the body: a hidden disease eating away at the entrails was replaced by one that was manifest.

The patient's social status gives a clue to the metaphorical value of this tale. He is identified as one of the privileged class of ancien régime France – as a suitable object for the disdain of virtuous members of the Third Estate. His bodily corruption is the direct result of the degenerate manners of this caste. Like Thomas Quart this old man is beyond the bourgeois pale; but he represents an aristocratic rather than a proletarian Other. The resolution of the man's chronic illness coincides with the political crisis that swept away the privileges of his class. The cure is, however, achieved at the cost of gross disfigurement.

Most of Alibert's remarks on the effects of political disturbance upon the body form an undisguised polemic against the excesses of the Revolution and its results. Even in 1806 this was a safe – indeed, an officially approved – posture. After the Restoration Alibert made clear his royalist sympathies. The *Nosologie naturelle* of 1817 opens with an obsequious dedication to the king and to his august ancestors. The story of the gouty roué is more, however, than an anti-revolutionary diatribe. It recognizes the corruption of aspects of the ancien régime and it ascribes a salutary influence to the Revolution – albeit one achieved at a ghastly cost. Alibert's text therefore embodies a centrist rather than an ultra interpretation of the events of recent French history; as such it recalls, in muted form, his earlier Rousseauite sympathies.

Spiritual Healing

The motif of a religious dimension to illness and healing runs through Alibert's work. It forms a natural complement to his explicitly political statements: attitudes to religion and politics were inseparable in post-revolutionary France. Because the Revolution had challenged the privileges and denied the social value of the Catholic Church, any attempt to rehabilitate religion was also a repudiation of a central aspect of the revolutionary legacy. The Catholic revival during the Restoration was fostered by and identified with the forces of reaction.[52]

Alibert's identification with the movement to restore the former dignity of Catholicism took a number of forms. In the first place, he stressed the important beneficial role played by religion within the theatre of disease. Thus his description of the 'salle des agonisans' in the Hôpital Saint-Louis is redolent of incense:

> The interior of this chamber gives rise to the most heart-rending impressions, because of the long sighs that suffering elicits, by the murmur of prayers to the Deity at the bedside of the dying, by the presence of priests charged with purifying the conscience, by the religious motions impressed upon the soul during the last moments of life ...[53]

The services of the religious within the hospital were not, however, confined to comforting dying patients and preparing them for the next world. Alibert is full of praise for the part played by the nursing staff within the hospital; he did not repeat the conventional complaints of French doctors about meddling nuns who undermined medical authority and hindered effective treatment. Patients were, for instance, led to the lime-grove where clinical instruction took place by the 'helping hand of those sisters of charity wisely instituted to relieve the burdens of existence, of those incomparable virgins whose voice is so consoling, and whose attentions are so unsparing'.[54] There is an undisguised allusion here to Chateaubriand's eulogy in the *Génie du christianisme* to the 'femmes angéliques' of the Hôtel-Dieu.[55]

Alibert was reluctant to attribute any direct curative power to supernatural agencies; he was, however, more sympathetic to such claims than many of his colleagues. He noted that in parts of the country where scrofula was prevalent, 'there are fountains consecrated by popular piety where large numbers of sufferers go in search of some relief for their complaints'. Alibert did not deny that such fountains might have some benefit, but he endeavoured to find a rational physiological explanation for this effect:

> Undoubtedly the emotions experienced during these pilgrimages impress upon the lymphatic system a salutary activity. I have, besides, thought it useful to record here the local beliefs and customs which always contain some instructive fact for the observer.[56]

There is evidence of embarrassment and prevarication in Alibert's remarks about the healing power of religious pilgrimages. He seemed anxious not to seem to endorse practices that other members of the medical profession might dismiss as superstitious; at the same time he was loath to risk the charge of scepticism by dismissing them. The question of religious healing became especially sensitive when it was coupled to the political issue of the nature of kingship. The restored Bourbons were, according to the Charter of 1814, supposed to be constitutional monarchs. After his accession in 1824, however, Charles X revived the practice of touching for the king's evil as part of his efforts to reinstate the doctrine of divine-right kingship.[57]

While dismissive of various popular remedies for scrofula, Alibert was altogether more respectful of the thaumaturgic claims of the French monarchy. Some, he reported,

> think that [scrofula] is of so malignant a nature that we must regard it as the result of celestial anger. They have even believed that this

supernatural affection is beyond all human power, and that God had delegated the ability to cure it to kings alone. Clovis is considered the first to have been invested with so august a privilege, and to have transmitted it to his successors.[58]

This account of the royal touch is scrupulously non-committal. Alibert makes clear that he is reporting the views of others, not stating his own opinion. Neither, however, does he express any scepticism about the alleged healing powers of royalty: he leaves open both the possibility that divine agency may be effective in the cure of certain diseases and the claim that members of the royal family might be God's chosen agents for the exercise of this prerogative.

By 1832 Alibert's attitude had apparently hardened. In an amended version of the passage quoted above he declared that 'there are individuals, misled by superstition, who think that [scrofula] is of so malignant a nature that it must be considered the result of divine anger'. The notion of the royal touch is thus apparently relegated to the category of other irrational popular beliefs about the disease. Alibert was, however, then obliged to confront a discrepancy between his stated views and what might be inferred from his recent actions. 'At the time of the consecration of Charles X', he conceded,

> in my capacity as his first physician-in-ordinary, I assisted at one of these solemn ceremonies at the hôpital Saint-Marcou in Reims. All those suffering from scrofula in the region had flocked, as if vying with one another, to place themselves under the eyes of the new sovereign. Several members of the court took the view that it was advisable to abolish this outdated custom, as being no longer in harmony with the philosophic ideas of the age. But the villagers who had mostly come long distances demanded with the most urgent solicitations a visitation from which they expected the greatest benefit. For beings who suffer, a great hope is almost health itself. It was therefore necessary to condescend to their wishes. The ceremony was most touching; it had the great advantage of being the occasion of royal generosity. Besides, according to the profound Stahl, it is always useful to make use of the mediation of the spirit to cure the ills of the body.[59]

There is a tension evident in these remarks. On the one hand, Alibert was anxious to appear faithful to the canons of rational medicine; by these standards, the concept of thaumaturgical kingship was at best risible and at worst a pernicious survival from an age of superstition. But he was also reluctant wholly to disown a practice so loaded with

Pious Pathology

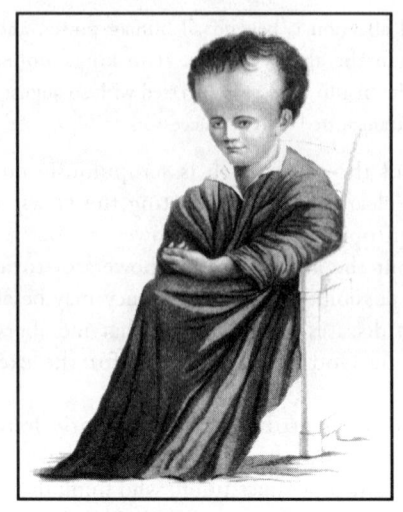

Figure 10
Alibert, *Nosologie naturelle*, f.p. 386, pl. A.
Reproduced with the permission of the
Wellcome Institute for the History of Medicine Library.

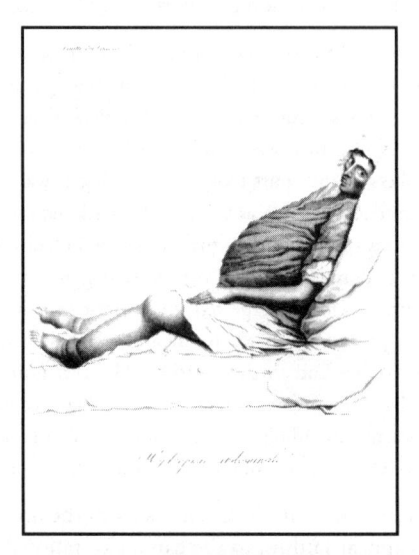

Figure 11
Alibert, *Nosologie naturelle*, f.p. 400, pl. B.
Reproduced with the permission of the
Wellcome Institute for the History of Medicine Library.

Pious Pathology

political significance. The royal touch symbolised a sacred conception of kingship that transcended arid Enlightenment theories of government. It imbued the monarch with a numinous quality, instead of depicting him as a mundane magistrate whose power depended ultimately on the popular will. Alibert's solution to this dilemma was to argue that it was safe – indeed, expedient – to let the masses believe in such things. They might derive some benefit from the experience of the royal touch. Moreover, through the spectacle of this ceremony something of the much-tarnished sanctity and authority of the French monarchy might be restored.

The religious dimension to Alibert's pathology was not, however, restricted to these explicit discussions; theological subtexts run through his work. One trope is especially persistent and prominent: namely, a concern to imply a dualist or spiritualistic understanding of human nature. Despite his early association with Cabanis, Alibert came to repudiate the *idéologue* doctrine that the moral and the physical could be conflated: 'to understand man', he declared, 'it is necessary to explore his soul, and not the material organs of his corporeal envelope'.[60] To the medical materialist no such distinction between *soma* and *psyche* was possible. Alibert, however, insinuated the truth of dualism into the texture of his case histories.

Thus he thought worthy of record the case of Jean-Auguste Chevalier, a 17-year-old who had since infancy suffered from hydrocephalus. At the age of nine months he became paralysed on the left side of the body, although he later regained some of the lost muscular power. He was also subject to occasional attacks of epilepsy. Nonetheless,

> his physiognomy was spiritual, and his responses extremely sound. He liked to read and took pleasure in exercising his memory; in short, everything about him indicated much intelligence.[61] (Fig. 10)

Despite the gross deformity of his brain, therefore, Chevalier retained his intellectual functions; he was living proof that the human spirit was autonomous of the body.

Alibert also told the tale of a woman who had died in the Hôpital Saint-Louis. This patient

> had a beloved daughter who, playing on the bank of the Seine, fell into the water. With no thought for her menstrual condition, she threw herself into the waves, and snatched her child from the danger that menaced her. Her periods were, however, immediately

Pious Pathology

suppressed, and she contracted an ascites that took her life after three years of agony and despair.

Despite these prolonged sufferings,

> The mind [*moral*] of this unfortunate woman was not ... in any way enfeebled. Her soul shone in her wasted body, and seemed to free itself from the physical chains of existence; she exhorted her children with a vivacious eloquence, which was undoubtedly the result of her morbid irritability. She was removed from their love after having passed through all the nuances of bodily decline, to arrive at a death as painful as it was inevitable.[62] (Fig. 11)

Although he ascribes the woman's eloquence to her morbid state, Alibert's account makes clear that the manner of her death should not be regarded merely as a species of delirium signifying nothing. On the contrary, her final agony was the occasion of a revelatory event; it demonstrated the vitality of the soul within a moribund body. The case might take as its moral Julie's words: 'it is my body and not my spirit that suffers'.[63] There is nothing idealized about the illustration that accompanies this narrative: indeed, Alibert emphasized its verisimilitude. The grimness of the representation is an incitement for the observer to express Christian compassion for the woman's suffering.[64] But at the same time the accompanying narrative conforms to many of the conventions of

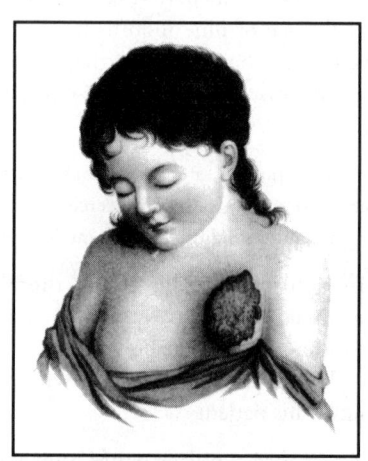

Figure 12
Alibert, *Nosologie naturelle*, f.p. 338, pl. C.
Reproduced with the permission of the
Wellcome Institute for the History of Medicine Library.

Pious Pathology

the 'beautiful death'.[65]

As well as the discursive religious element to Alibert's pathology, attention must also be paid to the figural aspects of some of his representations of disease, which make use of standard images derived from the rich tradition of western religious painting. Figure 12, for example, is less of an earthly child than of an angelic form. The effect is achieved chiefly by the composition of the features – note the cherubic lips; and in part by the bowed head and the downcast eyes. The overall impression is of transcendent composure and reverence.

A typical site for the display of these physiognomic conventions is in images of the Madonna. According to Lavater's description of a painting by Raphael (Fig. 13) embodying these characteristics, the Virgin 'bears the ineffaceable characters of calm, of simplicity, of gentleness, and of modesty; she combines the decency [*pudeur*], the humility, and the benevolence, that become her sex'.[66] The same qualities are denoted in some of Alibert's female figures: in one case even the head-dress recalls conventional representations of the virgin (Fig. 14). The same physiognomic signs are displayed in another figure (Fig. 15), only now reinforced by the overall posture of the body. This is the attitude of the nursing mother; the place of the infant is, however, taken by the grossly distended abdomen.

It is easier to identify such allusions to religious imagery within Alibert's iconography of disease than to offer any satisfactory interpretation. We need, in particular, to understand their place within a pathological text where such references might appear blasphemous. The first point to make is that the presence of the stigmata of suffering on a sacred body was an accepted feature of canonical religious art; Christianity is, after all, a religion that celebrates martyrdom. Such images usually signify the triumph of faith and grace over the tribulations of the body. On this analogy, Alibert's depictions suggest that disease is a form of martyrdom; that it can have a transfiguring effect upon the sufferer. Images that superimpose lesions upon beatified features indicate the soul's transcendence of pain and death (Figs 16 and 17): they assert the same spiritualist view of human nature found in Alibert's verbal text.

A second important characteristic of this class of image is that they are all of women; devotional texts are deemed to be more easily read on the female body. The presumption of an asymmetry between male and female was a common feature of nineteenth-

Pious Pathology

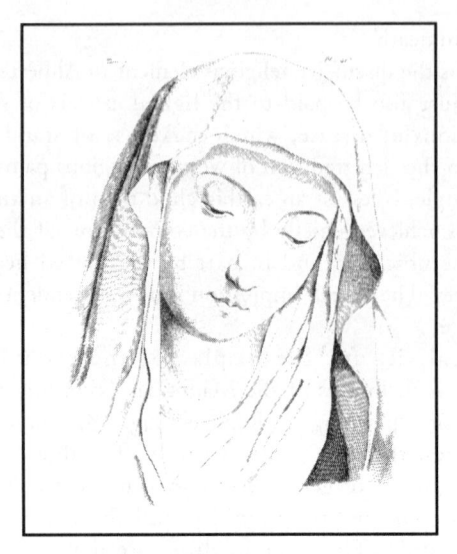

Figure 13
Lavater, *L'art de connaitre les hommes par la physionomie*, tome VII, f.p. 202, pl. 423. Reproduced with the permission of the Wellcome Institute for the History of Medicine Library.

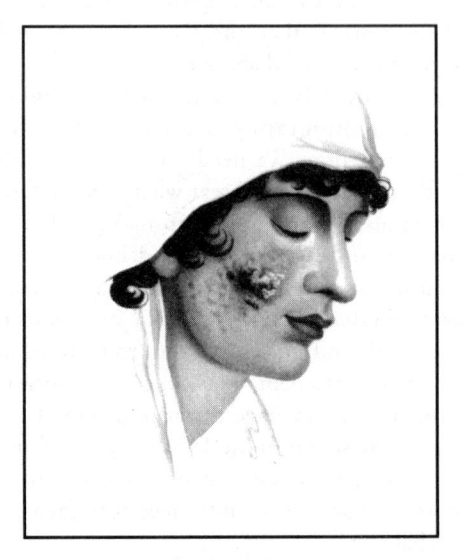

Figure 14
Alibert, *Descriptions des maladies de la peau*, pl. 16.
Reproduced with the permission of the Wellcome Institute for the History of Medicine Library.

Pious Pathology

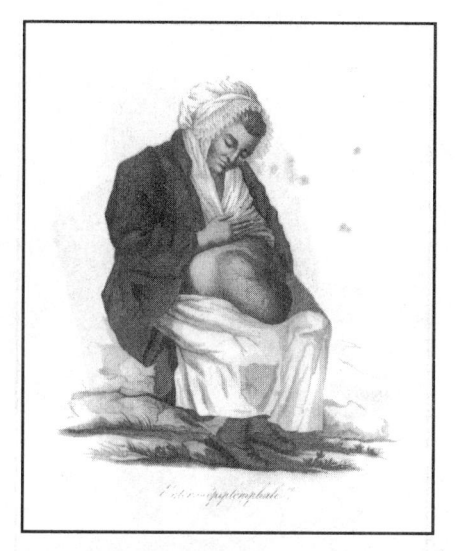

Figure 15
Alibert, *Nosologie naturelle*, f.p. 122, pl. C.
Reproduced with the permission of the Wellcome Institute
for the History of Medicine Library.

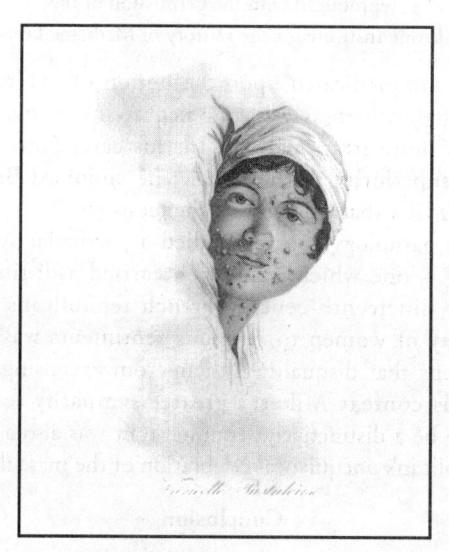

Figure 16
Alibert, *Clinique de l'Hôpital Saint-Louis*, pl. 9.
Reproduced with the permission of the Wellcome Institute
for the History of Medicine Library.

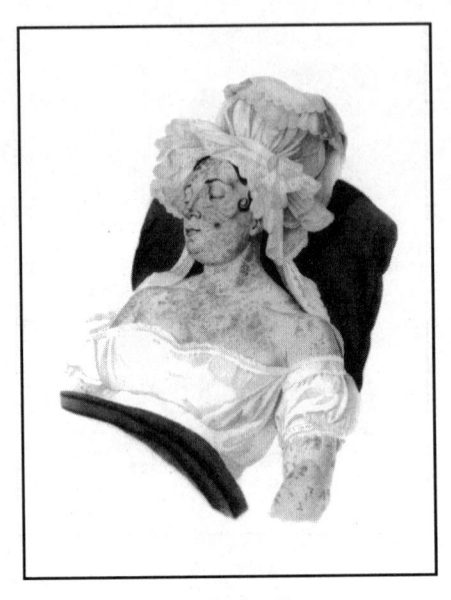

Figure 17
Alibert, *Clinique de l'Hôpital Saint-Louis*, pl. 12, 'Scarlatine Normale'.
Reproduced with the permission of the
Wellcome Institute for the History of Medicine Library.

century culture predicated upon the notion of the 'otherness' of woman.[67] Often 'otherness' was equivalent to inferiority: woman was the weaker, more irrational sex. In this case, however, Alibert imputed a superiority to the female; he endorsed Bernardin de Saint-Pierre's view that woman was 'the pious sex'.[68]

Alibert's pathology thus embodied a particular stereotype of femininity[69] – one which, moreover, carried a distinct political charge. For nineteenth-century French republicans the greater susceptibility of women to religious sentiments was one of the considerations that disqualified them from exercising a full civic role. In this context Alibert's greater sympathy for what was supposed to be a distinctively feminine trait was also a repudiation of the republican's unequivocal celebration of the masculine.

Conclusion

The representation of disease found in Alibert's texts embodies social, political, and religious discourses.[70] Put crudely, it can be seen as another document from the archives of the Christian, conservative reaction to the materialism and radicalism of the eighteenth century.

But as well as moral truths Alibert also, and to us unexpectedly, finds the beautiful and the sublime in disease; his opus represents an 'aestheticization' of pathology.[71] In these works, disease is represented visually 'in the manner of the great painters'.[72] The verbal elements of these works similarly approximated to literary rather than scientific models: Alibert prided himself on being a writer with an animated and eloquent style. Aesthetic considerations seem even to have influenced Alibert in his choice of patient; he noted that there were 'many authors and artists in the hospital'.[73]

The incorporation of an aesthetic sensibility into a medical text may seem incongruous; for Alibert, however, the roles of physician and artist were less distinct. He concluded a fulsome letter to a Parisian playwright by begging her to accept the 'felicitations of a child of Aesculapius. For Apollo, whom you love, was also the god of medicine…'.[74]

Alibert's is an aesthetic of the grand gesture, whether verbal or pictorial, of the spectacular. I have already noted the prevalence of the metaphor of the theatre in Alibert's texts. On one particularly hyperbolic occasion he declared that: 'the entire universe is no more than a vast theatre of sorrow and destruction'.[75] This figure is worth pursuing because it raises two key questions: who or what was the true spectacle to which Alibert sought to draw attention; and who was the audience for which this performance was intended?

The most obvious audience for books devoted to branches of pathology is, of course, the medical profession; and there is no doubt that Alibert did seek the approval of his professional peers both at home and abroad. But he also made it plain that he sought a wider readership. His books were directed not only at 'les gens de l'art' but also 'les gens du monde'.[76] Educated men, and possibly women, were supposed to derive edification if not entertainment from a perusal of these volumes. In particular, after the Restoration Alibert presented complimentary copies of his works to the aristocratic patrons who acted as arbiters of taste in the choice of medical practitioner as well as in matters of literature and painting.[77]

Alibert took great pains to ensure that his books were reviewed not only by the professional press but also in journals directed at the general reader. So anxious was he to ensure that these notices redounded to his credit that when possible he wrote the review himself.

This leads to the other question, of the identity of the spectacle to which the attention of this diverse audience was so insistently drawn. The most obvious answer might appear to be the patients who provided the 'material' for Alibert's narratives and depictions.

But occasionally Alibert insisted that it was the location within which these individuals acted out their roles that was the true centre of attention. In the words of one of Alibert's auto-reviews, 'M. Alibert has procured a European reputation for the Hôpital Saint-Louis. His book is in effect a lasting monument to the glory of this vast and useful establishment.' On another occasion the *Nosologie naturelle* is described as the Hôpital Saint-Louis transported into a book.[78]

But the question of where the audience's gaze is expected to rest is by no means simple. Consider another product of the Alibert publicity machine:

23 May 1818

> On the 20th of this month, at nine in the morning, Dr Alibert, physician to the Hôpital Saint-Louis, opened his clinical course in the confines of this vast and magnificent establishment. He improvised his first lesson in the open air and under the beautiful bowers which shade the avenue of the pavilion of the Angel Gabriel. The audience was immense. The patients themselves on whom the professor was to discourse found themselves at the session and seemed to take pleasure in hearing the history of their long sufferings, as well as the remedies appropriate to their cure. They were distributed into separate groups according to the class of disease to which they belonged, which provided a sight which was as instructive as it was interesting for the spectators. M. Alibert will continue the course during the summer.[79]

Where does the real centre of attention lie? The hospital forms a mere picturesque backdrop to the proceedings; one should, however, take note of the carefully sketched outdoor setting.[80] Although in this case the sick are overtly present in the garden for purposes of scientific instruction rather than spiritual edification, there may well be an allusion here to a devotional text.[81]

The students are mere extras whose purpose is to impress by weight of numbers. The role of the patients is more ambivalent; they are at once spectacle and audience. But all these characters are assembled to hear one man whose discourse is the *raison d'être* of the entire tableau. Alibert is the true centre of attention. I would suggest that this identification applies more widely. The Prospero-like figure visibly presiding over all the grotesque revels of the theatre of disease is none other than the good doctor himself. Alibert's iconography of disease is, along with much else, an opportunity for the portraiture of the self.

Notes

1. Sander L. Gilman, *Disease and Representation: Images of Illness from Madness to AIDS* (Ithaca: Cornell University Press, 1988), 147–8.
2. Review of 'Description des maladies de la peau' by J.L. Alibert, *La revue philosophique, littéraire et politique* (1806), no. 14: 338–9. A later instalment of this review makes clear that despite their subject matter, Alibert's illustrations were thought to have an aesthetic appeal as well as an instructive quality: 'one looks upon the most hideous evils that afflict humanity with as much pleasure and interest as one regards the flowers drawn by van Spaendonck or Redouté', *ibid.*, no. 28: 1–2.
3. M.A. Everett, 'Jean-Louis Alibert', *International Journal of Dermatology*, xxiii (1984), 351–6.
4. Elizabeth A. Williams, *The Physical and the Moral: Anthropology, Physiology, and Philosophical Medicine in France, 1750–1850* (Cambridge: Cambridge University Press, 1994), 90–2; for Alibert's later move to the political and philosophic right, see 122–34.
5. Susanne Dahm, *Frühe Krankenbildnisse: Alibert, Esquirol, Baumgärtner* (Köln: Institut für Geschichte der Medizin, 1981), 4.
6. Barbara Maria Stafford, *Body Criticism: Imaging the Unseen in Enlightenment Art and Medicine* (Cambridge, Mass.: MIT Press, 1991), 300.
7. Norman Bryson, *Word and Image: French Painting of the Ancien Régime* (Cambridge: Cambridge University Press, 1981), 6, 36.
8. J.L. Alibert, *Nosologie naturelle, ou les maladies du corps humain distribuées par familles* (Paris: Caille et Ravier, 1817), 448.
9. Gaspard Lavater, *L'art de connaître les hommes par la physionomie*, edited by J.-L. Moreau de la Sarthe, 10 vols (Paris: L. Prudhomme, 1806–9), vol. 5, 381.
10. Erwin H. Ackerknecht, *Medicine at the Paris Hospital, 1794–1848* (Baltimore: Johns Hopkins Press, 1967).
11. J.L Alibert, *Description des maladies de la peau observées à l'Hôpital Saint-Louis. Et exposition des meilleures méthodes suivies pour leur traitement* (Paris: Crapelet, 1806), i.
12. *Ibid.*, 234.
13. J.L. Alibert, *Clinique de l'hôpital Saint-Louis, ou traité complet des maladies de la peau, contenant la description de ces maladies et leurs meilleurs modes de traitement* (Paris: B. Corman, 1833), i. Alibert reiterated this trope even in his private correspondence; writing to request some books relevant to his researches from the Librarian of the Paris medical school, he declared that 'my work does not require

any kind of erudition, since I merely report what I observe'. Wellcome Institute for the History of Medicine (WIHM) London MS 7037, no. 13.
14. Alibert, *op. cit.* (note 11), 49.
15. *Ibid.*, x–xi.
16. *Ibid.*, 49.
17. *Ibid.*, xxii.
18. An association between medicine, disease and the theatrical had been well established in early-modern European culture: see Natsu Hattori, 'Performing Cures: Practice and Interplay in Theatre and Medicine of the English Renaissance', Oxford D.Phil. Dissertation, 1995. It may be that Alibert's text alludes to some residual traces of this tradition.
19. Alibert, *op. cit.* (note 11), 66.
20. *Ibid.*, xxi.
21. *Ibid.*, 211.
22. In his discussion of the aetiology of this condition Alibert's environmentalism recalls the contemporary official discourse dealing with the effects of milieu on regional character. See M.-N. Bourget, 'Race et folklore: L'image officielle de la France en 1800', *Annales*, xxxi, no. 2 (1976): especially 805–6, 813.
23. Alibert's attempts to engage the sympathy of his readers in the clinical stories he tells suggest an affinity between his writings and the emergence of a 'humanitarian narrative' in eighteenth-century medical texts to which Thomas Laqueur has drawn attention: 'Bodies, Details, and the Humanitarian Narrative', in Lynn Hunt (ed.), *The New Cultural History* (Berkeley: University of California Press, 1989), 176–204. But in Alibert's case there is no suggestion that these sentiments are provoked as a prelude to some form of remedial action; the arousal of compassion is an end in itself.
24. For an account of this process drawing upon British materials see: Mary E. Fissell, 'The disappearance of the patient's narrative and the invention of hospital medicine', in Roger French and Andrew Wear (eds), *British Medicine in An Age of Reform* (London: Routledge, 1991), 92–109.
25. Alibert, *op. cit.* (note 11), 77–8.
26. *Ibid.*, 239.
27. Alibert, *op. cit.* (note 8), vi.
28. On the central role of the passions within the discourse of 'anthropological medicine', see: Williams, *op. cit.* (note 4), especially 126–8.
29. Alibert, *op. cit.* (note 11), 9.

30. *Ibid.*, 10.
31. *Ibid.*, 12.
32. J.L. Alibert, *Monographie des dermatoses ou précis théorique et pratique des maladies de la peau* (Paris: Daynac, 1832), 803.
33. *Ibid.*, 804.
34. *Ibid.*, 798.
35. Alibert, *op. cit.* (note 11), 28.
36. *Ibid.*, 29.
37. *Ibid.*, 32–3.
38. See Georges Vigarello, *Concepts of Cleanliness: Changing Attitudes in France since the Middle Ages* (Cambridge: Cambridge University Press, 1988), 192–4.
39. 'Writing', according to Peter Stallybrass and Allon White, 'made the grotesque visible whilst keeping it at an untouchable distance'. *The Politics and Poetics of Transgression* (Ithaca: Cornell University Press, 1986), 139. The same consideration applies, perhaps *a fortiori*, to pictorial means of representation. The discursive separation of 'respectable' from debauched members of society appears to have been reproduced in the practical arrangements obtaining at the Hôpital Saint-Louis where a 'paternal' separation of 'vice and virtue' was enforced among female patients. J.L. Alibert, *op. cit.* (note 32), xii–xiii. There is more than a hint here of a fear that the moral as well as the physical corruption of the poor might prove contagious to other members of society.
40. Alibert, *op. cit.* (note 11), 28.
41. For a discussion of the redefinition of the scope of the political in Revolutionary France, see Lynn Hunt, *Politics, Culture, and Class in the French Revolution* (Berkeley: University of California Press, 1986), 1–3.
42. J.L. Alibert, 'De l'influence des causes politiques sur les maladies et la constitution physique de l'homme', *Magasin encyclopédique*, v (1795): 298.
43. *Ibid.*, 301.
44. *Ibid.*, 301–3.
45. Alibert, *op. cit.* (note 13), vii, xiv.
46. Alibert, *op. cit.* (note 11), ix.
47. *Ibid.*, 54–5.
48. Michèle Root-Bernstein, *Boulevard Theater and Revolution in Eighteenth-Century Paris* (Ann Arbor: UMI Research Press, 1984), 118.
49. On the revolutionary attack on traditional notions of servitude, see Sarah C. Maza, *Servants and their Masters in Eighteenth-Century*

France: The Uses of Loyalty (Princeton: Princeton University Press, 1983), 309–14.
50. See Cissie Fairchilds, Domestic Enemies: Servants and their Masters in Old Regime France (Baltimore: Johns Hopkins University Press, 1984), 242.
51. Alibert, op. cit. (note 11), xix.
52. See Gérard Cholvy and Yves-Marie Hilaire, Histoire religieuse de la France contemporaine. 1800/1880 (Toulouse: Bibliothèque historique Privat, 1985), 20–7.
53. J.L. Alibert, Physiologie des passions, 2 vols. (Paris: Béchet, 1825), vol. 1, 139.
54. Alibert, op. cit. (note 8), vi.
55. François-René, Vicomte de Chateaubriand, Génie du christianisme (Paris: Gallimard, 1978), 1038–9.
56. Alibert, op. cit. (note 11), 210. There is something strangely contemporary about Alibert's desire to be fair but not credulous to such popular beliefs: cf. Judith Devlin, The Superstitious Mind: French Peasants and the Supernatural in the Nineteenth Century (New Haven: Yale University Press, 1952), 53–7.
57. See Marc Bloch, The Royal Touch: Sacred Monarchy and Scrofula in England and France (London: Routledge, 1973), 226–8; Matthew Ramsey, Professional and Popular Medicine in France, 1770–1830 (Cambridge: Cambridge University Press, 1988), 246–7.
58. Ibid., 209.
59. Alibert, op. cit. (note 32), 623–4.
60. Alibert, op. cit. (note 53), i.
61. Alibert, op. cit. (note 8), 385–6.
62. Ibid., 400–1.
63. Jean-Jacques Rousseau, Julie ou la nouvelle Héloïse: Lettres de deux amants habitants d'une petite ville au pied des Alpes (Paris: Garnier Frères, 1960), 694.
64. A purely aesthetic reaction to this stark image was not, however, excluded. A manuscript notice of the Nosographie naturelle among Alibert's papers remarks that 'from an artistic viewpoint, what will attract surprise and admiration in this collection is the depiction of the last moments of the dropsied woman'. WIHM MS 7037, no. 156.
65. Expression taken from Philippe Ariès, The Hour of our Death (London: Allen Lane, 1981); see also John McManners, Death and the Enlightenment: Changing Attitudes to Death among Christians and Unbelievers in Eighteenth-Century France (Oxford: Clarendon, 1981), esp. 256.
66. Lavater, op. cit. (note 9), vol. 7, 202.

67. See Ludmilla Jordanova, *Sexual Visions: Images of Gender in Science and Medicine between the Eighteenth and Twentieth Centuries* (New York: Harvester Wheatsheaf, 1989), 14–15.
68. Jean-Jacques Bernardin de Saint-Pierre, *Études de la Nature*, 3 vols (Paris: Didot, 1784), vol. 2, 241.
69. A more extended analysis of Alibert's preoccupation with female nature is beyond the scope of this paper. See his 'Éloge historique of Pierre Roussel', in P. Roussel, *Système physique et moral de la femme. Suivi d'un système physique et moral de l'homme, et d'un fragment sur la sensibilité* (Paris: Caille, 1809).
70. For an example of a similar interweaving of medical, religious, and political tropes within a single body of texts, see Colin Jones, 'Plague and its Metaphors in Early Modern France', *Representations*, liii (1996): esp. 108.
71. I take this expression from Janet Beizer, *Ventriloquized Bodies: Narratives of Hysteria in Nineteenth-Century France* (Ithaca: Cornell University Press, 1994), 254 where it is applied to Charcot.
72. WIHM MS 7037, no. 156.
73. WIHM MS 7037, no. 259.
74. WIHM MS 7037, no. 276.
75. Alibert, *op. cit.* (note 42), 298.
76. WIHM MS 7037, no. 42.
77. For examples of such donations see WIHM MS 7037, nos. 22, 23.
78. WIHM MS 7037, nos. 37, 156.
79. WIHM MS 7037, no. 33.
80. As Richard Sennett has recently shown, the ecclesiastic garden possessed a venerable status as a refuge for the sick and destitute: *Flesh and Stone: The Body and the City in Western Civilization* (London: Faber and Faber, 1994), 179–82. Unlike other Parisian hospitals the Saint-Louis was not a converted monastery; it was built in the seventeenth century as a refuge for the sick. It was, however, staffed by priests and nuns who gave the establishment a religious character.
81. In a further religious allusion Alibert refers to the hospital as a 'sanctuary': Alibert, *op. cit.* (note 32), xiii. The distinction between the devotional and the pedagogic should not be pressed too far. One hostile observer complained that Alibert discriminated against students in whom he detected a lack of 'profound sentiments of devotion and piety'. [Joseph Morel de Rubempré], *Biographie des médecins français vivans, et des professeurs des écoles; par un de leurs confrères, docteur en médecine* (Paris: Les Marchands de Nouveautés, 1826), 9–10.

5

Corvisart and Broussais: Human Individuality and Medical Dominance

W. R. Albury

Introduction

The more one tries to capture what was the truly distinctive element in Parisian medicine of the early nineteenth century, the more elusive the quarry seems to become. Both Ackerknecht and Foucault in their respective seminal works acknowledge 'antecedents' of the Paris school's clinical teaching, and in the present volume the contribution by Brockliss explores this issue in great depth.[1] Moreover, Keel has mounted a decisive challenge to the notion that such concepts and practices as tissue theory, diagnostic percussion and the study of pathological anatomy can be uniquely associated with the clinical school of Paris.[2] But if clinical teaching, tissue theory and other such putative touchstones of Parisian medicine prove inadequate, how then should we characterize the importance of the Paris clinic?

One of the themes in Foucault's analysis of the clinic that seems to have been of less interest to historians of medicine than to other readers of his work, is the relationship between medical developments in early nineteenth-century Paris and the establishment of a new concept of human individuality.[3] As Foucault notes in his opening sentence, *The Birth of the Clinic* 'is about space, about language, and about death; it is about the act of seeing, the gaze'.[4] Much critical attention has been given to the idea of the clinical 'gaze', but to treat this element in isolation is to miss a fundamental point of Foucault's account. For it is the relationship among all these elements that is at issue here, much more than the novelty or uniqueness of any one of these elements in itself. The 'new medicine' of Paris, according to Foucault, arose from a systematic reorganization of this relationship and, in so doing, constituted one of the foundations of modern medical thought.

> It is this *formal* reorganization, *in depth*, rather than the abandonment of old theories and systems, that made *clinical experience* possible; it lifted the old Aristotelian prohibition i.e., that nothing below the level of the species could become an object of scientific knowledge: one could at last hold a scientifically structured discourse about an individual.[5]

The theme of the present discussion, then, is the medical knowledge of human individuality – what form the concept of such knowledge took for two of the Paris clinical school's most prominent figures, how it was systematically related to other concepts in their work, and how it differed from the classical Hippocratic–Galenic concept of the diversity of human constitutions.

Idiosyncrasy and Health

The recognition of constitutional variations between different persons was a central feature of Hippocratic–Galenic medicine, something for which the physician had to make due allowance when recommending measures for the preservation or restoration of any individual's health.[6] Everyone, according to this doctrine, was literally 'idiosyncratic' (ιδιος – pertaining to oneself; συν – with; κρασις – mixture, blending of constitutional elements). These idiosyncratic differences in anatomy and in 'temperament' or 'complexion' were not in themselves seen as pathological. On the contrary, they played an important role in the definition of the healthy state; for 'good complexion – that is, good health – lay somewhere within a range, or latitude, that differed in each individual and could never be precisely measured'.[7] Idiosyncrasy fell within the domain of the medical art, but it was not an object of medical science.

This doctrine of individual variation and the 'relativistic definition of health'[8] that went with it was still prominent in eighteenth-century medical thinking. As the article, 'Health', written for the *Encyclopédie* by the Montpellier medical graduate Arnulfe d'Aumont, maintained:

> *Health* does not consist ... in a precise point of perfection which is common to all persons in the exercise of all their functions; but it admits of a kind of latitude of extension ... which establishes many variations in the manner of being in good *health* ....

Hence it follows that there does not exist a state of health which can be appropriate for everyone; each person has their own manner of well-being, because this state results from a certain proportion in the [body's] solids and fluids, in their actions and their movements, which is specific to each individual. Just as one cannot find two faces exactly alike, as Boerhaave says on this subject, ... so too there are always differences between the heart and lungs of one man, and the heart and lungs of another.[9]

The fact that the Montpellier vitalist d'Aumont could cite the Newtonian mechanist Boerhaave as an authority on this point suggests just how uncontroversial the medical doctrine of individuality was at the time.

This doctrine did not imply that all healthy constitutions would be equally strong. The different ways of being in good health, d'Aumont says, include all the variations 'between the robust state of the athlete who is the furthest from the state of illness, and the state which comes nearest to that disposition in which health is entirely lost because of the lesion of some function'.[10] But all constitutions on this continuum of health, even the weakest, were capable of being maintained by a combination of the healing power of nature and a judicious application of the rules of hygiene.[11] Thus human art and the natural disposition of the body would work together to produce a beneficial result.

Of course the cultivation of one's health in this way was a time-consuming and often expensive activity, so only the wealthy could be expected to have the leisure and resources needed for this purpose.[12] Such persons, indeed, were the traditional focus of medical attention in the ancien régime,[13] and it was not surprising that physicians treated them with a certain amount of deference, placing great weight on the subjective experience of the patient as a measure of health or illness.[14] Thus, as d'Aumont wrote,

> it is by the ease which one feels when the functions of body and soul are exercised; by the satisfaction which one takes in one's physical and moral existence; by the agreeableness and constancy of this exercise; by the outward manifestations of this feeling and the relations of all these effects, that one can know that one is enjoying a life as healthy and as perfect as possible.[15]

The social conditions of medical practice were easily integrated here with the cognitive conditions of medical theory, which identified health and disease as matters of lived experience rather than objects of scientific knowledge. The individual's own sense of well-being, rather than the physician's determination, was thus the fundamental element for the diagnosis of good health in the present, just as it was for the prognosis of good health in the future: 'the signs by which one can forecast a long and healthy life are also usually the marks of a solid and well-established state of *health* in the present'.[16]

The Clinical Context

The ideal of 'a life as healthy and as perfect as possible' was not lost from sight during the revolutionary transformation of French medical institutions at the end of the eighteenth century. One of the goals explicitly set down for the new, clinically oriented *École de Santé* of Paris at the time of its establishment was that its teaching should show how 'one can preserve one's life for a long time, as free from ills as men may hope to be'.[17] The language of this statement would have been quite acceptable to a mid-eighteenth-century neo-Hippocratic physician such as d'Aumont, but how was its meaning affected by the changed circumstances of medical theory and practice? What role did the recognition of individual anatomical and constitutional differences play in the medical thinking of early nineteenth-century France? And how free from illness could one hope to be, and to remain, according to this new medical perspective?

If we examine the work of J. N. Corvisart, the first professor of clinical medicine (*la clinique interne*) at the Paris *École de Santé*, we enter a different conceptual world from that of the *Encyclopédie* and the Hippocratic–Galenic tradition.[18] We can find, to be sure, some familiar landmarks: Corvisart, like d'Aumont, draws attention to the vast range of human constitutional differences; but the emphasis is strangely inverted. His point of departure is not the physical perfection of the athlete's body but the teratological organization of a fœtus so severely malformed that it dies at birth.

> Now from the physical impossibility of independent life due to a monstrous conformation, to that precision of organization which makes the rarest longevity possible, the degrees of the defects in precision are probably incalculable, but they are no less real on that account.
>
> A necessary death for the immense majority of beings, those who occupy all the intermediate positions between these two extremes, is thus a sad but inescapable truth.[19]

Where d'Aumont sets out a continuum of health from the most perfect physique to the point just before disease supervenes, Corvisart gives us a continuum of defective constitutions from the least viable to the point of greatest (and rarest) longevity. And although Corvisart's continuum overlaps d'Aumont's, while moving in the opposite direction and extending further, none of the incalculable number of constitutions which Corvisart envisages is described by him as healthy. They are all just better or worse ways of postponing death.

Moreover, where d'Aumont calls upon the healing power of nature, assisted by human art, to help maintain the different constitutions in their respective idiosyncratic states of health, Corvisart rejects any concept of nature as a beneficial force.

> It is claimed that ... nature continually tends ... to strengthen the overly weak organ and to weaken the overly strong one; in a word, to establish equilibrium where it does not exist. But ... impartial observation gives the lie to this exaggerated solicitude of nature, this restorative and corrective spirit of the vital principle, if I may so express myself; and the errors of nature are perhaps both more frequent and more fatal than those constant, fortunate and seemingly deliberate efforts about which people all too often enjoy preaching ....
>
> One could even defend the contrary opinion with very plausible arguments, and prove that the strong organ triumphs over the weak one in such cases and makes the latter its victim.[20]

It would be easy to characterize the contrast between d'Aumont and Corvisart on this point rather simply, in terms of an optimist and a pessimist viewing the same object – the one seeing the proverbial glass of water as being half full and the other seeing it as being half empty.[21] Corvisart himself may be thought to have provided support for this kind of interpretation by contrasting his own attitude with that of the one-eyed porter in Voltaire's story, who was born without the eye which would have allowed him to see the bad side of life and whose other eye could only see what was good.[22] For his own part, Corvisart is reported to have said, 'I am one-eyed like him, but it is the other eye that I have lost: I have a rather peevish spirit and I always see things from a bad angle'.[23]

But however entertaining this anecdote may be, we cannot reduce Corvisart's position on individual constitutional variations to a matter of personality, for two important reasons: firstly, because it was shared by another leading medical figure of the period, a generation younger than Corvisart, whose personality was very different – François Broussais; and secondly, because this shared position had important links with the cognitive and institutional transformation of French medicine at the beginning of the nineteenth century. In the following pages I will try to justify these claims.

Corvisart and Individual Variations[24]

According to Corvisart, the systematic study of pathological anatomy, which had been made possible by the recent establishment of hospital-based medical teaching, had revealed that organic lesions – or pathological alterations of the solid parts of the body – were 'far more frequent than the majority of physicians have believed until now'.[25] In fact, he wrote, 'the organic diseases of all kinds' which result from these lesions 'have been so common that it has been rare to open a cadaver that did not present one of them'.[26] This virtual ubiquity of organic diseases was caused, in Corvisart's view, by the functioning of the body itself; its organs are pathologically altered 'by the very fact of their action'.[27] And even admitting a healing tendency in nature 'which ceaselessly repairs, *in so far as it can*, the damage caused',[28] this tendency is bound ultimately to fail because of the effect of individual variations.

> The causes which can make the organs degenerate from their natural condition are extremely numerous; the force of life can combat some of them, but it cannot resist them all; it can overcome them for a while, but it cannot vanquish them forever. ...
>
> The perfect concurrence of the regular action of all the organs constitutes life and health in the most desirable degree; but each organ takes a more or less active role in the execution of life. The augmented natural activity of an organ, by making it play a more energetic role, renders it, in spite of its appropriate organisation, more exposed to the common law of the alteration of organised bodies by the very fact of their action.[29]

It is because of this imbalance that a body composed entirely of healthy organs must nonetheless become diseased: 'each organ can be good in itself, and nevertheless be too strong or too weak in relation to the other organs ...'.[30] Only if there were no individual variations in anatomical structure and constitutional forces could human beings expect to retain their health; but such a dream of the perfect constitution is never realized.

> This ideal temperament is far from the actual temperament of each living being. No one is born with this degree of perfection. Each of us comes into the world more or less vitiated, from which there follows some defect in the equilibrium of our functions.[31]

The doctrine of individual variations has not just been viewed by Corvisart 'from a bad angle'; idiosyncrasy has been qualitatively transformed into a principle of destruction. The metaphorical glass of water is not only half empty, but the half-measure still remaining in it has been poisoned.

> What I have just said is sufficient, I think, to prove that ... *the very fact of life is the cause of death*, after having produced organic diseases in most cases. Long ago it was said – but in a more abstract sense than I say it here – that the first day of life is the first step towards death.[32]

If the natural propensities of the body do not, in themselves, tend toward a state of health, what of the human art which d'Aumont called upon to second the alleged healing power of nature? For d'Aumont the rules of hygiene were chiefly concerned with the proper management of the six 'non-naturals' of Galenic theory: air, food and drink, movement and rest, sleep and wakefulness, excretion and retention, and the passions of the soul.[33] Corvisart, on the other hand, without using the term 'non-naturals', saw most of the factors listed under this heading as damaging, especially to the heart and lungs.[34] The activities associated with the professions, the arts and the trades, the turmoil of the moral affections – all of these are sources of organic lesions. To prevent them from destroying human health would require two impossibilities: 'to bring about the dissolution of society ... [and] ... to deprive men of their passions...'.[35] Thus, with the exception of a very small number of people who might combine independent wealth, a good physical constitution and a placid disposition with a willingness to submit themselves to the 'wise counsels' of the medical art, it is the lot of humans to develop incurable organic lesions.[36] Here medicine is helpless: 'one finds almost everywhere the fatal prognosis of death...'.[37]

Finally, what is the status of the individual's sense of well-being, which figured so prominently in d'Aumont's discussion of health? For Corvisart, diseases are identified with organic lesions hidden within the body, rather than with the experience of illness. It is therefore possible to have diseases without symptoms, which only the physician can detect: 'it is evident that organic diseases have, in general, already established very deep roots when they become perceptible, either to the most delicate tact[38] or by means of the subtlest perception of the slightest derangement of the injured organ's function ...'.[39] For this reason the active diagnostic examination, including such techniques as palpation and percussion, must replace the older reliance on verbal reports of subjective illness or well-being.[40] And even with these active techniques being employed by the physician, some diseases will never reveal themselves during the life of the patient. 'In the cadaver one frequently finds traces of inflammation, of which one had not perceived any trace and which had not in fact presented any sign during life.'[41] Such a circumstance helps to explain the therapeutic limitations of medicine in dealing with organic diseases. 'However sagacious the physician may be, the art [of medicine] cannot furnish any means of perceiving an internal derangement which is not manifested by any sign and, consequently, cannot apply any treatment to it.'[42]

For the range of benign idiosyncratic variations which Hippocratic–Galenic thought recognized in the constitutions of different individuals, Corvisart substituted a range of pathological deviations from an unattainable ideal of organic equilibrium. For the concept of a diversity of ways of being healthy, each one uniquely appropriate to a different constitution, Corvisart substituted a generic process of lesional development which occurs with an intensity proportional to the degree of each individual's deviation from the ideal organic norm.[43] And for the providential notion of the healing power of nature which assists each constitution to achieve its appropriate state of health, Corvisart substituted a vision of nature as a blind force, sometimes repairing organic damage but more often powerless to overcome it or even contributing further to its destructive effects.[44]

Broussais and Individual Variations

I would now like to show that the main features of Corvisart's position as I have just outlined it were shared by another leading figure of French clinical medicine, François Broussais.[45] The personalities of Corvisart and Broussais were markedly dissimilar: where Corvisart was reserved and taciturn, Broussais was flamboyant and pugnacious. But more importantly for our present discussion, if we consider their respective approaches to therapeutics we would have to describe Corvisart as a pessimist and Broussais as an optimist. For while both agreed that there was nothing medicine could do to cure an organic lesion once it was well established in some part of the body, Broussais did not share Corvisart's therapeutic scepticism about other conditions.[46] On the contrary, he believed that he had found the secret of preventing organic lesions from occurring in the first place, by the active treatment of local inflammations, especially by bloodletting.[47] But despite this important difference between Corvisart and Broussais, their positions had much in common.

Like Corvisart, Broussais understood the range of individual human variations primarily in pathological terms: every temperament derives from the predominant exercise of a particular functional system in the body and therefore gives rise to its characteristic diseases.[48] The 'gastric' temperament originates in the dominance of the digestive system; the 'bilious' temperament in the hypertrophy of the liver, etc.[49] Different environments and ways of life may have some effect in modifying the propensity of each system toward disease,[50] but 'the physical and moral causes of infirmities'[51] are destined to prevail.

The reason for this pathological tendency is that '[h]ealth supposes the regular exercise of the functions; disease results from their irregularity ...'. This pathogenic irregularity of the functions is further explained as follows: 'The functions are irregular when one or more of them are exercised with too much or too little energy'.[52] So when any function predominates, as happens in each of the temperaments, irregular activity results. The energy of a function – that which makes it predominate at any given time – is produced, according to Broussais, by external stimulation or excitation;[53] and it is ultimately this variation in excitation that is most commonly responsible for disease.

> Excitation is never uniform in the animal economy; it is always excessive in certain parts and deficient in several others, and it predominates successively in various regions [of the body]. This inequality often ends up deranging the equilibrium of the functions.[54]

Once the equilibrium of the functions is deranged, 'one or more of the organs which are charged with the exaggerated function, and with the functions which have been disturbed, are threatened with destruction'.[55]

Can one hope that the organs thus threatened by the formation of organic lesions might be protected from this destruction by the healing power of nature? In the most minimal sense, Broussais does recognize a natural restorative power in the body, but he limits its beneficial activity to the repair of minor damage after the cause of that damage has been removed. Nature succeeds here in what might be called passive healing, after the event, rather than in actively opposing the pathological process itself.

> Intermittent inflammations which are left to nature heal themselves when they are slight and when their determining causes no longer exist. In the contrary cases, they either intensify into the continuity of acute inflammations, or else they degenerate into a chronic continuity which is ultimately accompanied by *obstructions* and by hydropsy. ...
>
> Hydropsy brought on by the sympathetic influence of a chronic phlegmasy is rarely curable, because this phlegmasy almost never brings on hydropsy until after it has disorganised the part in which it is situated.[56]

On the other hand, when nature does actively oppose the development of an inflammation, the means by which it does so – producing what Hippocratic–Galenic medicine called a crisis – is more likely to be harmful than beneficial:

> It is always dangerous not to halt an inflammation when it begins, because crises are violent and often dangerous efforts which nature deploys in order to remove the [animal] economy from a great danger; it is therefore useful to prevent them and imprudent to wait for them.[57]

From this point Broussais' therapeutic activism follows, not in supporting the processes of nature but in opposing them as destructive tendencies: 'one will always conserve the patient's forces by calming an irritation; because a prolongation of the febrile movement for twenty-four hours will destroy more of these forces than will a bleeding or two'.[58]

This therapeutic activism is also required because it is virtually impossible, according to Broussais, to conduct one's way of life so as to avoid the development of diseases. Broussais' *Traité de physiologie appliquée à la pathologie* may well have been written for 'the man who wants to learn how to employ his life well, with the aim of preserving or re-establishing his own health and that of his fellows',[59] but it consists, for the most part, of a catalogue demonstrating how each functional system can become a source of disease. Consider, for example, the discussion of respiration.

It may at first seem as if a well-regulated manner of respiration could maintain one in a state of health: 'As long as one's inhalation and exhalation are regular, they cannot bring on any pathological state. Thus only the modifications of these movements are capable of producing such states ...'. As the passage continues, however, one sees that these modifications are of such a kind that no one could reasonably expect to avoid them: 'now these modifications are found ... in the voice, in speaking, in singing, in laughing, in sighing, in sobbing, in coughing and in sneezing'.[60]

In a similar fashion, all the other physical activities of the body,[61] as well as 'the exercise of the intellect, the emotions and the passions ...',[62] are identified as causes of diseases. And just as Corvisart highlighted the cardio-pulmonary system, and especially the heart, as a particularly vulnerable focus of disease, so too did Broussais highlight the gastro-intestinal system, and particularly the stomach, in the same way.

> [The] stomach is a singular organ; its destiny is to be always irritated .... If, therefore, it is not irritated by the presence of food and drink, it becomes irritated by their absence; it contracts, it is irritated, it attracts the blood, it draws toward itself the fluids secreted by its annexes.[63]

Moreover, most other diseases are nothing but sympathetic displacements of gastro-intestinal inflammations: 'The knowledge of gastritis and of gastro-enteritis is thus the key to pathology'.[64] So it was clearly not possible within Broussais' conceptual world, any more than it was within Corvisart's, for the individual to maintain a state of health by careful management of the 'non-naturals'.

Neither was it possible, according to Broussais, for individuals to identify their own sense of well-being with health. While Broussais located diseases in the physiological processes of irritation and inflammation rather than in the resulting lesions, as Corvisart had done, he nevertheless shared with Corvisart the concept of symptomless disease. 'It has been ... proven that the irritations which begin in an insensible manner and persist at an obscure level always have the same outcome, *disorganization*.'[65] Indeed, to support his contention that every organic lesion was caused by an inflammation, he appealed to constitutional variations as part of the proposed explanation of how symptomless inflammations could occur.

As for the cases in which organs deteriorate without this having been preceded by exterior signs of that violent and sanguine irritation which is called inflammation, to discover their origin it is indispensable to return to physiology and hygiene, to observe how external agents modify the vitality of our organs, to appreciate the susceptibility of each one of our systems and tissues *according to our different ages and constitutions* ....[66]

The diversity of constitutional variations, rather than valorizing the individual's subjective experience of health and well-being, becomes in this programmatic statement a part of the reason why that experience cannot be trusted.

Some False Continuities

Corvisart and Broussais offer a similar picture of life under threat from destructive disease. In this picture, both individual constitutional variations and the type of factors previously characterized as 'non-naturals' are portrayed as inevitably pathogenic. The body's own natural tendency toward healing is too weak to resist the development of serious diseases, and in many cases it does more harm than good. Moreover, the disease process can be so insidious that a person's health may be fatally undermined before he or she experiences any symptoms of illness.

Notwithstanding some apparent continuities with the older Hippocratic–Galenic doctrine of life and health, this picture represents a qualitatively different vision of human existence. Certainly it had been recognized before the nineteenth century that some constitutions were intrinsically defective. The Chevalier de Jaucourt, for example, a prolific contributor to the *Encyclopédie* who had studied medicine under Boerhaave,[67] wrote:

> Since it has seemed that each man has his own proper [state of] health, and that all bodies differ one from the other, both in their solids and in their fluids, although they may each be healthy, that constitution of each body which makes it differ from other equally healthy bodies has been named *idiosyncrasy*, and the vices which derive from it have sometimes passed for incurable, because they have been thought to exist from the first moment of the body's formation ....[68]

But after introducing the notion of inherent constitutional deficiencies, the main thrust of Jaucourt's brief article, 'Idiosyncrasy', is to emphasize how rare such defects are, and how often it is that diseases caused by mismanagement of the 'non-naturals', especially in the upbringing of children, 'are ... inappropriately considered to be innate diseases ...'.[69] This is a very different proposition from the treatment of individual variation by Corvisart and Broussais as a pathogenic deviation from a rarely attainable organic norm – a treatment quite in keeping with the pejorative tone which the term 'idiosyncrasy' has for us today, but which was utterly foreign to it in earlier times.

In d'Aumont's articles, too, there are some darker passages in which he concedes, for example, that 'it is extremely difficult to conserve one's good health and to preserve oneself from disease during a long life'.[70] His primary reference here is to the ageing process, however – the longer one lives the more difficult it becomes to retain one's good health: 'such is the sad condition of humankind, that the disposition necessary to produce the most perfect health possible, which is a high degree of mobility in the organs, cannot be exercised for long without destroying itself'.[71] In the article, 'Old Age', which d'Aumont cross-references to this passage, Jaucourt elaborates on the kind of destruction involved in this process.

> [A]s one advances in age, the bones, the cartilages, the membranes, the flesh and all the fibres of the body dry up and solidify; all parts become constricted, all movements become slower and more difficult ....
>
> In *old age*, the calibre of the vessels shrinks, the secretory filters are obstructed; the blood, lymph and other humours must consequently thicken, alter, become extravasated and produce all the vices of the liquids which lead to destruction. Such are the causes by which the machine naturally goes to ruin.[72]

It is clear that this natural deterioration of all the bodily parts, this 'decrepitude of advanced age',[73] is to be understood as a generalized effect of senescence and not as the localized, pathological destruction of specific organs due to constitutional imbalance, as envisaged by Corvisart and Broussais.[74]

Strategies for Medical Dominance

Broadly speaking, for the first quarter of the nineteenth century the medical profession in France was faced with the problem of reasserting its dominance in the area of health and healing after the disestablishment of its institutional base during the Revolutionary period.[75] The reorganization of the hospitals, the development of systematic clinical teaching from the founding of the *écoles de santé*, the political manœuvring associated with the law of 1803 which reintroduced legal control of medical practice and recognized the *officier de santé* – these and other practical measures were evaluated by physicians, and either supported or opposed, in the light of their effect on the professional standing of medicine, in addition to whatever other considerations may have applied.

There is ample evidence that both Corvisart and Broussais were concerned with the enhancement of medicine's professional stature and took an active role in supporting practical measures directed toward that end.[76] The focus of the present discussion will be on a different level, however, where medical theory and professional ideology intersect. It is here, as I hope to show, that the pursuit of truth and the legitimation of power reinforce one another in the writings of Corvisart and Broussais, and the linkage is provided between their shared conception of the body's vulnerability to disease, on the one hand, and the professional status of French medicine, on the other.[77]

The two general approaches adopted by French physicians to bolster their professional position in the first decades of the nineteenth century can be called, respectively, the 'scientific research' strategy and the 'social engineering' strategy.[78] The first of these was based on the hospital as a privileged site of research, a source of medical truth from which competitors of various sorts (most of the *officiers de santé*; all of the 'unqualified' practitioners) could be excluded. The second strategy, oriented toward social engineering, sought to establish itself in the public health arena by extending the scope of medicine's usefulness to government authorities.

It should be clear that in arguing for the importance of these two overall strategies for our understanding of the medical profession at this time, I am not asserting that the profession acted in a monolithic way. Broussais, more perhaps than anyone else during this period, was involved in attacks on medical colleagues who did not share his theoretical orientation. But there is no reason why the 'external politics' of the profession as a whole should rule out the existence of 'internal politics' within the profession, just as the pursuit of a country's 'national interest' in its foreign policy does not rule out the possibility of political divisions in its domestic affairs. What is to be expected, however, is that the exigencies of the profession's external political goals should serve as both a constraint upon and a resource for its internal political activities.[79]

To illustrate the shared approach of Corvisart and Broussais to the re-establishment of medical dominance, we can consider four principal claims which they both asserted; the first three relating to the scientific research strategy and the last one to the social engineering strategy.

1. The Certainty of Medical Knowledge

Attacks on medicine as a tissue of uncertainties, a purely conjectural art and a haven for charlatanry appear to have been common enough in early nineteenth-century France to be a matter of great concern to leading members of the profession.[80] Corvisart seems to have been particularly exercised over this issue, perhaps because as First Physician of the Emperor he so often had to contend with sarcastic comments from Napoleon in this vein.[81] In his *Essai* Corvisart laments the fact that society continues to repeat 'that outdated accusation, that *medicine is a conjectural art*', and 'that sophism of J.-J. Rousseau, that *medicine would be better off without physicians*'.[82] And Broussais, too, in his *Examen* complains that there are even some physicians who 'glory in doubting the reality of medicine ... in order to evade the railleries of those savants who reproach them – and not without reason – for the uncertainty of their art and the incoherence of their theory'.[83]

Both Corvisart and Broussais address the issue of the uncertainty of medical knowledge by denouncing the errors of their predecessors and by insisting that their own discoveries have now brought medicine to a new level of certainty. It was the failure of previous generations of physicians to study pathological anatomy and physiology, according to Corvisart, which led them into 'frequent and I dare say gross errors, by often substituting effects for their causes, and by mistaking one disease for another'.[84] With the systematic pursuit of this study by Corvisart and his colleagues, however, medicine has already begun to achieve its goal of diagnostic certainty, 'recognising [organic] diseases by signs which are certain and by symptoms which are constant'.[85]

Likewise Broussais asserted that medical 'ontologists', who reified diseases instead of acknowledging that '[t]he nature of diseases results ... from the appreciable physiological modification of the organs', were responsible for the fact that 'medicine has remained vague and uncertain until our own day'.[86] If you follow the approach of the ontologists, 'in the majority of internal affections, you will not obtain a diagnosis of the affection which presents itself until after the death of the patient: this is all too frequently proven by the errors into which physicians fall daily...';[87] whereas Broussais' own approach, 'that of studying the organs in relation to their modifications, will always be ... a fertile and inexhaustible source of new truths...'.[88]

2. The Valorization of the Hospital

As Corvisart's protégé, Horeau, points out, the study of pathological anatomy and physiology, on which Corvisart based his claims to diagnostic certainty, 'necessarily required a large hospital in which the patients could be noted and selected, and a physician could be obstinate in his research, never hesitating to interrogate the cadavers of the patients who succumbed'.[89] This situation is sharply contrasted with that of 'busy [private] practitioners in large cities, who are rarely presented with the opportunity to conduct autopsies; permission for which is, in any case, difficult to obtain ...'.[90] These latter practitioners, without access to hospital patients, must become consumers of medical knowledge and defer to colleagues with hospital-based expertise. The hospital is thus doubly valorized as the source of medical certainty for the external politics of the profession and as the source of cognitive authority for the internal politics of the profession.[91]

To appreciate the importance of the hospital in both these regards it is only necessary to consider the way in which Broussais, who as an army doctor is unable to call upon the resources of the civilian hospitals of Paris, seeks to establish his military medical experience as a competing source of knowledge. 'It is in the midst of camps and armies, and in the military hospitals, that I have rectified my first medical ideas.'[92] Civilian physicians criticized the value of this experience as a basis for medical discovery: 'According to them, the only people one treats there are wretches exhausted by fatigue, harsh weather and bad food'.[93] But Broussais countered not only that the troops were often in very good condition, well fed and rested after their victories, but in addition that many other people were also examined by the army medical staff, since the civilian inhabitants of the areas where the army was camped often came for treatment as well.

When these considerations were combined with the fact that the Napoleonic armies had been deployed throughout Europe, Broussais concluded that the experience of the military doctors was medically more informative than that of physicians in the civilian hospitals.

> There are few among us who have not had occasion to combine civilian and military medicine, and who have not observed diseases

in people of all ages and both sexes, throughout the different latitudes of Europe. Thus to the advantages of seeing the most powerful causes of human infirmities – such as cold, heat, fatigue, violence, famine, noxious emanations – acting upon large numbers of people at the same time, we have joined the privilege of comparing the temperaments and the common diseases of different climates, and of obtaining from local physicians their precious teachings on the methods of treatment which have procured for them the most constant success.[94]

In his polemic against the researches of G.-L. Bayle on pulmonary phthisis,[95] Broussais turned the tables on the civilian critics of his military medical experience and argued that it was in fact the Parisian hospitals, such as the *Charité* where Bayle had worked, that inherently limited one's opportunities for observation. Contesting Bayle's claim that in all seasons phthisis is one of the most frequent and most deadly diseases, Broussais asks,

> Should one judge this disease on the basis of facts observed in Paris, where the temperature is never consistently warm enough for people not to be endlessly exposed to pectoral phlegmasies? Is it on the basis of the practice of the Charité, where only those wretches who have no way of protecting themselves from the influence of the cold are received, that one should make pronouncements on the relative frequency of the phthises?[96]

Bayle had been misled on this matter by the intrinsic narrowness of his Parisian clinical experience, despite some 900 autopsies conducted in the course of his research; whereas Broussais, who is able to judge the matter 'on the basis of twelve years of practice and of autopsying cadavers in the hospitals of the armies' throughout Europe,'[97] sees more clearly the causal relationship between phthisis and cold weather.

> I have said – and physicians who have had a breadth of vision, and who have not over-generalised from observations made in one small locality or in one particular establishment, have said it before me – that pulmonary phthisis is incomparably more common in the cold and the temperate countries than in the hot countries; and that men who would have been the victims of this disease in France or Holland have been free of it in Italy and Spain.[98]

The principle of the hospital as the privileged source of information about the true nature of diseases is not compromised by this dispute between Bayle and Broussais; it in fact provides the ground on which this dispute takes place. The issue is only to determine *what sort of hospital*, or even *whose hospital*, produces the most authoritative knowledge. Broussais, as a matter of the internal politics of medicine, seeks to establish the dominance of the military hospital as a more comprehensive and thus more reliable source of medical information than the civilian hospital; but he does so within the constraints of the profession's external politics of valorizing the hospital itself as a research institution.

3. The Ubiquity of Lesions

The lesson of the hospital autopsy table, both for Broussais and for Corvisart, is that organic lesions (and, for Broussais, the inflammations that produce them) are so frequent in cadavers that the formation of these lesions may be considered a universal characteristic of the human body. The fact that many of these destructive processes found at autopsy could not be detected while the patient was alive, allows one to generalize from 'the sick' to include 'the apparently healthy' as well.[99]

Under these circumstances, it becomes difficult to accept that most human constitutions are sound and that an inherent healing power of nature acts to maintain each of these constitutions in its own idiosyncratic state of health. But something more than naïve induction is involved in this rejection of the Hippocratic–Galenic doctrine of individual variations. A cognitive change has occurred in which the autopsy of the cadaver has become the focal point around which medical knowledge is now to be organized.

> It is when death is epistemologically integrated into medical experience that disease could detach itself from the contra-natural and *become embodied* in the *living bodies* of individuals. ... [F]rom the positioning of death within medical thought is born a medicine which presents itself as a science of the individual.[100]

This change in medical thinking did not take place in isolation from contemporary developments in related fields. At the same time as medicine was valorizing the autopsy of cadavers as the key to truth about disease, the comparative anatomy developed by Georges Cuvier and others was valorizing the dissection of animal species as the key to truth about the living organism.[101] The monopoly of the hospital in the production of pathological knowledge was paralleled by the monopoly of research centres like the *Muséum national d'histoire naturelle* in the production of biological knowledge. Just as

Horeau insisted on the superiority of Corvisart's hospital-based research over the autopsies of the 'busy practitioner', so too did Cuvier insist on the superiority of his own style of 'sedentary' research at the *Muséum* over the studies of field naturalists such as Alexander von Humboldt.

> The field naturalist passes through, at greater or lesser speed, a great number of different areas, and is struck, one after the other, by a great number of interesting objects and living things. ... But he can only give a few instants of time to each of them .... He is thus deprived of the possibility of comparing each being with those like it, of rigorously describing its characteristics .... If the sedentary naturalist does not see nature in action, he can yet survey all her products spread before him. He can compare them with each other as often as is necessary to reach reliable conclusions. He can bring together the relevant facts from anywhere he needs to ... [and not] leave a subject until, by observation, by a wide range of knowledge, and connected thought, he has illuminated it with every ray of light possible in a given state of knowledge.[102]

The most characteristic feature of this new biological way of understanding the living body and its activities was the priority given to the concept of functional organization as a way of meeting the threat of death. The functional integrity of the organism provided, in Cuvier's terms, its internal conditions of existence.[103] In every species the organs must form a harmonious functional unity, without which the species could not exist. An animal with a carnivorous digestive system could not survive with hooves and flat teeth, for it could neither seize nor devour its prey. Every organ in a given species had, therefore, to be well integrated in a balanced totality. Variety in the animal kingdom was represented by its many different species, which could be classified according to four great divisions. But within any particular species, only the most trivial variation was compatible with survival.

By transferring this biological outlook into the domain of human pathology, one could conclude that idiosyncratic variations within the human species are anything but benign.[104] Rather than providing the basis for each individual constitution to achieve its own uniquely appropriate state of health, these variations instead make the state of health virtually unattainable. Health thus becomes a normative ideal from which each individual, *qua* individual, deviates in his or her own distinctive, and scientifically determinate, way.[105]

4. The Medicalization of Life

At this point the scientific research strategy of the medical profession overlaps with its social engineering strategy, for the scientific lesson of the autopsy table is that every constitution provides the formative conditions of disease, and thus everyone in principle, whether apparently healthy or not, requires constant medical surveillance and intervention. Active diagnostic investigation must be undertaken in order to discover, 'by the subtlest perception of the slightest derangement of the injured organ's function',[106] those diseases which are imperceptible to the patient who harbours them – or, to put the matter in terms consistent with Foucault's analysis of 'the confession' as a privileged source of truth in Western society,

> the body must be subjected to a medical examination which will allow it to confess its pathological secrets to the physician, even while concealing them from the patient. ... As the confessional subject has arisen in the modern era, so too has the confessional body ....[107]

According to Corvisart, it is usually too late to cure the patient of organic diseases, once they have been detected in this way. Broussais, more optimistic, offers a therapeutic programme for curing these diseases in their early stages of inflammation: 'Local bleedings, [dietary] abstinence and watery drinks always abort incipient phlegmasies, when the inflammation has not yet spread extensively through the viscera'.[108] Thus he promises a cure if the inflammation is stopped 'before the stage of *disorganization*';[109] but like Corvisart he cautions that 'from the moment when this disorganization is consummated, all hope of cure is lost'.[110]

From this perspective, any possibility of relying on the individual's experience of well-being as a measure of the healthy state, or on the healing power of nature as a way of maintaining that state, is excluded. Regardless of whether the patient can be cured or not, constant medical attention will be necessary. Even if medicine cannot cure an organic lesion, as in Corvisart's view, the patient will nevertheless require a continuous program of palliative treatment and medical management:

> [Medicine] ... can be of major utility in mitigating the effects and minimizing the accidents that this lesion can produce, by teaching the sick those rules of conduct and of regimen which they cannot infringe without compromising or abridging their existence.[111]

On the other hand, if medicine can produce a cure for most diseases, as in Broussais' view, it sets two conditions for doing so. Firstly, it must be able to intervene therapeutically on an almost continuous, 'directive' basis:

> The physician who cannot direct the irritability of the stomach will never be able to treat any disease.[112] ...
>
> [B]ut the stomach is a singular organ; its destiny is to be always irritated ....[113]

And secondly, it must be able to carry out its therapeutic interventions for as long a time, and with as many delicate adjustments, as it requires. For example, in the case of certain irritations of the stomach, '[t]his cure sometimes requires several years, but it is the only one which is lasting; it can even succeed when a certain degree of disorganization has occurred'.[114] Thus for Broussais, just as for Corvisart,

> [t]he *vis medicatrix naturae* is replaced by a *vis medicatrix scientiae*, and the old therapeutic goal of responding to particular episodes of disease is replaced by the programme of an open-ended 'management' of life.[115]

Conclusion

In presenting an analysis of the position taken by Corvisart and Broussais on the question of individual variations, I hope to have shown that their view of this matter was strikingly different from that represented by the Hippocratic–Galenic tradition which had extended from antiquity to the eighteenth century. I have argued that the particular conceptual constellation made up of (a) constitutional idiosyncrasy, (b) the relativistic definition of health and (c) the respective roles of the healing power of nature and the management of the 'non-naturals' in maintaining an individual's health, was transformed in the work of Corvisart and Broussais into a constellation consisting of (a) pathogenic constitutional imbalances, (b) a definition of health as an ideal organic norm, unattainable in practice, and (c) the respective roles of the body's harmful natural tendencies and the inherent unhealthiness of most human activities and surroundings. If Broussais' writings do not convey the same flavour of medical dystopia as do Corvisart's, this is not because they fail to share the same underlying vision of the pathogenicity of life, but only because they are so aggressively optimistic in their therapeutic outlook.

In stressing the thoroughness with which the position of Corvisart and Broussais on 'the science of the individual' repudiates the benevolent interpretation of individual variation found in classical Hippocratic–Galenic thought, I do not wish to suggest that no element of their shared position can be found in earlier medical texts. As foreshadowed in the introduction to this chapter, my purpose is not to argue for the absolute novelty of any element in isolation, but to illustrate the systematic relationship uniting individuality, death and disease in the work of Corvisart and Broussais, and to ground this relationship both in the cognitive framework of Paris clinical medicine and in the 'external politics' of the French medical profession during the early nineteenth century.

Nor do I wish to suggest that the position taken by Corvisart and Broussais on human individuality was the only one possible within the context of French medicine during this period. A consideration of figures such as Laennec and Alibert makes it clear that more than one option was available for the development of medical theory within the same cognitive and professional environment.[116] But what particularly attracts our attention in the position of Corvisart and Broussais is the sense of its coherence with a deep change in the relationship between medicine and the individual which transformed the 'experiencing subject' into 'clinical material' – a change which the Paris clinical school did much to inaugurate and which still structures, and limits, our present perceptions of 'medical dominance'.[117]

Notes

1. Erwin H. Ackerknecht, *Medicine at the Paris Hospital, 1794–1848* (Baltimore: Johns Hopkins Press, 1967), ch. 3, 'Antecedents'; Michel Foucault, *Naissance de la clinique: Une archéologie du regard médical* [1963], 2nd edn (Paris: Presses Universitaires de France, 1972), translated from the first edition by A. M. Sheridan Smith as *The Birth of the Clinic: An Archaeology of Medical Perception* (New York: Pantheon, 1973), ch. 4, 'The Old Age of the Clinic'; and L. W. B. Brockliss, 'Before the Clinic: French Medical Teaching in the Eighteenth Century', in this volume.
2. See, for example, Othmar Keel, *La généalogie de l'histopathologie* (Paris: Vrin, 1979); *idem*, 'Percussion et diagnostic physique en Grande Bretagne au 18e siècle: l'exemple d'Alexander Monro secundus', *XXXI Congresso Internazionale di Storia Della Medicina: Atti* (Bologna: Monduzzi, 1988), 869–75; and *idem*, 'Was Anatomical and Tissue

Pathology a Product of the Paris Clincal School or Not?', in this volume.
3. See, for example, Clare O'Farrell, *Foucault: Historian or Philosopher?* (London: Macmillan, 1989), 81–3 and 103.
4. Foucault, *Birth of the Clinic*, ix.
5. *Ibid.*, xiv. Here, and throughout this chapter unless otherwise indicated, all italics in quoted passages are given as in the original.
6. See, for example, the Hippocratic texts, *Tradition in Medicine* [usually translated as *Ancient Medicine*], ch. 23, *The Nature of Man*, ch. 9, and *A Regimen for Health,* ch. 2, in G. E. R. Lloyd (ed.), *Hippocratic Writings* (Harmondsworth: Penguin, 1978), 86, 267, 273; Ludwig Edelstein, 'The Dietetics of Antiquity', in *idem, Ancient Medicine* (Baltimore: Johns Hopkins Press, 1967), 304; and Nancy G. Siraisi, *Medieval and Early Renaissance Medicine* (Chicago: University of Chicago Press, 1990), 102, 121.
7. Siraisi, *Medieval and Early Renaissance Medicine,* 123.
8. William Coleman, 'Health and Hygiene in the *Encyclopédie*: A Medical Doctrine for the Bourgeoisie', *Journal of the History of Medicine* 29 (1974), 406.
9. Arnulfe d'Aumont, 'Santé (*Œcon. anim.*)', in Denis Diderot and Jean LeRond d'Alembert (eds), *Encyclopédie, ou dictionnaire raisonée des sciences, des arts et des métiers* (Paris/Neuchâtel/Amsterdam, 1751–80), vol. xiv, 629. All translations in this chapter are mine unless otherwise indicated. For a general assessment of d'Aumont's contributions to the *Encyclopédie* on matters of health and hygiene, see Coleman, 'Health and Hygiene', 399–421.
10. d'Aumont, 'Santé', 629.
11. *Ibid.,* 629–30; *cf. idem* [?], 'Hygiène (*Médecine*)', in Diderot and d'Alembert, *Encyclopédie,* vol. viii, 385–8.
12. See Edelstein, 'The Dietetics of Antiquity', 303–16, for the Greek tradition, and also the application of Edelstein's argument to the eighteenth-century French context in Coleman, 'Health and Hygiene', 416–17.
13. This traditional, 'private' focus of medical practice would soon be challenged by the newer 'public' focus of medicine represented by the Société Royale de Médecine, founded in 1778. See Caroline C. Hannaway, 'The Société Royale de Médecine and Epidemics in the Ancien Régime', *Bulletin of the History of Medicine* 46 (1972), 257–73; and T. D. Murphy, 'The French Medical Profession's Perception of its Social Function between 1776 and 1830', *Medical History* 23 (1979), 259–62.
14. *Cf.* the interpretation of English medicine during this same period

offered in N. Jewson, 'Medical Knowledge and the Patronage System in Eighteenth-Century England', *Sociology* 8 (1974), 369–85.
15. d'Aumont, 'Santé', 629.
16. *Ibid.*
17. *Plan général de l'enseignement dans l'Ecole de Santé de Paris* (Paris, An III), 1, quoted in Foucault, *Naissance de la clinique*, 72. My translation here differs somewhat from that given in Foucault, *Birth of the Clinic*, 72.
18. W. R. Albury, 'Heart of Darkness: J. N. Corvisart and the Medicalization of Life', *Historical Reflections/Réflexions historiques* 9 (1982), 17–31, reprinted in Jean-Pierre Goubert (ed.), *La médicalisation de la société française, 1770–1830* (Waterloo: Historical Reflections Press, 1982), 17–31. See also Ackerknecht, *Medicine at the Paris Hospital*, 83–5.
19. J. N. Corvisart, *Essai sur les maladies et les lésions organiques du cœur et des gros vaisseaux* [1806], 3rd edn (Paris: Méquignon-Marvis, 1818), xxi–ii.
20. *Ibid.*, 376.
21. See, for example, the description of Corvisart's 'philosophy' as the product of 'the life-long personal melancholy of a divorced, childless, noble, embittered, and stoical man' in Ackerknecht, *Medicine at the Paris Hospital*, 85.
22. [François-Marie Arouet de] Voltaire, 'Le crocheteur borgne', in *idem, Romans et contes* (Paris: Gallimard, 1954), 647–52. I wish to thank my colleague, Michael Freyne, for identifying this reference.
23. Joseph Reveillé-Parise, 'Éloge de Corvisart', *Gazette médicale de Paris,* 27 novembre 1837, quoted in Paul Ganière, *Corvisart, médecin de l'Empereur,* new edn (Paris: Librairie Académique Perrin, 1985), 211.
24. The material in this section summarizes and expands upon the discussion in Albury, 'Heart of Darkness'.
25. Corvisart, *Essai,* vii.
26. *Ibid.,* xvi.
27. *Ibid.,* xvii.
28. *Ibid.,* xviii.
29. *Ibid.,* 367–8. See also *idem,* 'Commentaire', in Leopold Auenbrugger, *Nouvelle méthode pour reconnaître les maladies internes de la poitrine par la percussion de cette cavité ... [1763]; ouvrage traduit du Latin et commenté par J. N. Corvisart* (Paris: Migneret, 1808), 158.
30. Corvisart, *Essai,* 375.
31. *Ibid.,* 371.
32. *Ibid.,* 381 (emphasis added).
33. d'Aumont, 'Non-Naturelles, Choses', in Diderot and d'Alembert,

Encyclopédie, vol. xi, 217–24. The 'non-naturals' were distinguished in Galenic theory from the 'contra-naturals', or diseases; *cf.* Siraisi, *Medieval and Early Renaissance Medicine*, 101.
34. Corvisart, *Essai*, xxiv–vi; *cf. idem*, 'Commentaire', 180–91.
35. Corvisart, *Essai*, xxxiv.
36. *Ibid.*, xxxv.
37. *Ibid.*, xxxiii.
38. Corvisart defines *tact* as that combination of skilled observation and clinical judgement which allows the medical practitioner to understand, almost instantaneously, the essential features of a patient's condition. See Corvisart, 'Préface du traducteur', in Auenbrugger, *Nouvelle méthode*, x.
39. Corvisart, *Essai*, 367 (mispaginated as 637); *cf. idem*, 'Commentaire', 124. It is also possible, conversely, to have symptoms without diseases; see *idem*, *Essai*, xiv–v.
40. Corvisart, 'Commentaire', 37; *cf.* Foucault, *Birth of the Clinic*, 162.
41. Corvisart, *Aphorismes de médecine clinique* (Paris: Masson, 1929), 110, § CCCIV.
42. Corvisart, *Essai*, 367.
43. *Cf.*, on this general issue, Georges Canguilhem, *Le normal et le pathologique* (Paris: Presses Universitaires de France, 1966), translated by Carolyn R. Fawcett as *On the Normal and the Pathological* (Dordrecht: Reidel, 1978).
44. Corvisart, 'Commentaire', 272.
45. For sharply contrasting overviews of Broussais' work, see Ackerknecht, *Medicine at the Paris Hospital*, ch. 6; and Foucault, *Birth of the Clinic*, ch. 10. Also of interest is Jean-François Braunstein, *Broussais et le matérialisme: Médecine et philosophie au XIXe siècle* (Paris: Méridiens Klincksieck, 1986).
46. For Corvisart's attitude to therapeutics, see, for example, *idem*, *Aphorismes*, 24, §§ XXXIII–IV, and *idem*, 'Commentaire', 273.
47. F.-J.-V. Broussais, *Examen des doctrines médicales et des systèmes de nosologie*, 3rd edn, 4 vols (Paris: Delaunay, 1829–34), vol. i, lix, § CCLXIV. See also Albury, 'Ideas of Life and Death', in W. F. Bynum and Roy Porter (eds), *Companion Encyclopedia of the History of Medicine*, 2 vols (London and New York: Routledge, 1993), vol. i, 260–1.
48. Broussais, *Traité de physiologie appliquée à la pathologie*, 2 vols (Paris: Delaunay, 1822–3), ch. xii [mislabelled as ch. xi], vol. ii, 518ff.
49. *Ibid.*, 539.
50. *Ibid.*, 563.
51. *Ibid.*, 550.

52. Broussais, *Examen des doctrines médicales*, vol. i, xvii–iii, §§ LXVII–III.
53. *Ibid.*, vol. i, i, § I.
54. *Ibid.*, vol. i, xvi, § LXI.
55. *Ibid.*, vol. i, xviii, § LXIX.
56. *Ibid.*, vol. i, xciv, xcvi, §§ CCCLXXXV, CCCXCIII.
57. *Ibid.*, vol. i, lix, § CCLXII.
58. Broussais, *Examen de la doctrine médicale généralement adoptée, et des systèmes modernes de nosologie* (Paris: Méquignon-Marvis, 1816), 216.
59. Broussais, *Traité de physiologie appliquée*, vol. i, 4.
60. *Ibid.*, vol. ii, 69; *cf.* the similar list in Corvisart, *Essai*, xxix–xxx.
61. Broussais, *Traité de physiologie appliquée*, vol. ii, *passim*.
62. *Ibid.*, vol. i, 275.
63. *Ibid.*, vol. ii, 145.
64. Broussais, *Examen des doctrines médicales*, vol. i, lxix, § CCCVII.
65. Broussais, *Histoire des phlegmasies ou inflammations chroniques*, 4th edn, 3 vols (Paris: Gabon, 1826), vol. iii, 458.
66. Broussais, *Examen de la doctrine médicale généralement adoptée*, 407–8 (emphasis added).
67. John Lough, *The Encyclopédie* (London: Longman, 1971), 73.
68. Louis, chevalier de Jaucourt, 'Idiosyncrase (*Médec.*)', in Diderot and d'Alembert, *Encyclopédie*, vol. viii, 497.
69. *Ibid.*
70. d'Aumont, 'Non-Naturelles, Choses', 224.
71. *Ibid.*
72. Jaucourt, 'Vieillesse (*Physiolog.*)', in Diderot and d'Alembert, *Encyclopédie*, vol. xvii, 260.
73. *Ibid.*
74. *Cf.* Albury, 'Ideas of Life and Death', 257.
75. Murphy, 'The French Medical Profession's Perception', 262–78; Jacques Léonard, *La médecine entre les pouvoirs et les savoirs* (Paris: Aubier Montaigne, 1981); and Matthew Ramsey, *Professional and Popular Medicine in France, 1770–1830* (Cambridge: Cambridge University Press, 1988), esp. 71–125. See also the discussion in Albury, 'Heart of Darkness', 24–5, and the lengthy quotation from this discussion, inadvertently unattributed, in Dorinda Outram, *The Body and the French Revolution* (New Haven, Connecticut, and London: Yale University Press, 1989), 61–2.
76. For Corvisart, see Ganière, *Corvisart*, 68–70; and for Broussais, see Léonard, *La médecine entre les pouvoirs et les savoirs*, 207–8.
77. See John Harley Warner, *The Therapeutic Perspective: Medical Practice, Knowledge, and Identity in America, 1820–1885* (Cambridge,

Mass., and London: Harvard University Press, 1986) for a stimulating account of the cognitive commitments and professional politics of nineteenth-century American physicians which led them to develop and maintain a quite different set of relationships between individuality and disease during the *ante-bellum* period in the United States. American medical visitors studying in France during this period evaluated Parisian medicine in the light of their own cognitive and professional background, and so their experience of the Paris Clinical School was different from that of French students, as Warner shows in 'Paradigm Lost or Paradise Declining? American Physicians and the "Dead End" of the Paris Clinical School', in this volume.

78. The present paragraph summarizes the discussion in Albury, 'Heart of Darkness', 26; *cf.* Murphy, 'The French Medical Profession's Perception', 271.
79. For a fuller discussion of this point, see Albury, 'The Politics of Truth: A Social Interpretation of Scientific Knowledge, with an Application to the Case of Sociobiology', in Michael Ruse (ed.), *Nature Animated* (Dordrecht: Reidel, 1983), 115–29; and *idem, The Politics of Objectivity* (Geelong: Deakin University Press, 1983), 34–51.
80. See, for example, P.-J.-G. Cabanis, *Du degré de certitude de la médecine* [1797], in C. Lehec and J. Cazeneuve (eds), *Œuvres philosophiques de Cabanis*, 2 vols (Paris: Presses Universitaires de France, 1956), vol. i, 92; and Philippe Pinel, *Nosographie philosophique*, 2 vols (Paris: Richard, Caille et Ravier, 1798), vol. i, i.
81. Ganière, *Corvisart*, 54, 116–20.
82. Corvisart, *Essai*, xv, xxiii.
83. Broussais, *Examen de la doctrine médicale généralement adoptée*, 152–3.
84. Corvisart, *Essai*, xvi.
85. *Ibid.*, ix; *cf. idem*, 'Commentaire', 33–4.
86. Broussais, *Examen des doctrines médicales*, vol. i, cxvii, cxix, §§ CDLXII–III, CDLXVIII.
87. Broussais, *Examen de la doctrine médicale généralement adoptée*, 405.
88. Broussais, *Traité de physiologie appliquée*, vol. i, 6.
89. C. E. Horeau, 'Préface de l'Éditeur', in Corvisart, *Essai sur les maladies et les lésions organiques du cœur et des gros vaisseaux; extrait des leçons cliniques. ... Publié, sous ses yeux, par C. E. Horeau* (Paris: Migneret, 1806), xiv.
90. *Ibid.*, xi.
91. By contrast, the status of the hospital as a source of medical knowledge remained very low in the United States until the last third

of the nineteenth century. Warner, *The Therapeutic Perspective*, 265.
92. Broussais, *Examen de la doctrine médicale généralement adoptée*, xi.
93. *Ibid.*, xii.
94. *Ibid.*, xii–xiii.
95. Gaspard-Laurent Bayle, *Recherches sur la phthisie pulmonaire* (Paris: Gabon, 1810).
96. Broussais, *Examen de la doctrine médicale généralement adoptée*, 313.
97. *Ibid.*, 318.
98. *Ibid.*, 324–5.
99. '[A]n apparent state of good health can, to a certain extent, co-exist for several months, and even longer, with an obstruction in some part of the thorax, and this obstruction will, in time, become a cause of fatal organic disease'. Corvisart, 'Commentaire', 124.
100. Foucault, *Naissance de la clinique*, 200–1. My translation here differs from that given in Foucault, *Birth of the Clinic*, 196–7, in part because of revisions in the second French edition of *Naissance* which are not reflected in the English edition.
101. On the importance of Cuvier's work in this area, see William Coleman, *Georges Cuvier, Zoologist* (Cambridge, Mass.: Harvard University Press, 1964), chs 2–3; Foucault, *Les mots et les choses* (Paris: Gallimard, 1966), translated anonymously as *The Order of Things* (New York: Pantheon, 1970), 263–79; and François Jacob, *La logique du vivant: Une histoire d'hérédité* (Paris: Gallimard, 1970), translated by Betty E. Spillmann as *The Logic of Life: A History of Heredity* (New York: Pantheon, 1973), 100–11. Cuvier took a direct interest in medical matters, joining the *Société de santé* in 1797, the *Comité d'administration de l'école de médecine de Paris* in 1800 and the *Société de médecine de Paris* in 1803. Outram, *Georges Cuvier: Vocation, Science and Authority in Post-Revolutionary France* (Manchester: Manchester University Press, 1984), 211.
102. Georges Cuvier, 'Analyse d'un ouvrage de M. Humboldt intitulé: *Tableaux de la nature* ...' [1807], manuscript quoted in Outram, 'New Spaces in Natural History', in N. Jardine, J. A. Secord and E. C. Spary (eds), *Cultures of Natural History* (Cambridge: Cambridge University Press, 1996), 259–61; original French quoted in Outram, *Georges Cuvier*, 62–3. Ironically, in the same year that Cuvier wrote this defence of 'sedentary' naturalists, he embarked on his own fieldwork programme to study fossils in the geological formations around Paris. *Ibid.*, 153.
103. See, for example, Cuvier, *The Animal Kingdom* [1817] (London: Bohn, 1863), 2–3.
104. It was of course possible to recognize Cuvier's biology as a scientific

model for medicine without necessarily drawing this negative conclusion about individual variations – especially after the first quarter of the nineteenth century, when the professional context of French medicine had changed, and even more so if one had never been part of that professional context. See, for example, the comments of the American physician Jacob Bigelow, visiting Paris in 1833, as reported in Warner, *The Therapeutic Perspective,* 27.

105. Just as the Hippocratic doctrine of the individual constitution was replaced in early nineteenth-century France by the biological principle of the internal conditions of existence, so too was the Hippocratic doctrine of the 'epidemic constitution' – that is, a particular conjunction of climatic conditions thought to be responsible for a given epidemic – replaced by the biological principle of the external conditions of existence. See François Delaporte, *Disease and Civilization: The Cholera in Paris, 1832,* translated by Arthur Goldhammer (Cambridge, Mass.: MIT Press, 1986), 78–86.

106. Corvisart, *Essai* (1818), 367.

107. Albury, 'The Production of Truth: Body and Soul. Part 2: Displaying the Truth of the Body', in O'Farrell (ed.), *Foucault: The Legacy* (Kelvin Grove, QLD: Queensland University of Technology, 1997), 359–60; *cf.* Dirk Meure, 'The Production of Truth: Body and Soul. Part 1: "Telling Truths": Truth Telling in the Judicial Process', *ibid.,* 346–55, and the analysis of confession in Foucault, *Histoire de la sexualité, 1: La volonté de savoir* (Paris: Gallimard, 1976), translated by Robert Hurley as *The History of Sexuality, Volume 1: An Introduction* (London: Penguin, 1979), 58–60.

108. Broussais, *Examen des doctrines médicales,* vol. i, lxxxviii, § CCCXXXIII.

109. Broussais, *Histoire des phlegmasies,* vol. iii, 459.

110. *Ibid.,* 458.

111. Corvisart, *Essai* (1818), 430.

112. Broussais, *Examen des doctrines médicales,* vol. i, lxxi, § CCCVII.

113. Broussais, *Traité de physiologie appliquée,* vol. ii, 145.

114. Broussais, *Examen des doctrines médicales,* vol. i, lxviii–ix, § CCXCVIII. In view of Broussais' reputation as an advocate of excessive bleeding and starvation, it is worth noting that this passage continues with the following admonition: 'Above all it is important not to debilitate the patient too much by sanguine evacuations or by abstinence, which could cause the viscera to lose their assimilative faculty'.

115. Albury, 'Heart of Darkness', 29.

116. On Laennec, see Jacalyn Duffin, 'Vitalism and Organicism in the Philosophy of R.-T.-H. Laennec', *Bulletin of the History of Medicine*

62 (1988), 525–45, and especially *idem,* 'Laennec and Broussais: The "Sympathetic" Duel', in this volume, which delineates both similarities and differences in the positions of Laennec and Broussais. On Alibert, see L. S. Jacyna, 'Pious Pathology: J. L. Alibert's Iconography of Disease', in this volume.

117. On the limitations of the concept of 'medical dominance', see William Ray Arney and Bernard J. Bergen, *Medicine and the Management of Living: Taming the Last Great Beast* (Chicago: University of Chicago Press, 1984).

6

Laennec and Broussais: The 'Sympathetic' Duel

Jacalyn Duffin

Renaudot and Patin, Magendie and Bell, Pasteur and Pouchet, Gallo and Montagnier – medical names linked by competition, controversy, and polemic. René-Théophile-Hyacinthe Laennec (1781–1826) and François-Joseph-Victor Broussais (1774–1838) were also great rivals and during their 'duel célèbre', waged in the amphitheatres and publications of post-Revolutionary Paris, each accused the other of sloppy pathology, plagiarism, and excessive self-love. Laennec died before his opponent, but the battle continued for twelve more years until Broussais too was dead.[1] Posterity counted Laennec the victor, as it elevated his reputation;[2] Broussais, with his injurious style, was relegated to the ranks of the mediocre systematists. Ackerknecht's assessment is telling: Broussais may have been [M. F. X.] Bichat's 'only legitimate offspring', but 'medically speaking', he was 'an abortion'.[3] The late assignation of glory to Laennec does not explain why their dispute took place. If Laennec saw in Broussais no more than the crude polemicist later historians have tried to make of him, why did he stoop to fight? And there should be no doubt that Laennec fought too.

The medical revolution of early nineteenth-century France owed much to Broussais's iconoclasm and radical localism, a contribution recognized by some contemporaries and re-discovered by twentieth-century historians.[4] Laennec, too, understood the power of Broussais's ideas. In this essay, I will attempt to show that these legendary foes shared more than mutual contempt. They challenged each other to think and write; Broussais's criticism of Laennec stimulated his later research. Their 'best of enemies' hostility, like the non-medical sparring of Hollywood actors Spencer Tracy and Katharine Hepburn, reflected grudging but profound respect and sometimes even tacit agreement. Finally, in a 'vulgar' attempt to offer an explicit explanation,[5] I hope to reconcile this dispute with recent work in the sociology of science by demonstrating that it arose within an intellectual form of anomie, product of the recent triumph of anatomo-clinical medicine in the Paris school.

Laennec

Laennec invented the stethoscope in 1816 and, with this tool, altered the conceptualization of disease. Before his invention, diseases were viewed as constellations of symptoms, identified by consideration of the nature and sequence of various subjective events. Pathological anatomy was only rarely applied to bedside medicine, since it was impossible to detect the organic changes in a cadaver before the patient died. Specific organic lesions had been described for at least a century, but, for several reasons, practising physicians were unfamiliar with anatomical changes. Lesions were identified with the cadaver and it seemed they may have been artefacts of death. Lesions could only rarely be detected in the living patient and even when they were detected, lesions could not be corrected surgically or medically. The doctor's purpose was to relieve symptoms, not to remove structural alterations.[6]

With auscultation, it became possible to detect internal changes in the living patient. Laennec's treatise introduced a new diagnostic instrument, but it also presented discoveries in the pathological anatomy of the chest, especially with respect to tuberculosis, pneumonia, pleurisy, emphysema, bronchiectasis, and pulmonary oedema.[7] In fact, his English translator initially considered the pathological anatomy to be more important than the technique of auscultation.[8] Laennec revised his work for a second edition that appeared in 1826, the year of his death.[9] In the seven years between editions, however, stethoscopy had spread through Europe and to America.

Laennec is also credited with 'unifying' tuberculosis, from the several different diseases it had been, into a single entity.[10] Both auscultation and pathological anatomy contributed to this unification. He followed the changes over time in the chests of his patients and carefully dissected their bodies after they had died. This allowed him to link the progress of the tubercle from its inception as a tiny granule to softening and evacuation or to dissemination. From these observations, he was able to hypothesize the possibility of spontaneous cure – an idea that met with immediate derision.

These achievements were the basis of Laennec's enduring fame.

They were of such importance in the future of medicine that he became a 'hero' to some eyes and was awarded glowing epithets: the 'French Hippocrates', 'a sort of Newton or Galileo', the 'crowning glory' of the Charité Hospital, or the 'Founder of Modern Medicine'.[11] Yet during his life, Laennec was, if anything, somewhat infamous.

Born in Finistère, the 'Land's End' part of Lower Brittany, Laennec considered himself more Breton than French. A devout Catholic during the atheism of the Revolution and a royalist during the Napoleonic Empire, his attitudes were unusual for a physician in the post-Revolutionary Paris school. Some have concluded that his political and religious opinions were the main reason for his lack of popularity. Others interpret them as evidence of his moral rectitude and strength of character, further supported by his patient endurance of chronic ill-health, poverty, and isolation, and romanticized by his love of art, music, and classical authors.

Broussais

Broussais was also Breton, but not from the peasant land of Lower Brittany. He was born in St Malo, like the writer and statesman, René de Chateaubriand (1768–1848). Broussais's parents had been brutally massacred by the royalist Chouans in the post-Revolutionary Terror of 1794. The tragedy has been used as an explanation for much of his subsequent behaviour. Unlike either Laennec or Chateaubriand, Broussais was anti-royalist and anti-Church. His political sentiments, though not bonapartist, were liberal.[12]

Broussais began his medical training, like Laennec, as a surgical cadet in the revolutionary armies. He was already married when he went to Paris in 1798, to complete his studies with Philippe Pinel (1745–1826), François Chaussier (1746–1828), and Xavier Bichat (1771–1802). Broussais claimed Bichat as a friend. Although he would later condemn Pinel for the sin of 'ontology', his medical thesis on 'hectic fevers' was pervaded with Pinelian nosology.

Broussais founded a system of medicine which he called 'la médecine physiologique', first presented in his work *Histoires des phlegmasies*, published in 1808 (Figure 1).[13] He complained that all systems of medicine were too abstract and too complicated to be practical. He deplored the absence of discussion, first, concerning the causes of disease, and second, concerning the relationships between cause, organic change, and symptoms. His physiological medicine was the study of causes and their connections to the body, which he labelled 'sympathies'. Without rejecting symptom-based nosology or anatomical pathology, he reduced them to what he

Figure 1
Broussais's 'doctrine physiologique'

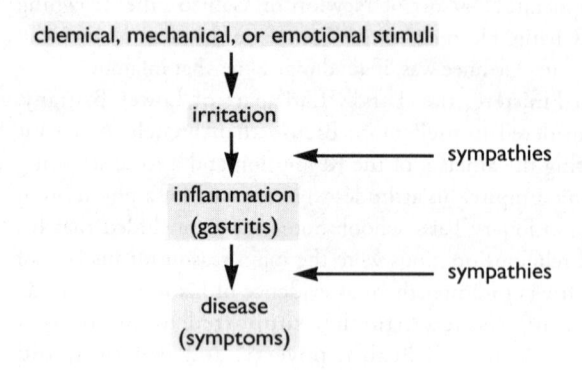

chemical, mechanical, or emotional stimuli
↓
irritation
↓ ← sympathies
inflammation
(gastritis)
↓ ← sympathies
disease
(symptoms)

considered to be their essential features. Most diseases were due to 'irritation', itself the result of chemical, mechanical, or emotional stimuli (such as cold, heat, contagion, or depression). This 'irritation' most commonly (although not always) led to inflammation, which in turn could lead to other organic changes such as tubercles or cancer. The first site of inflammation was usually the stomach and intestine.

Localization to the gastrointestinal tract was not Broussais's own idea. It had first been described by P. A. Prost in 1804.[14] Prost may have observed the erosions, now called stress ulcers (or Cushing's gastritis), or he may simply have had an unusual opportunity to observe the tissues as they appear in life. The healthy stomach mucosa appears brilliant red in health or in the immediate post-mortem state, but fades rapidly after death. Thus, every soldier, whose wounds allowed close inspection, appeared to have an 'inflamed' stomach.[15] Gastritis and superficial ulceration are frequent complications of any acute illness, even if no other organic lesion is present. In addition, Broussais recognized the 'rapport', described by Cabanis, between the moral and the physical aspects of the organism. The stomach seemed to be a logical location for this property, as anxiety, fear, and desire result in digestive symptoms.

Broussais did not pretend that the concept of irritation could explain all causes, but he thought it was more scientific than symptom-based nosology or pathological anatomy: at least, it acknowledged the importance and existence of a cause preceding the onset of symptoms and organic change. Causal relationships must become known, he maintained, if medicine ever hoped effectively to treat and cure disease. For precisely this reason, Auguste Comte (1798–1857) endorsed the notion of irritation as a 'positive' improvement over the metaphysical and theological vitalism ('psychology') that had become a 'vague and chimerical pursuit' of 'the young generation of France'.[16]

Unlike his colleagues in the Paris school, Broussais emphasized therapy. English and American medical students, who ventured into post-Revolutionary Paris, complained that French doctors were interested more in diagnosis than in treatment.[17] Broussais was an exception. His success as a practitioner stemmed from his enthusiastic embrace of vigorous therapy, dominated by 'la saignée', bleeding by leeches or phlebotomy. Sigerist and Ackerknecht characterized his impact on French medicine in terms of a transformation in the French leech trade, from a nèt export of over a million to a net import of over twenty million leeches per year.[18] Some have suggested that Broussais's patients may have enjoyed a better outlook than those of other doctors, because his therapy protected them from the noxious concoctions of doctors who used pharmaceuticals. His confident presence may have had a powerful psychosomatic effect.[19]

From Laennec's point of view, Broussais practised poor pathological anatomy. His examinations were incomplete, his records too brief, if not falsified, and his conclusions were the product of expectation not observation.[20] This opinion was not shared by medical students, who paid special fees to attend Broussais's private courses, since he did not have a University appointment. Laennec's lectures at the Collège de France were sparsely attended, while Broussais spoke to a full house.[21] He was large and handsome, an impressive orator, gifted with a rare ability to see the truly ridiculous in the medical past and a tongue that knew how to take maximum advantage of his insights. Nothing was sacred, except his own vision of how things ought to be done. He attacked everything and everyone, living or dead, and mocked the contributions of his contemporaries by casting aspersions on their integrity. His insults have been quoted to emphasize his outrageous nastiness, as yet another cross-to-bear for the long-suffering Laennec. According to Broussais, Laennec was 'medico-jesuitique', a 'bad observer', a 'bad therapist', 'with a brain ... heated by an all-consuming fever that devoured him, who could be nothing in medicine if not a visionary'. He implied that Laennec and his friend,

Gaspard-Laurent Bayle (1799–1858), withheld treatment from their patients in order to augment their supply of autopsy material.[22]

These quotes are derived from the various editions of Broussais's *Examen des doctrines médicales et les systèmes de nosologie*. In the first edition of 1816, virtually all medical systems fell under attack, from Hippocrates to the Paris school, including Pinel. In the second edition of 1821, almost one hundred pages decried Laennec and the other 'fatalistic' pathological anatomists.[23] The third edition, swollen to four volumes of polemic, devoted 194 pages to Broussais's arch (but now defunct) foe.[24] He insinuated that Laennec had died of his own ignorance, as if 'la médecine physiologique' could confer immortality on its adherents.[25]

The *Examen* is a remarkable production both for its bombast and for its insight. Interspersed among the insults, are a number of fundamental criticisms that reveal their author to be the enemy of pretence and the champion of suffering patients and confused students. The later editions also display grandiosity and suspicion that hint at paranoia. At the end of his career, Broussais turned to the medically chic preoccupations of phrenology and psychiatry.[26] His reductionist theories were opposed by the faculty of medicine, by François Magendie (1783–1855), and by the medical beneficiaries of the royalist Restoration.[27] But to liberal students and professors, he symbolized anti-Restoration feeling. He finally was appointed to the University and the Académie de Médecine after the Revolution of 1830.

Populist factors were important but not the only reason for Broussais's success with students. He was respected for his intelligent clairvoyance, as much as he is now scorned for his diatribes. The ignominious reputation came later, endorsed by criticisms of his inaccuracies and as a by-product of the late glorification of Laennec. But Broussais had contributed to a rupture in medical thought. Almost through overstating his case, he helped to complete the work of organic localization, begun by the pathologists of the eighteenth century.[28] Unlike Laennec, he was recognized in his own time, for some significant if poorly understood contribution to the scientific destiny of medicine. Magendie seemed to avoid attacking Broussais's theories, although he described them as simplistic. On the other hand, Magendie joined in the posthumous 'Laennec-bashing'.[29] J. B. Bouillaud (1796–1881) supported the physiology of Broussais over the pathology of Laennec.[30] More than a generation after their deaths, a member of the Académie de Médecine observed that Laennec had been consumed with resisting Broussais 'systematically, even in opposition to the evidence'.[31]

Laennec and Broussais: The Rivalry

To a certain extent, the work of Laennec and Broussais represents a dialogue between formidable minds: each publication is a response to criticisms of the opponent. Laennec reworked, rethought, and revised his ideas in answer to Broussais's criticisms. He too made provocative insults. Broussais and Laennec brought out the worst in each other. If Broussais was scandalous, Laennec became ridiculous. By adopting awkward, nuanced positions, Laennec paid a price, in his immediate popularity, his health, and his work.

Many years before Broussais wrote his first book, Laennec had opposed the reduction of all disease to lesions of the digestive tract. In 1802–3, he had published a lengthy article on peritonitis, in which he questioned its relationship to intestinal disturbances.[32] Two years later, he had reviewed Prost's book on gastro-intestinal ulcers, criticizing the work for incoherence, neglect of prior authors, and theoretical assumptions:

> We must be grateful to M. Prost for drawing our attention to the great frequency of these alterations of mucous membranes in acute disease, especially fevers, but ... he ought to have limited his observations to noticing the frequent coincidence of the occurrence of these lesions of the intestinal mucosa with the existence of diverse diseases, without insisting on perceiving one as cause and the other as effect: proof of this association requires much longer and more careful observation.... One should never hasten to publish a scientific work, especially when one proposes to give it the pompous title of *Medicine*, enlightened by the opening of bodies.[33]

Four years later, Broussais's *Histoires des phlegmasies* supported and extrapolated on Prost where Laennec had criticized.[34] Rouxeau maintained that as early as 1808, Laennec recognized Broussais's debt to Prost and immediately rejected what he would later call the 'imprecise' notion, in this 'otherwise estimable' treatise, that inflammation could cause tubercles.[35]

In 1812, Laennec wrote an article on pathological anatomy for the new *Dictionnaire des sciences médicales (DSM)*.[36] He presented a classification of organic lesions, rather than diseases, based on a system involving previously unrecognized distinctions, which he had recognized while still a student.[37] Immediately following Laennec's article was an essay by Bayle concerning the methodological problems in identifying diseases solely on the basis of organic lesions.[38] Neither cited Broussais; neither named inflammation or irritation as a cause of organic change.

In the 1816 *Examen*, Broussais attacked Bayle, who had only just died, with a section entitled, 'M. Bayle n'a pas tout vu!' He criticized Bayle's six-fold classification of tuberculosis, because Bayle failed to mention that all types were caused by irritation and inflammation.[39] Broussais proclaimed himself the first to notice the failings of nosology and to promote localization of disease in organic lesions. Perhaps he had forgotten, or did not like to remember, that fourteen years earlier, Bayle had already challenged Pinel on these points, while Broussais was preparing his own 'Pinelian' thesis.[40]

Laennec did not object to the localism in the *Examen*, but he disapproved of the poor pathological anatomy and deplored the slights on Bayle. Broussais used the terms 'inflammation' and 'irritation' to express pathophysiological notions. At the same time, Laennec was laboriously refining the meaning of these words in the histological sense. 'Inflammation' for Laennec was becoming a well-defined pathological name; Broussais was invoking it for other purposes. The insults directed against his dead friend piqued Laennec, especially since, in his view, Broussais's much-touted localism was a debt owed to Bayle. Not only had Bayle seen and described local changes first, but he had described them better: his pathological anatomy had been more careful, more descriptive, and less simplistic.

In 1818, the editor of the *DSM* invited Broussais to write entries on 'irritation' and 'inflammation'. In protest, Laennec led a mass exodus from the cooperative editorial group, taking with him other important contributors, including Alard, Bouvenot, Cayol, Geoffroy, Guibert, Kergaradęc, Landré-Beauvais, Lullier-Winslow, Moutron, and Pétroz.[41]

Shortly after this resignation, Laennec published his treatise on auscultation. Without naming his adversary, he alluded to a clinical disagreement with Broussais. He also defended Bayle against the attacks of 'a doctor whose opinions appear to me to be poorly grounded only in that they are too general and exclusive'. He continued:

> No, without doubt, Bayle did not see everything, no one has that opportunity, but what he did see he saw very well and there are very few books with less to erase than his. One day, when the controversies incited by new ideas presented in too absolute a fashion have faded away, this doctor [Broussais] on calmly re-reading what he wrote, under the influence of necessary contradiction, will no doubt realize that he did not always keep himself within acceptable limits ... and, with me, will recognize [in

Bayle] a man of modest superiority ... who died without ever having inspired the slightest feeling of hate or aversion in anyone.[42]

One month after the publication of his book, Laennec retired to Brittany because of his poor health. He did not intend to return to Paris and the pressures of patients and teaching. In his native Brittany, he planned to cultivate his lands, study stethoscopic sound, paint, play music, and do a little clinical medicine. Even this retreat failed to bring peace with Broussais.

The second edition of the *Examen* appeared in 1821, accusing Laennec of condescension and of having plagiarized the notion of localization from *Histoires des phlegmasies*. Concerned over possible inadvertent influence, Laennec re-examined the earlier book and was reassured.[43] Nevertheless, Broussais's other criticisms did contain a degree of truth.

It was true that Laennec's anatomic descriptions were exceedingly long: the difficulty of their abundant adjectives and nuances exasperated his otherwise admiring translator, who boasted he had been able to shorten the text to half the original length with no loss of substance.[44] It was true, as Broussais claimed, that Laennec's loyal defence of Bayle was based not on the latter's work, but on his gentle personality and upright behaviour; Laennec too had been puzzling over some of Bayle's 'errors'.[45] It was true that Laennec often emphasized his stethoscope to the neglect of other modalities. It was also true that he had written little on therapy. Broussais's criticisms were expressed in immoderate language, but their validity was sufficient to 'irritate' Laennec.

In a letter to his uncle, Laennec reflected on the challenge Broussais offered and considered a return to Paris. His dismay mingled with delight that some of Broussais's intended insults could be taken as compliments:

> our new heretic ['hérésiarque'] Broussais ... pays me the honour of calling me the champion of Hippocratic, eclectic, and anatomic doctors. ... when I was a [student] journalist, I would have loved to skewer an author that offered me so much undefended flank and, although the taste for this activity has left me, although writing tires and agitates me, I smiled like a hunter who has just seen the coming hare.[46]

In the autumn of 1821, Laennec drafted a 66-page argument against Broussais, in the vain hope that it would appear in the *Bibliothèque médicale* early in 1822. He said,

> I didn't expect to be obliged to return to the medical 'carrière' for a combat. Nevertheless, it's unavoidable. M. Broussais provokes me without even knowing if I am still living or if his voice can reach a hermit lost in the rocks of Finistère. He defies me, he waits for me ... he addresses me by private name and collective name and in choosing me somehow as champion of doctors, who, like me, profess Hippocratic empiricism, that is enlightened by the observation of the living and the dead, by the relationship of facts and by the very reserved use of the inductive method.... Only an invalid could refuse to defend such a beautiful cause.[47]

Laennec seems to have abandoned his Breton retreat to defend his work from the onslaught of Broussais. He took the intended insult of 'eclecticism' and conspicuously allowed it to become the name of his own medical doctrine.[48] In engineering his return to the city, Broussais had unwittingly brought about the very circumstances which led to his rival's greatest honours: the Chair of medicine at the Collège de France, professorship at the Faculty, membership in the Paris Académie de Médecine, and the Légion d'honneur. These awards, given mostly as royalist favours, had the satisfying effect of angering Broussais even more.[49] Laennec's lectures and clinics were attended by many English students; Broussais was anti-English. This was further fuel to his anti-Laennec, anti-jesuit, anti-royalist fire. Braunstein and Valentin have vividly portrayed the vicious circle: the more Broussais was ostracized, the more violent he became.[50] The more he attacked, the more Laennec resisted, relishing the privileges that so annoyed Broussais.

Biographers have taken pains to show that Laennec was polite and kept his insults within the bounds of professional decorum.[51] These judgements notwithstanding, Laennec did indulge in verbal Broussais-baiting, the scope of which may never be known because, like the manuscript 'Réponse aux attaques', it did not fully appear in print. The Collège de France provided an ideal platform for the counter-attack. In his inaugural address of December 1822, Laennec deliberately compared Broussais to Paracelsus.[52] Some people attended the lectures only to hear the snide remarks against Broussais and his followers. A contemporary left this description:

> He [Laennec] began by reading the subject for the day, but often digressed, to make observations, to recount a few original anecdotes, to strike a few blows at, or knock a few edges off the physiological doctrine [of Broussais], which he debated in name ....

The assembly would greet these piquant shafts with a smile.[53]

Manuscript notes for four years of lectures have been preserved. They address all aspects of medicine, including psychiatric disorders and even gastroenteritis. At least a third of the lessons refer to Broussais and his physiological doctrine, lending credibility to his claim that friends had urged him to sue Laennec for defamation.[54]

Laennec's 1826 second edition of the *Treatise on Auscultation* answered Broussais. It began with a railing preface containing some of the material written in 'response to attacks',[55] but the later chapters show Broussais's specific criticisms were taken quite seriously. Complaints made in the second edition of the *Examen* about the first edition of the *Treatise on Auscultation* provoked additions and/or modifications in Laennec's later work.

Broussais had said that Laennec overemphasized the stethoscope; Laennec reorganized his treatise from one centred on auscultation to one based on chest diseases. Broussais had observed that Laennec did not address hydrops of the heart; Laennec added a section on hydrops with three case reports.[56] Broussais had ridiculed Laennec's imprecision about the heart sounds; Laennec removed the passages where he had equivocated and changed passages on heart murmurs in a fashion that has, more recently, been judged as 'retrograde'.[57] Broussais had scorned the ancient notions of coction and crisis and Laennec's retention of them; Laennec accused Broussais of plagiarizing Hippocrates and set about proving the utility of the ancient theories of coction and crisis by the new method of statistics.[58] Broussais had complained that the stethoscope (and its inventor) had done nothing for therapeutics; Laennec extolled the virtues of the antimonial drug, tartar emetic, in the treatment of pneumonia.[59] Did he turn his attention to this controversial remedy, because Broussais had accused him of therapeutic nihilism? It seems entirely possible.

Laennec died in 1826, shortly after the completion of his second edition. Broussais continued to repeat the old accusations with the new insinuation that his rival had died of his own ignorance.[60] He noticed the changes that Laennec seemed to have made in answer to his criticisms, and he complained that he had not been acknowledged for his useful suggestions.[61] He criticized the use of high-dose tartar emetic and recognized the absurd postures Laennec adopted in order to refute the physiological doctrine of irritation and inflammation.[62]

In becoming the sworn enemy of Broussais's irritation, Laennec had also become the enemy of inflammation as a cause of organic change. The result was a refusal to admit that inflammation could ever constitute an independent, causal mechanism. His explanations of disease became increasingly convoluted, as he strove to find an alternative organic association whenever inflammation became a possible candidate for causative process. This process is exemplified by his stance on the relationship between inflammation and tuberculosis. Laennec maintained that inflammation was never associated with tubercle, except as a secondary change.[63] He recognized pleurisy as an inflammatory condition, but (because it was inflammatory) said it had nothing to do with tuberculosis. Yet, pleurisy and pleural effusions occur frequently in tuberculosis. Laennec would have been offered many occasions to make the connection, which he seemed to resist. Broussais noticed. He said Laennec had cultivated a 'vicious habit' of elaborating 'specious' hypotheses designed to refute the possible influence of irritation and inflammation on the production of disease.[64]

Laennec and Broussais: Agreement

Despite their polemic, Laennec and Broussais often agreed, although they admitted it only grudgingly. Broussais used and praised the stethoscope. Laennec diagnosed gastroenteritis and used leeches more frequently than his biographers tend to admit. They both objected to the thesis of Bayle's nephew, Antoine-Laurent Bayle, who had linked the neurological condition called general paresis, to syphilitic inflammation of the meninges: Broussais, because irritation, not inflammation, was the cause;[65] Laennec, because inflammation could never be a cause.[66] Neither wanted to preserve Pinel's nosography, but they respected his work as an 'aliéniste' and embraced the notion of moral treatment, with a few modifications: Broussais would have added leeches; Laennec, a straitjacket.[67]

Evidence for qualified admiration can be found in their writings. Broussais said, 'I am far from disdaining M. Laennec. As a result, I will attack him very vigorously in the best interests of science and humanity';[68] and Laennec, 'I have the highest regard for the talent of M. Broussais in spite of all that I will say concerning his mistakes and his manner of presenting his ideas and attacking his opponents'.[69]

Their most important conceptual agreement, however, was on the limitations of pathological anatomy. Elsewhere, I have suggested that one reason for Laennec's unpopularity was his failure to jump on the band-wagon of 'organicism', a movement which sought to link all diseases to internal organic changes.[70] Laennec's stethoscope was an impetus to organicism, but it seemed to the new organicists that its inventor was peculiarly resistant to the logical extrapolation of his own discoveries. He viewed organicism as overly reductionist: many well-defined conditions simply did not have equally well-defined organic changes associated with them. He cited epilepsy, gout, angina, asthma and generalized fevers.

Broussais was opposed to the pathologists' preoccupation with the dead subject and their wordy descriptions, which had little to do with the living patient or with the pathogenesis of the lesions. Like Laennec, he was not an organicist, although he appeared to support a simplified version of their theory.[71] For him, pathogenesis, that is an abnormal physiological process, not the structural lesion, was the disease. Treatment had to be directed against the physiological process, not against the organic lesions secondary to it.

Broussais may have held a narrow view of lesions, but he did have a point. With his accusations, he evoked the intriguing problems of the unexplained causes of disease, their mysterious link with lesions and symptoms, and the uncertain ways in which to treat. To explode the theories of Broussais one required a better theory, capable of dealing with these unexplained problems. And that was precisely what was lacking.

In his own attempts to explain that which Broussais had shown needed explaining, Laennec could not do much better: he retained the ancient notion of a 'vital force'. The certain limitations of pathological anatomy had been brought to his attention by Bayle. As students, they had wondered how to explain fatal diseases that did not seem to

Figure 2
Laennec's 'doctrine'

The body has three components: solid (organs), liquids, and vital principle. Each can be altered to produce disease.

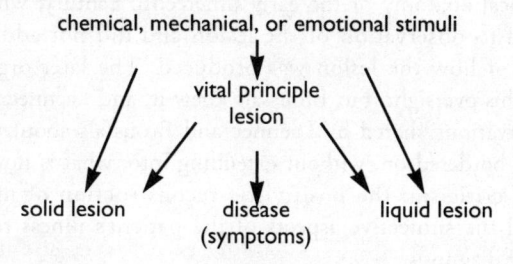

chemical, mechanical, or emotional stimuli

vital principle
lesion

solid lesion   disease   liquid lesion
                (symptoms)

be associated with any organic change. At first, the limitations did not dominate Laennec's thinking, nor did they enter into his conceptualization of disease; he concentrated on the solid ground of pathological anatomy. Years later, however, when he taught at the Collège de France, he was faced with defining diseases, not lesions. The old limitations became more apparent. To speak of all diseases, Laennec wished to retain the utility of pathological anatomy, without ignoring other unknown causes and effects. In his own view, 'vital principle' was the most neutral term to address the 'physiological sympathies' defined by Broussais (Figure 2; previous page).

Broussais had couched his concerns in jargon borrowed from pathology. Unable to use pathological terminology loosely, Laennec expressed his reservations in traditional, vitalistic words, borrowed from Hippocrates and Montpellier, via Bayle, and rendered scientific by chemistry, physics, and the experimental work of Magendie. Had he chosen his words deliberately to 'irritate' his enemy, the effect could not have been greater. Broussais said that Laennec was 'small and nasty in his theory just like he was in person'.[72]

Broussais noticed Laennec's concern about the over-emphasis of organic change and flattered himself that these ideas had been taken from his own physiological doctrine. He failed, however, to perceive their significance in Laennec's approach. Inaccurately reducing Laennec's method to a 'complete subjugation of medicine' to a nosology based on pathological anatomy, he portrayed Laennec as possessed of an extreme 'medical materialism', which he found impossible to reconcile with his apparent 'religious spiritualism'.[73] What Broussais mistook for 'religious spiritualism', or 'poorly defined notions of nervous influence', was Laennec's own version of the physiological doctrine.[74]

The words 'irritation' and 'sympathy' of Broussais dealt with the same notions as the altered 'principe vital' of Laennec: pathogenesis. Knowledge of pathogenesis was beyond the newly endorsed pathological anatomy of the early nineteenth century, which was restricted to observation of the lesion and did not address the problem of how the lesion was produced. The later organicists ignored this oversight, but Broussais knew it, and Laennec did too. The reservations shared by Laennec and Broussais about the new medicine bordered on, without extending into, what is now a new realm of criticism: the positivistic reconstruction of medicine distanced the subjective aspects of the patient's illness from the process of diagnosis.

Since Laennec's ideas about the vital principle were not

published, they have enjoyed the comparative advantage of historical invisibility. In his lifetime, however, these so-called 'errors' were known and ridiculed by contemporaries. The explanations appeared to be spiritual natterings, typical of a royalist-jesuit-opportunist with an exaggerated notion of the importance of his invention. How could a man of science continue to use such terms and expect to be taken seriously? Gabriel Andral (1797–1876) described Laennec's stance as a 'paradoxical' retreat from his own achievements.[75] Since Laennec was a practising Catholic, it was easy to place his vitalism with the retrograde 'theological' or 'metaphysical' categories in Comte's vision of knowledge, an indictment spared Broussais's physiological doctrine when Comte himself had declared 'irritation' to be 'positive'.[76] Broussais seemed to know what would happen:

> In spite of all his faults, the name of Laennec will remain in science and be honourable for his homeland. What he has done will be used to advantage and his mistakes, for which he will no longer be chastised, will fall into oblivion.[77]

Conclusion

According to sociologists of science, competition has both positive and negative implications. It encourages risk-taking and enthusiasm; however, intermediate failure can discourage future work, and lead to secrecy, precipitous publication, and 'deviant' behaviour, such as plagiarism or, more commonly, accusations of plagiarism.[78] Only a few case studies of scientific competition are taken from biological or medical sciences.[79] Most have focused on institutional, professional, or individual rivalry. In the latter category, priority disputes and closure have been given the greatest attention probably because they can be taken to signify 'discovery', sometimes even the violation and/or reconstruction of scientific norms that identifies a Kuhnian revolution. But closure does not always occur and individuals can compete for outcomes other than priority, especially in the more common situation when their research might eventually lead to the same discovery, but has not yet done so. In that case, they compete for the expression of the goal of their research – or, in other words, for the best description of the problem that motivates their investigations. A scientific fight that is neither institutional, nor personal, dwells within the conceptual heart of a matter; each opponent may be making plausible statements that the other is reluctant to admit. As a result, analysis of a seemingly social phenomenon might elucidate a philosophical problem.[80]

The rivalry of Laennec and Broussais displayed some sociological features of scientific competition, including precipitous publication and mutual accusations of plagiarism. Recognition of the conventional aspects of their competitive behaviour might be taken as further evidence of their common purpose. Did their competition stimulate other research? What would have happened to Laennec's reputation and to medical science if he had stayed home in Brittany in 1822? How did Broussais influence auscultation and the success of the anatomo-clinical method? What did Laennec accomplish with his return?

Had Laennec stayed home medical science would not have 'suffered': the most important auscultatory discoveries had already been made and the instrument was in the hands of enough dedicated users that its survival was assured. His last years of hard work were disappointing; in some areas, he seemed to move 'backward', rejecting some of his initial discoveries, such as heart murmurs, which were later to be revived by others. Had he not accepted the position at the Collège de France, he might even have avoided scorn for accepting royalist favours and for exposing his apparently metaphysical ideas.

Laennec's return produced the Collège de France manuscripts, which explicate his unpopular conception of disease. Aside from the light they shed on the conceptual dilemmas of his age, they reveal the dialogue Laennec conducted with himself and his opponents, as he sought an accord between clinical observations and the body of information that he recognized as medical science. In that sense, these papers permit the present 'rapprochement' of his thought with that of his arch-rival, whose constant goading was the ultimate reason they were written.

In the many differences between Laennec and Broussais, the common factor appears to be semantic. They tacitly agreed on a paradigm concerning the problems, as well as the advantages, of anatomic localization. They tried to draw attention to the aspects of disease that would continue to defy explanation by the anatomo-clinical method. Michel Foucault claimed the new method had resulted in a reorganization of medical discourse and characterized the clinical gaze as 'the paradoxical ability to hear a language as soon as it perceives a spectacle'.[81] However, the nascent clinic was still devoid of acceptable norms or terms with which to frame any seemingly threatening criticisms.

Thus, in an intellectual form of sociological 'anomie', Laennec and Broussais strove toward a common goal within a conceptual environment that favoured reduction and materialism and tolerated neither the preservation of ancient terms nor the creation of neologisms devoid of organic correlatives.[82] They chose radically different means to accomplish their task and barely succeeded in defining the problem in two different vocabularies that reflected their personal, political, and intellectual biases.[83] Neither definition survived, but they did manage to defeat each other's language.[84] When the dust settled, there emerged a calm, less prolix, medical community, purged, thanks to Broussais, of the words 'vital principle', 'crisis', and 'Hippocratism', but also free of the terms 'irritation' and 'sympathy' and wary of the expression 'gastroenteritis', thanks to Laennec.

Notes

I am grateful to Toby Gelfand, Mirko Drazen Grmek, Olga Kits, and Robert David Wolfe for their helpful comments on earlier versions of this chapter, which emerges from my book, *To See With A Better Eye: A Life of R.T.H. Laennec* (Princeton, New Jersey: Princeton University Press, 1998).

1. Erwin H. Ackerknecht, 'Broussais, or a Forgotten Medical Revolution', *Bulletin of the History of Medicine* 27 (1953): 320–43; Erwin H. Ackerknecht, *Medicine at the Paris Hospital, 1794–1848* (Baltimore: Johns Hopkins Press, 1967), 61–80; Erwin H. Ackerknecht, 'Laennec and Broussais', *Revue du Palais de la Découverte* no. spécial 22 (1981): 208–12; Alfred Rouxeau, *Laennec* [1912 and 1920], facsimile, 2 vols (Quimper: Editions de Cornouaille, 1978), 2: 315–41; Michel Valentin, *François Broussais, empereur de la médecine: jeunesse, correspondence, vie et oeuvre* (Cesson-Sévingé: Association des Amis du Musée du Pays de Dinard, 1988), 196–204; Henry E. Sigerist, *The Great Doctors* [1933] (Garden City, NY: Doubleday, 1958), 267–74.
2. George Weisz, 'The Posthumous Laennec: Creating a Modern Medical Hero, 1826–1870', *Bulletin of the History of Medicine* 61 (1987): 541–62. J. B. Bouillaud considered Laennec as 'la plus grande illustration médicale de son époch', after Broussais. Jean-Baptiste Bouillaud, *Essai sur la philosophie médicale et sur les généralités de la clinique médicale* (Paris: Rouvier et Bouvier, 1836), 87.
3. Erwin H. Ackerknecht, 'Elisha Bartlett and the Philosophy of the Paris Clinical School', *Bulletin of the History of Medicine* 24 (1950): 43–60, esp. 53.

4. Jean-François Braunstein, *Broussais et le matérialisme: médecine et philosophie au XIXe siècle* (Paris: Meridiens Klincksieck, 1986); Michel Foucault, *The Birth of the Clinic: An Archeology of Medical Perception* [1963], trans. A. M. Sheridan (London: Tavistock, 1973), 184–92.
5. 'Few historians do anything so vulgar as to advance an explanation': Steven Shapin, 'History of Science and Its Sociological Reconstructions', *History of Science* 20 (1982): 157–211, esp. 196.
6. Stanley Joel Reiser, *Medicine and the Reign of Technology* (Cambridge and New York: Cambridge University Press, 1979), 29–30; Russell C. Maulitz, *Morbid Appearances: The Anatomy of Pathology in the Early Nineteenth Century* (Cambridge: Cambridge University Press, 1987), 97–105; Ackerknecht, *Paris Hospital*, 88–99.
7. R. T. H. Laennec, *De l'auscultation médiate ou traité du diagnostique des poumons et du coeur*, 2 vols (Paris: Brosson and Chaudé, 1819).
8. Forbes, in R. T. H. Laennec, *A Treatise on the Diseases of the Chest*, trans. John Forbes (London: Underwood, 1821; facsimile New York: Hafner and the New York Academy of Medicine, 1962), ix–x, xxvi.
9. R. T. H. Laennec, *Traité de l'auscultation médiate et des maladies des poumons et du coeur*, 2nd edn, 2 vols (Paris: Chaudé, 1826).
10. Jacalyn Duffin, 'Unity, Duality, Passion, and Cure: Laennec's Conceptualisation of Tuberculosis', in Danielle Gourevitch (ed.), *Maladie et maladies, histoire et conceptualisation: Mélanges en l'honneur de Mirko Grmek* (Geneva: Droz, 1992), 255–71.
11. Léon Bernard, cited in Henri Duclos, *Laennec* (Paris: Flammarion, 1932), 11–12; Ackerknecht, *Paris Hospital*, 88.
12. Braunstein, *Broussais*, 15–16, 192–5; Valentin, *Broussais*, 119–40, 201–3.
13. F. J. V. Broussais, *Histoires des phlegmasies ou inflammations chroniques*, 2 vols (Paris, 1808).
14. A. Prost, *La médecine éclairée par l'observation et l'ouverture des corps* (Paris: Demonville, 1804).
15. Insight of the late Pierre Huard, seminar, Ecole Pratique des Hautes Etudes, 1984. The frequency of typhoid and the use of arsenic therapy (hence arsenic poisoning) may also have added to an increased incidence of gastritis in the early nineteenth century, Ackerknecht, 'Broussais', 331–2; Braunstein, *Broussais*, 37–9. In 1795, writing about his war experiences, Broussais told his father 'les cadavres ne manquent point', cited in Valentin, *Broussais*, 114.
16. Auguste Comte, 'Examination of Broussais' Treatise on Irritation [1828]', in Frederick Harrison (ed.), *Early Essays on Social Philosophy*, trans. Henry Dix Hutton (London: Routledge, 1911), 333–52, esp. 337–8.
17. Ackerknecht, 'Elisha Bartlett'; Ackerknecht, *Paris Hospital*, 135;

Russell C. Maulitz, 'Channel Crossing: the Lure of French Pathology for English Medical Students', *Bulletin of the History of Medicine* 55 (1981): 475–96; John Harley Warner, 'The Selective Transport of Medical Knowledge: Antebellum Physicians and Parisian Medical Therapeutics', *Bulletin of the History of Medicine* 59 (1985): 213–31; idem, 'Remembering Paris: Memory and the American Disciples of French Medicine in the Nineteenth Century', *Bulletin of the History of Medicine* 65 (1991): 301–25; idem, *Against the Spirit of System: The French Impulse in Nineteenth-Century American Medicine* (Princeton, New Jersey: Princeton University Press, 1998).

18. Ackerknecht, *Paris Hospital*, 62; see also Matthew Ramsey, *Professional and Popular Medicine in France, 1770–1830* (Cambridge: Cambridge University Press, 1988), 48, 122.
19. Ackerknecht, 'Broussais'; Sigerist, *Great Doctors*, 273.
20. Broussais claimed he lost only one in every thirty patients, but the Val de Grâce Hospital statistics revealed the death rate to be one in twelve. François-Joseph-Victor Broussais, *Examen des doctrines médicales et des systèmes de nosologie*, 2nd edn, 2 vols (Paris: Méquignon-Marvis, 1821), 2: 686, 700, *passim*; Laennec, *Auscultation*, 1819, 1: xxiin. See also Ackerknecht, 'Broussais', 326.
21. Notes on the lectures given by both Broussais and Laennec in 1823–4 by the American medical student, James Kitchen, are in the Archives of Hahnemann Medical College, Philadelphia. On Laennec's lectures, see n. 54 below.
22. Preoccupied with Broussais's 'brutalité', Rouxeau collected a large number of these insults, *Laennec*, 2: 324, 339–40.
23. Attacks on the 'fatalism' of pathological anatomy flowed into specific criticisms of Laennec. Broussais, *Examen*, 2nd edn, 1821, 2: 672–761, esp. 701–61; Braunstein, *Broussais*, 40–3.
24. François-Joseph-Victor Broussais, *Examen des doctrines médicales*, 3rd edn, 4 vols (Paris and Brussels: Delaunay, Librairie médicale française, 1829–34), 4: 141–335.
25. Broussais, *Examen*, 3rd edn, 1834, 4: 163, 251.
26. Maurice Genty, 'Le cerveau de Dupuytren', *Progrès médicale*, 1935, supplement 2: 16; François-Joseph-Victor Broussais, *De l'irritation et de la folie* (Brussels: Dr K. Comet, 1828); Valentin, *Broussais*, 255–68.
27. John E. Lesch, *Science and Medicine in France: The Emergence of Experimental Physiology, 1790–1855* (Cambridge, Mass. and London: Harvard University Press, 1984), 160–1. Other opponents of Broussais's reductionism included Thomas Hodgkin and Elisha Bartlett. Maulitz, *Morbid Appearances*, 205; Ackerknecht, 'Elisha

Bartlett'.
28. Ackerknecht, 'Broussais', 33; Foucault, *Birth of the Clinic*, 192.
29. Ackerknecht and Lesch both suggested that Magendie's attack in 1820 was against Broussais, but it could have been aimed at the armchair physiologists of the eighteenth century. Braunstein, *Broussais*, 60–1; Ackerknecht, 'Broussais', 333; Lesch, *Science and Medicine*, 160–1. Magendie criticized Laennec's cardiology at the Collège de France and in print. François Magendie, 'Mémoire sur l'origine des bruits normaux du coeur' [read 3 February 1834] *Mémoires de l'Académie Royale des Sciences* 14 (1838): 154–84, esp. 158, 162.
30. Bouillaud, *Essai*, 87–93; Foucault, *Birth of the Clinic*, 192.
31. Claude-François-Herman Pidoux, cited in *Bulletin de l'Académie Impériale de Médecine* 32 (1866–7): 1278 and in A. Lecadre, *Etude comparative: Laennec et Broussais* (Le Havre: Le Pelletier, 1868), 19.
32. R. T. H. Laennec, 'Histoires d'inflammation du péritoine recueilles à la clinique interne de l'école de médecine de Paris sous les yeux des professeurs Corvisart et J. J. Leroux', *Journal de médecine* 4 (An X [1802]): 499–547 and 5 (An XI [1803]): 3–59.
33. R. T. H. Laennec, 'Analyse de *La médecine éclairée par l'ouverture des corps*, par P. A. Prost', *Journal de médecine* 8 (An XII [1804]): 260–72, esp. 266, 271. Unless otherwise indicated, all translations are my own.
34. Broussais's *Histoires des phlegmasies*, 1808, was a collection of case observations (all diagnosed gastroenteritis) gathered during his army service.
35. Rouxeau, *Laennec*, 2: 316; Laennec, *Auscultation*, 1819, 1: 167n.
36. R. T. H. Laennec, 'Anatomie pathologique', in C. L. F. Panckoucke (ed.), *Dictionnaire des sciences médicales*, 60 vols (Paris: Panckoucke, 1812–22), 2 (1812): 46–61.
37. Laennec was accused of plagiarism by Guillaume Dupuytren. See Maulitz, *Morbid Appearances*, 73–8.
38. Gaspard-Laurent Bayle, 'Considerations sur l'anatomie pathologique' in *DSM*, 2 (1812): 61–78.
39. Broussais had been referring to Bayle's *Recherches sur la phthisie pulmonaire* (Paris: Gabon, 1810). He repeated the same criticism in the second edition of the *Examen*, 1821, 2: 715–6. See also Valentin, *Broussais*, 185–7.
40. During the defence of his thesis before Pinel himself, Bayle praised symptom-based nosology, but argued for organic-based pathology. The dialogue was preserved by Laennec who kept a shorthand record of the defence. Parts of G. L. Bayle's defence were reproduced in Antoine-Laurent-Jesse Bayle and Auguste Thillaye, *Biographie*

médicale par ordre chronologique, 2 vols (Paris: Delahaye, 1855), 2: 884–99.
41. Rouxeau, *Laennec*, 2: 318–9.
42. Laennec, *Auscultation*, 1819, 2: 114. For other references to Broussais including an error in consultation, see Rouxeau, *Laennec*, 2: 317–20. The case records also reveal their rivalry, when Laennec and Broussais shared patients. See manuscript records of Louise Boisot, Nantes MS Cl. III, ff. 156r–158r; Athanase Vorogides, Nantes MS Cl. 1, lot j [X], f. 245v–246v. On the Laennec papers, see Lydie Boulle, Mirko D. Grmek, Catherine Lupovici and Janine Samion-Contet, *Laennec: catalogue des manuscrits scientifiques* (Paris: Masson, 1982).
43. Rouxeau, *Laennec*, 2: 325.
44. John Forbes, 'Translator's Preface', in Laennec, *A Treatise on the Diseases of the Chest*, x, xxv–xxvi.
45. Laennec, *Auscultation*, 1819, 1: 20–1, 36, 310–11.
46. Laennec, letter to his uncle Guillaume Laennec, 16 October 1821, cited in Rouxeau, *Laennec*, 2: 325–6.
47. Laennec, cited in Rouxeau, *Laennec*, 2: 326. See also Laennec, 'Matériaux d'une réponse aux attaques de Broussais', Nantes MS Cl. 7, lot d [A], ff. 1–56.
48. Braunstein, *Broussais*, 102–9; Jacalyn M. Duffin, 'The Medical Philosophy of R. T. H. Laennec', *History and Philosophy of the Life Sciences* 8 (1986): 195–219, esp. 209–10n.
49. Braunstein, *Broussais*, 190–2; Rouxeau, *Laennec*, 2: 341–57.
50. Braunstein, *Broussais*, 185; Valentin, *Broussais*, 198–203.
51. For example, 'au moins sait-il toujours garder … la correction du *gentleman* qu'il restera jusqu'à sa dernière heure', Rouxeau, *Laennec*, 2: 338. 'Laennec resta courtois et ferme', Duclos, *Laennec*, 253.
52. The first lecture was published. R. T. H. Laennec, 'Extraits du discours prononcé par M. Laennec à l'ouverture de son cours de médecine au Collège de France', *Archives générales de médecine* 1 (1823): v–xx.
53. Lecadre, cited in Rouxeau, *Laennec*, 2: 307.
54. Broussais, *Examen*, 3rd edn, 1834, 149n. Laennec's Collège de France lecture notes are divided in two parts and held in two archives: Bibliothèque interuniversitaire de médecine, Paris, and the Musée Laennec, Nantes. For a detailed guide, see Boulle *et al.*, *Catalogue*.
55. Laennec, *Auscultation*, 2nd edn, 1826, 1: xx–xxii.
56. Broussais, *Examen*, 2nd edn, 1821, 2: 739; Laennec, *Auscultation*, 2nd edn, 1826, 2: 228–32.
57. Broussais, *Examen*, 2nd edn, 1821, 2: 751; Jacalyn M. Duffin, 'The Cardiology of R. T. H. Laennec', *Medical History* 33 (1989): 42–71.

Roger Rullière, 'Laennec cardiologue: le bon grain et l'ivraie', *Revue du Palais de la Découverte*, 1981, special no. 22: 130–7.

58. Broussais, *Examen*, 2nd edn, 1821, 1: 6–39; Laennec, *Auscultation*, 2nd edn, 1826, 1: xxix–xxxn; Jacalyn Duffin, 'L'Hippocrate de Laennec repris; la fièvre à l'ombre de l'anatomie pathologique', in Paul Potter, Gilles Maloney, and Jacques Desautels (eds), *La Maladie et les maladies dans la Collection hippocratique. Actes du VIe Colloque International Hippocratique* (Québec, Québec: Sphinx, 1990), 433–61.
59. Broussais, *Examen*, 2nd edn, 1821, 2: 710, 717; Laennec, *Auscultation*, 2nd edn, 1826, 1: 492–516; Rouxeau, *Laennec*, 2: 324.
60. Broussais, *Examen*, 3rd edn, 1834, 4: 163, 251.
61. Broussais, *Examen*, 3rd edn, 1834, 4: 160–2, 189.
62. Broussais, *Examen*, 3rd edn, 1834, 4: 165, 171, 176, 185, 189–90. Broussais also recognized Laennec's tendency to relate each disease to one stethoscopic sound and vice versa. *Examen*, 3rd edn, 1834, 4: 169–75.
63. Laennec, *Auscultation*, 1819, 1: 31–2; *Auscultation*, 2nd edn, 1826, 1: 562–80.
64. Broussais, *Examen*, 3rd edn, 1834, 4: 151, 214–18.
65. A. L. Bayle, 'Recherches sur les maladies mentales', thèse de médecine (Paris no. 247, 1822); F. J. V. Broussais, *De l'irritation et de la folie*, 2nd edn, 2 vols (Paris: Baillière, 1839), 2: 333–43, esp. 413–14. See also Braunstein, *Broussais*, 49, 52.
66. See Laennec's notes for his Collège de France lecture 8, 1823–4, on 'vesania' and his annotation, 'lésions organiques rapport du prix Esquirol', Nantes MS Cl. 2 lot a (B), ff.174, 183r–v; Laennec, *Auscultation*, 2nd edn, 1826, 2: 528–9n. On the Prix Esquirol see Jan Goldstein, *Console and Classify: The French Psychiatric Profession in the Nineteenth Century* (Cambridge: Cambridge University Press, 1987), 140–1, 253.
67. Broussais, *Irritation*, 2: 504–6, *passim*; Laennec, 'si obligé de lier avec la camisole ne pas hâter de rendre à la société'. Laennec, Nantes MS Cl. 2 lot a (B), 181v; Braunstein, *Broussais*, 45–52, 77–81.
68. Broussais, *Examen*, 2nd edn, 1821, 2: 716.
69. Laennec, cited in Rouxeau, *Laennec*, 2: 326.
70. Jacalyn Duffin, 'Vitalism and Organicism in the Philosophy of R. T. H. Laennec', *Bulletin of the History of Medicine* 62 (1988): 525–45.
71. Braunstein, *Broussais*, 244–7.
72. Broussais, *Examen*, 3rd edn, 1834, 4: 334.
73. Broussais, *Examen*, 3rd edn, 1834, 4: 142.
74. Linking theology and vitalism, Broussais said that all the forces of the

Montpellier doctors were 'petites divinités'. He was slightly more tolerant of Gall's use of 'lésions vitales', but maintained it was simply an out-dated way of expressing irritation. Broussais, *Irritation*, 2: 424–5, 433n.

75. Gabriel Andral in the 'Preface', to his edition of R. T. H. Laennec, *Traité de l'auscultation médiate et des maladies des poumons et du coeur*, 4th edn, 3 vols (Paris: Chaudé, 1837), 1: viii.
76. Comte, 'Examination'; Braunstein, *Broussais*, 203–26.
77. Broussais, *Examen*, 3rd edn, 1834, 4: 334–5.
78. Jerry Gaston, *Originality and Competition in Science: A Study of the British High Energy Physics Community* (Chicago and London: University of Chicago Press, 1973), 69–77; Warren O. Hagstrom, *The Scientific Community* (New York: Basic Books, 1965), 85–98; Robert K. Merton, *The Sociology of Science* (Chicago and London: University of Chicago Press, 1973), 283–4.
79. Exceptions include John Farley and Gerald Geison, 'Science, Politics, and Spontaneous Generation in Nineteenth-Century France', *Bulletin of the History of Medicine* 48 (1974): 161–98; Mirko D. Grmek, *History of AIDS*, trans. Russell C. Maulitz and Jacalyn Duffin (Princeton, New Jersey: Princeton University Press, 1990), 60–77; David Harley, 'Honour and Property: the Structure of Professional Disputes in Eighteenth-Century English Medicine', in Andrew Cunningham and Roger French (eds), *The Medical Enlightenment of the Eighteenth Century* (Cambridge: Cambridge University Press, 1990), 138–64; Paul Cranefield, *The Way In and the Way Out* (Mount Kisco, New York: Futura, 1974), 44–54; Elizabeth Labrousse and Alfred Soman, 'La querelle de l'antimoine: Guy Patin sur la sellette', *Histoire, économie et société* 5 (1986): 31–45.
80. On the need for (and obstacles to) reconciliation between philosophical and sociological studies of cognitive aspects of science see Nico Stehr, 'Robert K. Merton's Sociology of Science', in Jon Clark, Celia Modgil, and Sohan Modgil (eds), *Robert K. Merton: Controversy and Consensus* (London, New York, Philadelphia: Falmer Press, 1990), 285–94.
81. Foucault, *Birth of the Clinic*, xix, 108.
82. The much-discussed term, anomie, has been used to describe a multitude of settings, both cognitive and social, desirable and undesirable, by a host of authors from Thucydides to Merton. I use it here to designate an unintended, social and cognitive result of the adoption of anatomo-clinical medicine, a state of 'normlessness' with respect to discourse and the possibilities of discourse concerning the failings of the new method. Laennec and Broussais both tried to

criticize, but the lack of acceptable terms (norms) for the expression of criticism fostered their 'deviant' behaviour. On anomie, see Marco Orrù, *Anomie: History and Meanings* (Boston: Allen and Unwin, 1987); *idem*, 'Merton's Instrumental Theory of Anomie', in Jon Clark *et al.* (eds), *Robert K. Merton*, 231–40.

83. On the relationship between language and science see Karin D. Knorr-Cetina, *The Manufacture of Knowledge: An Essay on the Constructivist and Contextual Nature of Science* (Oxford, New York, Toronto: Pergamon, 1981), 49–67 and 94–135; Michael Mulkay, Jonathan Potter, and Steven Yearley, 'Why an Analysis of Scientific Discourse is Needed', in Karin D. Knorr-Cetina and Michael Mulkay (eds), *Science Observed: Perspectives on the Social Study of Science* (London, Beverly Hills, New Delhi: Sage, 1983), 171–203.

84. See also Braunstein on Broussais's 'anti-ontologisme', *Broussais*, 250–2.

7

Dichotomy or Integration? Medical Microscopy and the Paris Clinical Tradition[*]

Ann La Berge

French leadership in science and medicine was unchallenged in the first third of the nineteenth century. Paris was the scientific and medical capital of the Western world. By mid-century a major shift had occurred, and German pre-eminence in science and medicine was widely recognized, especially by French scientists. The standard interpretation of what happened to French medicine between 1830 and 1850 is well known. Erwin Ackerknecht has summed it up for us in a chapter in his book on Paris medicine entitled 'The Dead End' in which he suggested that by ostracizing physiology, chemistry, and microscopy 'French medicine had maneuvered itself into a dead end'. Thus Ackerknecht contended that by the 1840s the creativity and vitality of the Paris clinical school with its emphasis on observational hospital medicine, pathological anatomy, and medical statistics had worn itself out. In their overemphasis on the clinical approach and their failure to embrace laboratory medicine, specifically experimental physiology, chemistry, and microscopy, French clinicians and pathological anatomists had been shortsighted and narrowminded. One of the oft-cited examples of this was the reluctance of many French clinicians to adopt the microscope, in spite of the fact that, as Ackerknecht points out, 'France possessed a whole phalanx of outstanding microscopists'.[1]

At the outset we are confronted with an apparent contradiction. Why would French clinicians be reluctant to employ a new technique, given such available expertise? Ackerknecht suggested that the main problem was clinicians' conceit and conservatism.

---

[*] Many thanks to Caroline Hannaway, Joy Harvey, Muriel Lederman, and Doris Zallen for their comments on this and earlier drafts of this chapter.

And surely this is part of the explanation. But Ackerknecht had not studied the Parisian microscopy community or early French medical microscopy, nor did he attempt to examine the development of medical microscopy within the context of French clinical medicine. We should not accept uncritically the dichotomy that Ackerknecht has set up between clinical and laboratory medicine without looking at the role of microscopy within the Paris school.[2]

I will argue that although the Paris school did not embrace microscopy, neither did its leaders reject it. Some clinicians were apathetic, seeing microscopy as unrelated to their daily work. But many of the leading physicians used the microscope in their research and teaching, cooperated with microscopists by sending them specimens for pathological examination, and acknowledged the utility of the instrument in some areas of diagnosis even while questioning its use in others. By mid-century two principal points of view emerged: the clinical, which found its strength in dichotomy, and the microscopical, which emphasized integration. The clinical viewpoint juxtaposed clinical, that is, hospital-based, patient-oriented medicine with scientific or laboratory medicine (just as Ackerknecht did), French with German medicine, clinicians with microscopists. Proponents of the microscopical viewpoint urged the integration of microscopy into clinical medicine and pathological anatomy and the acceptance of microscopists as clinicians. The problem with such a neat categorization is the same as the problem with the clinical point of view: our categorization and clinicians' dichotomization do not accurately reflect the reality and complexity of Paris medicine. Understanding clinicians' dichotomies and why microscopists did not share them is, I believe, the key to understanding the relationship of medical microscopy to Paris clinical medicine.

Although scientists and amateurs had used the microscope since the seventeenth century, Parisian physicians did not employ the instrument for medical research until the 1830s. They were slow to adopt the microscope for several reasons. First, within the context of the dominant theories of disease causation in the eighteenth century, the humoral and environmental theories, the microscope seemed to contribute little to an understanding of disease. Second, a philosophy of radical empiricism which emphasized the use of the unaided senses in medical observation was predominant in the early era of Paris medicine. Xavier Bichat and René-Théophile Laennec, for example, rejected the microscope in both medical research and practice. Bichat saw it as interfering with naked-eye observation, the principal method of medical research. His objection reflected both the 'sensualist' point of view and the reality of the instrument's inadequacies when he said: 'Let us neglect all these idle questions where neither inspection nor experience can guide us. Let us begin to study anatomy there where the organs begin to fall into the range of our senses.'[3] For his part, Laennec rejected the use of the microscope in medical practice, because he believed the instrument would distract the physician from his most important task, which was patient observation and care.[4] In the first two decades of the nineteenth century Parisian physicians considered microscopical observation neither factual nor empirical, but illusory and imaginary, not the stuff of which science, as they understood it, was made.

A final reason why Parisian physicians rarely used microscopes in medical research and practice before the 1830s was that until the 1820s they were hard to make, hard to use, and expensive. Images were often blurred, and coloured fringes encircling the visual field distorted the image. Microscopy required considerable skill and training and a very delicate handling of specimens. Technical inadequacies posed problems for scientists (naturalists) as well as physicians. For example, before the 1820s (though actual details are lacking) most specimens were mounted dry. According to Brian Bracegirdle, a historian of microtechnique, with dry mounts not much detail is visible and such specimens have little resemblance to life. Scientific research, he concluded, was almost impossible for all but the most extremely skilled investigators until the techniques of wet mounts, fixing, and staining were developed.[5]

Technically superior microscopes became available in the 1820s, when microscopist Joseph Jackson Lister in England and instrument maker Charles Chevalier in France introduced compound achromatic microscopes in which the distortion factor was reduced from about 19 to 3 per cent, and in which the fringes of colour around the object being observed were removed.[6] Some French scientists began using the new microscopes in their research. Most notable was François Raspail, regarded as the father of histochemistry, who began to use Chevalier's new microscope, along with chemical analysis, to study plant tissue. Raspail, along with Chevalier and the naturalist A. C. M. Le Baillif, greatly improved techniques of specimen preparation. By 1830 they were mounting specimens in a fluid medium, and Chevalier introduced glass cover slips. By the 1830s better and cheaper instruments and new techniques of mounting specimens made microscopes more accessible as research tools.[7]

Historian of microscopy Brian Ford does not share the general consensus that technical superiority was the main factor in the increasing acceptance of microscopy after the 1820s. Instead, he argues that scientists and physicians embraced the new achromatic, compound microscopes for aesthetic, social, and professional reasons. He maintains that the simple microscopes were small and unattractive instruments, whereas the new microscopes were works of art. A principal factor in acceptance, he claims, was the prestige associated with the instrument. Compound microscopes were socially and professionally acceptable in a way that simple microscopes were not. Nor does Ford think that the simple microscope was as difficult to use and unreliable as some historians have claimed, and he argues that, in the hands of a skilled microscopist, it was a reliable scientific instrument. Ford's analysis may apply better to the British than the French situation. First, few French physicians were skilled microscopists. For them the instrument was hard to use. Second, although British instruments were fancy and expensive, by contrast, many of the French microscopes were inexpensive tools. There is no indication that Parisian physicians adopted the microscope because it lent prestige to either their practices or their research or that they embraced microscopy for aesthetic reasons.[8]

By the 1830s Paris medicine was changing. Although pathological anatomy, exemplified by the earlier work of Laennec, François Broussais and others and by the ongoing research of Jean Cruveilhier, remained a central focus of Paris medicine, physicians investigated new diagnostic approaches. The notion that one could dissect and analyze organs, tissues, and body fluids to find disease provided an atmosphere in which the microscope could become an important tool in the physician's research arsenal. One question that emerged was whether the microscope could extend and enrich pathological anatomy or whether it challenged that approach and its findings.[9] The microscope also reinforced a renewed interest in the causes of disease. Although early in the century Bichat and other researchers had abandoned the search for causes of disease, Broussais and his followers had recognized the need to return to the pursuit of disease causation. The microscope held out the possibility of identifying specific microorganisms that caused specific diseases and also of pinpointing more precisely the seat of disease.

A few Parisian physicians, such as Jean-Baptiste Bouillaud, Pierre Rayer, and Alfred Donné, began using the microscope in their research in the early 1830s. Donné undertook the microscopical analysis of body fluids; Rayer performed microscopical and chemical analysis of urine; and Bouillaud encouraged Donné and others in the use of the instrument, which he himself began to use as early as 1830. More widespread interest in medical microscopy dated from 1837, when a professor at the University of Brussels, Gottlieb Gluge, sent his microscopical work on tumours to the Academy of Sciences, and Donné began offering the first public microscopy course in Paris. Gluge's paper opened for the Parisian medical and scientific community a debate on tumours which lasted well into the 1850s and Donné's course made it possible for French and foreign physicians and medical students to learn to use the new technology. By the late 1830s François Magendie was using the instrument as a teaching tool in his physiology classes at the Collège de France, and Gabriel Andral and Jules Gavarret were analyzing blood with the microscope.[10] By the 1840s, in addition to Donné, there were three other microscopy teachers in Paris: a German, Hermann Lebert, and two Hungarians, David Gruby and Louis Mandl. In addition to their teaching, all were active in medical research. Together with the clinicians and surgeons with whom they collaborated and the students they taught, Donné, Lebert, Gruby, and Mandl formed the Parisian microscopy community and began to develop their own integrative point of view regarding the role of microscopy in Paris clinical medicine.[11]

From 1837 to the mid-1840s some physicians displayed widespread acceptance of and support for most applications of medical microscopy; for others, benign neglect prevailed. Leading physicians and surgeons, such as Velpeau, Rayer, Bouillaud, Andral, Magendie, studied and collaborated with Donné, Gruby, and Lebert and used the microscope in their teaching and research. Some who did not use it nevertheless recognized the instrument's usefulness for certain areas of diagnostic medicine, such as the identification of the animal and vegetable parasites which caused common skin diseases. One issue that became controversial by the mid-1840s was the nature of cancer – or of malignant and benign tumours in general – and somewhat later, the use of the microscope to diagnose cancer. A major debate on tumours of the breast took place in the Academy of Medicine in 1843–4.[12] The publication of Lebert's *Physiologie pathologique* in 1845, in which he proposed his theory of the specific cancer cell, broadened the controversy over cancer, the microscope, and the microscopy community.[13] The debate over the microscope and microscopists, indeed the whole Paris clinical tradition, came to a head in the thirteen-session debate in the Academy of Medicine in 1854–5. The debate brought into the open the main tensions between microscopists and clinicians.[14]

The Introduction of Microscopy into Paris Medicine: Clinical Medicine and Pathological Anatomy in the 1830s

Medical microscopy developed within the context of Paris clinical medicine, whose dominant research method in the 1830s was pathological anatomy. In the first decades of the century, pathological anatomy was taught in private and public courses outside, but complementing, the regular courses of the Faculty of Medicine. Only in 1835 did the speciality become institutionalized when a chair was created at the Paris Faculty for Jean Cruveilhier.[15] This extracurricular education was one of the principal characteristics of Paris medicine and a main attraction for foreign medical students, as John Warner's essay in this volume demonstrates. It was in extracurricular courses that microscopy was introduced into Paris medical education, first by Donné in 1837, and in the 1840s by Lebert, Mandl, and Gruby.

In the 1830s clinicians and physiologists, calling themselves eclectics, and including Andral, Rayer, Bouillaud, and others, embraced new methods, namely, animal experimentation, the numerical method, medical chemistry, and microscopy.[16] Animal experimentation and medical chemistry, with traditions going back several hundred years, seem to have provoked little controversy. The numerical method and medical microscopy were more vexing. Both challenged clinical medicine and pathological anatomy as they were being practised in the 1830s.[17] At the heart of the controversy over each new method were differing perceptions of clinical medicine. The microscopical, or integrationist, point of view, held that clinical medicine should include laboratory methods and new medical technologies. The other point of view, a narrower version of clinical, held that a move to incorporate unproved methods and technologies threatened to undermine the integrity of the Paris school with its focus on patients and hospitals, its emphasis on practical training at the bedside and pathological anatomy. Microscopy also aroused epistemological concerns: what counted as reliable and legitimate knowledge and how could it best be acquired? It was not clear that microscopy provided a trustworthy account of reality, but it was clear that the new instrument and its practitioners challenged established interests and clinicians' authority. In order to understand both views of clinical medicine, we must examine the reality behind the rhetoric and the agendas of the proponents of both positions.

Trained in the clinical tradition in Paris, Berlin, and Vienna, the early medical microscopists practising in Paris saw microscopy as a way to improve clinical medicine by strengthening medical research and diagnostic medicine. Alfred Donné introduced microscopy into French medicine in the early 1830s and dominated the field for more than a decade. Donné received his M.D. from the Paris Faculty in 1831. He opened what became a successful private practice, worked as *chef de clinique* under Bouillaud at the Charité hospital, and began a research programme in medical microscopy. Having failed in his attempt for the *agrégation* in medicine at the Paris Faculty in 1835, he never held a faculty position. He continued his medical research and private practice, and in 1837 started teaching a public microscopy course in the evenings in one of the amphitheatres of the Faculty of Medicine.[18]

In his thesis, *Recherches physiologiques et chimico-microscopiques sur les globules du sang, du pus, du mucus, et de ceux des humeurs de l'oeil*, Donné announced the centrality of microscopy for anatomy, while noting that few Parisian physicians had incorporated the instrument into their research:

> The use of the microscope applied to the observation of tissues and liquids of the system is still rarely used by physicians; it would seem, however, that in an epoch in which anatomy has made such progress, that everything which we can directly observe with our senses in the various organs of the human body and that everything which can be attained by the thin blade of the scalpel is almost completely understood, observers ought rapidly to adopt an instrument which, doubling the power of their means [of observation] reveals to them an unknown world, and permits them to see and analyze that which up to now has escaped their detailed investigation.[19]

Donné suggested two reasons why some rejected the new technology: a healthy scepticism for new techniques and the practical difficulties involved in using the instrument. On the first point, echoing Bichat's radical empiricist position, he commented:

> Microscopical observations generally inspire little confidence from anatomists; this instrument appears to them more proper for procuring troublesome illusions than for precisely retracing the truth. They are sceptical of anything that they cannot see with their [naked] eyes and touch with their finger; they leave this type of research [microscopic] to botanists, who have made good use of it

for several years, to clarify plant physiology, and they do not believe they ought to include the microscope among the numerous useful apparati of their amphitheatres.[20]

The second reason Donné believed anatomists were reluctant to use the microscope in their research arsenal was that they found it hard to use. Microscopy required practice, patience, and skill, and beginners were easily discouraged:

> Even though it seems, at first glance, that it suffices just to look [through the microscope] in order to see, it is certain that untrained people begin by seeing nothing when they are not well directed; their patience wears thin, runs out, and they reject the instrument which they do not at all know how to operate.[21]

Donné made a similar comment thirteen years later (1844), by which time he had been teaching microscopy for seven years:

> It is wrong to imagine that all it takes is to look into the microscope and [that] consequently everybody is capable of using this instrument as one uses opera glasses. Microscopical observation really constitutes a science which has its principles and its rules, its difficulties and its methods, whose knowledge cannot be improvised any more than that of any other science.[22]

By the early 1840s some Parisian physicians were using the instrument as an aid in diagnosing diseases of the skin, blood, kidneys, and urogenital system. Andral and Rayer used microscopic and chemical analysis to examine blood and urine.[23] Donné discovered the parasitic protozoon that causes one common form of vaginal infection, making the aetiology and diagnosis of that problem more precise.[24] He also identified the disorder characterized by an excess of white blood cells, which later became known as leukaemia.[25] David Gruby and Onésime Delafond used the microscope to discover plant and animal parasites that caused some skin and blood diseases in humans and animals.[26] Clinicians and microscopists such as Andral, Rayer, Donné, Mandl, and Lebert sought to broaden pathological anatomy by incorporating microscopy and a neohumoral approach. They believed the instrument would allow pathological anatomists to achieve new levels of analysis and understanding, continuing the progression of events which had first focused on the organ, then tissues, now body fluids and globules/cells. Microscopists argued that the instrument was a natural extension of pathological anatomy and physiology, requiring some new skills but no major conceptual adjustments. Microscopical examination, they contended, fell well within the pathological-anatomical tradition.

The advantages of microscopical pathological anatomy and physiology were not immediately self-evident, however. It was debatable whether microscopical observation of tumours, for example, revealed any more than naked-eye observation. Alfred-Armand Velpeau, chief surgeon at the Charité hospital, who cooperated with microscopists by sending them tumour sections for examination, argued that the microscope revealed no more than could be discerned with the naked eye.[27] Unless the microscope offered clear advantages for the practice of medicine and surgery, it was easy for physicians and surgeons to conclude that there was no compelling reason for them to spend the time and effort needed to learn to use the instrument.

Writing in 1866 in his two-volume *Traité des tumeurs*, Paul Broca, a student of Lebert and leading spokesman for the second generation of Parisian medical microscopists, told the story of the early years of medical microscopy and its relationship to pathological anatomy. Referring to the late 1830s, Broca explained:

> A means of investigation hitherto neglected by physicians, the microscope, suddenly enlarged the field of pathological anatomy. A great number of new facts from an order not in common use came suddenly, without [any] transition to invade the classic ground, threatening to altogether overturn classification, doctrines, even language. It was too much at one time. While the most receptive people resisted an invasion, the most progressive men guarded against innovations [which were] too general and too rapid. This reserve is not only legitimate, it is the safeguard of science, which would be, without it, open to all sorts of dangers. There was, then, owing to the force of circumstances, a resistance proportional to the importance of the debate.[28]

Broca thus saw the initial resistance of clinicians to microscopy as a positive factor, demonstrating a sceptical attitude toward the introduction of any new theory or technique. Such scepticism, according to Broca, was a built-in safeguard of the practice of scientific medicine, in keeping with the tradition of the Paris school.

Broca suggested an interest theory analysis to explain pathological anatomists' reluctance to adopt the microscope. He argued that pathological anatomists, with their reputations established, did not welcome the intrusion of the microscope, which required them to acquire new skills and to rethink the limits and utility of their method. Were the microscopical approach to dominate, these practitioners of gross pathological anatomy, ensconced in their positions of authority, might see their power base threatened, their authority challenged.[29]

The Microscopy Community and its Goals in the 1840s

An active microscopy community thrived in Paris in the 1840s in spite of the misgivings and resistance chronicled by Broca. Early in the decade the Parisian microscopy community expanded as three foreigners came to Paris seeking fame and fortune, but mainly employment. The microscope was their entrée into the 'Paris hospital', to borrow Ackerknecht's useful term referring to the whole battery of medical institutions in early nineteenth-century Paris. David Gruby, Hungarian by birth, came to Paris in 1840 after receiving an M.D. from the University of Vienna, where he studied pathological anatomy under Karl Rokitansky and Joseph Berres and wrote a thesis on the application of microscopy to pathological anatomy. He engaged in intensive scientific research in the first five years after his arrival in Paris and began teaching microscopy in his private laboratory. His principal research contribution was to identify microscopically the plant parasites that caused several common skin diseases, such as thrush and tinea (ringworm). Gruby and veterinarian Onésime Delafond, with whom he collaborated in his research, introduced microscopy studies at the Veterinary School at Alfort.[30]

Some specialists in diseases of the skin, such as Cazenave, were initially reluctant to accept Gruby's discoveries, creating tensions within the nascent speciality of dermatology.[31] Gruby's findings did not fit with prevailing beliefs about the aetiology and treatment of skin diseases, according to which moral and environmental considerations were dominant. L. S. Jacyna's essay on Alibert, in this volume, illustrates the kind of thinking that made attributing causality to a microorganism difficult.[32] Controversy over Gruby's microscopical discoveries was shortlived, however, and by the early 1850s, clinicians recognized the utility of the microscope in the diagnosis of skin diseases. Once microorganisms were shown to be the cause of several common skin diseases, some of the most troublesome could be prevented – or at least managed – and often cured.

Louis Mandl, a Hungarian like Gruby, also came to Paris in 1840. He conducted microscopical research in a number of areas, specializing in the study of tumours. He began teaching a public microscopy course in 1846 and made microscopical technique accessible to physicians by publishing one of the three popular microscopy manuals available at the time. Such how-to books contributed to the diffusion of microscopical technique by allowing physicians and others to acquire microscopy skills without formal attendance at classes.[33]

Hermann Lebert, a Prussian, studied medicine and natural science in Berlin and Zurich, receiving his M.D. from the University of Zurich in 1834. He then attended clinics of leading physicians and surgeons first in Paris, then in Berlin. After this postdoctoral study he found employment as a cantonal physician in Switzerland. Beginning in 1842 he began spending his winters in Paris and his summers working as resident physician at the water-cure establishment at Lavey-les-Bains, Switzerland. In 1846 he settled in Paris permanently, and by the late 1840s had become the leading microscopist in the city, succeeding Donné, who left Paris in 1848 to pursue a career in academic administration. Lebert opened a private practice, taught microscopy to a few students in his private laboratory, engaged in extensive microscopical research, and achieved a certain notoriety for his theory of the specific cancer cell.[34]

Lebert's introduction to the atlas which accompanied his influential two-volume *Physiologie pathologique* (1845) was the text that came the closest to a programmatic statement of the microscopical position. Here we find the clearest account of the theory and practice of early medical microscopy and its relationship to pathological anatomy and clinical medicine. Although Lebert accepted pathological anatomy as the central research component of Paris clinical medicine, he also pointed out its limitations, namely, its focus on the solid parts of the body, to the exclusion of body fluids. Thus Lebert argued for a neo-humoral approach to emphasize the study of vital secretions and the morbid alterations of body fluids after death. Andral's research on blood and Rayer's on urine exemplified the direction he thought pathological anatomy should take – moving toward a science of pathological physiology, as the title of his book made clear.[35] Lebert criticized the still-dominant gross anatomical approach of the Paris school, advocating the application of chemistry and microscopy to pathology. He argued that clinicians should avail themselves of new techniques to supplement, but not replace, the existing ones. Lebert emphasized the complementary nature of scientific practice, asserting that for medicine to progress, clinical study, animal experimentation, and microscopical observation should be pursued together:

> For my part, I realized early that, if one wanted to arrive at more precise notions in pathological physiology, it was necessary, in addition to chemical research, to have the concurrence of three other methods of investigation, namely: clinical study, animal experimentation, and microscopical observation.[36]

For Lebert, clinical observation was the basis of scientific medicine and pathological physiology. The microscope had to be used in conjunction with patient observation and physical examination:

> The microscope can be a great help in pathology, but its role only begins after the use of other methods capable of unveiling the nature of disease. Thus clinical observation will always be the basis of pathology. It will remain the centre of activity and the goal of all the efforts of the true physician...[37]

In Lebert's programme, the clinician maintained his privileged and dominant position in the study of disease, assisted by chemists and microscopists:

> The chemist who will analyze a product of secretion, the microscopist who will study the details of a morbid tissue, will be able to provide valuable information, but this information – by itself – would only have a secondary value. Both can provide materials for medical doctrines, but only the clinician is capable of coordinating them [the information] in a regular manner.[38]

Chemists and microscopists assisted clinicians, functioning as laboratory technicians, but only the clinician had the judgement and experience to put all the information together and interpret it. For Lebert new techniques did not challenge the authority of clinicians, but increased it. He reasserted the clinician's authority based on the centrality of his judgement and expertise to clinical medicine and of the latter to the larger medical enterprise.

Donné and Lebert: Microscopy as an Entrée to Paris Medicine

Lebert's approach to pathological anatomy and clinical medicine served his professional interests. In his emphasis on the complementary nature of microscopy and clinical medicine and his goal of integration, Lebert sought to carve out a niche for himself within the Parisian medical community. At a time when the supply of physicians in Paris was far greater than the demand and when there were only a limited number of hospital and academic positions, a promising new area like microscopy could serve as a point of entry to the 'Paris hospital'. The careers of Donné and Lebert illustrate how microscopy and the microscopical point of view could be used to create professional opportunities within the Paris school.[39]

Donné was the first French clinician to acquire a reputation as a medical microscopist. Having failed in his bid for the *agrégation*, he sought other teaching options. One was to offer public and private courses outside the Faculty, and this is what Donné did when he inaugurated his public microscopy course (1837). Donné saw offering a public course in a speciality as one way to gain access to the system, by supplementing the established curriculum. These courses – called public because they were open to the public free of charge – and private courses, for which one paid the instructor – were one of the great strengths of Paris medicine, augmenting the regular medical curriculum.[40]

In order to achieve professional recognition, microscopists had to convince the Parisian medical community of the centrality of microscopy to clinical medicine and pathological anatomy, and then to provide opportunities for colleagues and students to acquire microscopical skills by offering courses. Early in his career Donné made limited, but important, claims for the instrument, suggesting that microscopy was not a science in its own right, but a technique fundamental to many branches of medical science, including anatomy, physiology, pathology, chemistry, natural history, and legal medicine.[41] Donné and Lebert did not envision microscopy's ever assuming separate disciplinary status or think that a chair in microscopy would be established at the Faculty of Medicine as had been the case with pathological anatomy. They founded neither a journal of microscopy, nor a professional society.[42] Their pronouncements and actions indicate their desire to see microscopy as complementing and enriching the established clinical tradition rather than challenging it. Their strategy was integration of microscopy into the institutional and theoretical framework of Paris medicine.

To be accepted within the 'Paris Hospital', microscopists sought legitimation and professional recognition by publicizing the benefits of microscopy and the latest research accomplished with the instrument. They sent letters and research papers to the Academy of Sciences, published their research in professional journals such as the *Archives générales de médecine*, and published books on microscopy – ranging from how-to manuals like Mandl's *Traité pratique du microscope*, to textbooks, like Donné's *Cours de microscopie*, to scholarly treatises, such as Lebert's *Physiologie pathologique*.

One way to gain professional recognition was to stake out a particular area and become the recognized expert in it. Both Donné and Lebert employed this strategy. Donné set out to be the French authority on the microscopical analysis of human milk. Milk studies allowed him to combine two areas of expertise: proto-paediatrics and microscopy. A specialist in diseases of infants and children, Donné saw an opportunity to make an important public health contribution while establishing his reputation in microscopy by proposing that microscopical analysis was a scientific way to measure the quality and quantity of human milk. Parents would know how to choose a good wet nurse, and mothers would know if their milk was satisfactory. Donné contended that by using the microscope good milk could be distinguished from bad, pathological situations identified, and both quality (the richness) and quantity of milk determined. With regard to quality, for example, Donné reported that if milk was examined with a magnification of 300x, milk globules swimming in transparent liquid could be observed. Then by using chemical agents, the observer could detect if globules were fatty (buttery) matter. Richness could be determined by the number and density of globules. In a satirical article, 'Le Médecin' (1841), discussed by Joy Harvey in her paper in this volume, the author suggested ways an aspiring physician could advance professionally by referring to Donné (without naming him): 'One could use the microscope to prove there were organisms in the milk of wet nurses.'[43]

Donné sought to determine if microscopical observation of milk was a reliable way to detect disease in the nurse. Thus he examined milk for possible alteration by organic products, such as colostrum, or morbid products, namely pus. He published the initial results of his research on milk in a work titled *On Milk, and in Particular That of Nurses* in 1837, which established his reputation as a milk specialist. By 1839, Donné's work on the microscopical analysis of human milk was being discussed in the Royal Academy of Sciences.

Donné also increased his scientific reputation by introducing photomicrography. In 1840 he applied Louis Daguerre's invention of photography to microscopical observations. Just a few months after Daguerre's announcement to the Royal Academy of Sciences, Donné presented a photomicrograph, a photograph taken through a microscope, to that august institution. Photography had clear advantages for microscopy by providing an objectivity heretofore lacking. Compared with hand-drawn illustrations, now the image could be fixed, reproduced, published, and studied.[44]

Donné's contemporaries recognized his contributions to microscopy, especially his public course, his introduction of photomicrography, his work on blood and mucus, and his discovery of the pathogenic protozoon *Trichomonas vaginalis*.[45] Some of his work, however, provoked controversy within the medical/scientific community, fuelling the fire of the anti-microscopy, or the so-called clinicians' "camp". By the early 1840s, Donné was, in the estimation of some of his contemporaries, an opportunist, a man eager to use microscopy as a way to make a name for himself at any cost. He came to personify what some clinicians feared: microscopy might be mainly an avenue for personal aggrandizement, or even worse, a gimmick, a pseudo-science. While the charges were personal ones directed at Donné, the debates surrounding his work that took place in the Academy of Sciences and the Academy of Medicine decreased confidence in microscopical endeavours more generally and led some critics, such as Velpeau, and even proponents, such as Bouillaud, later to argue that the main problem was not the microscope but the microscopists.[46] If Donné was representative of the microscopy community in the 1840s, then those who were sceptical of microscopists could easily see the latter as a group of self-serving opportunists, not physicians whose main goal was caring for patients – the clinical ideal. Within this analytical framework, microscopy was antithetical to the norms of the clinical tradition, exemplified by physicians such as Philippe Pinel or René-Théophile Laennec.[47]

The first, and less important, incident involved Donné's run-in with François Arago, the perpetual secretary of the Academy of Sciences, over Donné's invention and demonstration of a purportedly new instrument, the lactoscope. Donné was persistent in sending his work to the Academy of Sciences, submitting a number of research papers, reports of which were published in the *Comptes-rendus*. In this case he sent an instrument for the Academy to examine. The purpose of the lactoscope was to detect the richness of milk. When the committee from the Academy examined the instrument, two problems emerged: first, the lactoscope did not appear to committee members to be superior to a regular microscope, and second, Arago accused Donné of plagiarism, a far more serious charge, claiming that such an instrument had already been developed.[48] Donné's reputation was tarnished by this episode, but in 1842 even more serious charges were levelled against him at the Academy of Medicine.

Dichotomy or Integration?

The occasion was the submission by Alphonse Devergie, a candidate for a vacant place in the hygiene section of the Academy and legal medicine specialist, of an essay entitled 'On the Value of Microscopical Examination of Milk in the Choice of a Wet Nurse'.[49] Now Donné had staked much of his scientific reputation on the utility of the microscope to improve infant hygiene and public health by a scientific analysis of human milk, and he was considered the reigning French expert on the topic, when Devergie decided to do his own study. Devergie had previously held a variety of medical positions (among them, director of the Paris morgue), but was employed as a medical inspector at the Paris wet-nursing office in 1837 when Donné's work on milk appeared. Although other investigators had performed chemical analyses of milk, Donné wanted to establish his exclusive pre-eminence in the microscopical analysis of milk. Devergie attempted to reproduce Donné's results to determine if Donné was right in his contention that microscopical and chemical analysis of milk could help in the choice of a wet nurse. Devergie performed 172 observations at the wet-nursing office. His findings did not support Donné's argument and led the Academy committee to conclude that the microscope was less useful in choosing a wet nurse than Donné had claimed. With Donné and Devergie, the committee was confronted with diametrically opposed opinions.[50]

The case raised broader questions about the limits of microscopical utility and the nature of scientific investigation. Donné was portrayed as having made overarching and unsubstantiated claims for the utility of the microscope, whereas Devergie was seen as more circumspect. Donné appeared to reject all previous empirical knowledge about choosing a wet nurse in favour of the microscopic evidence, whereas Devergie contended that the microscope was of only secondary utility. The committee rejected Donné's claims and sided with Devergie, concluding that in the choice of a wet nurse the new scientific methods really did not help that much. The traditional methods, such as the age, stature, complexion, and disposition of a wet nurse were adequate. The microscope complemented other forms of enquiry, but its utility was limited. The committee members urged a balanced view, contending that in the present state of science physicians should not ask more of microscopy than it could give. What the committee implied was that Devergie was the real scientist, working in the open-minded spirit of scientific enquiry, providing a realistic assessment of the utility of the instrument. By contrast, Donné appeared to be a self-serving opportunist, making unsupportable

Dichotomy or Integration?

claims for the instrument on which he had staked his professional reputation.[51] For the Academy of Medicine committee, Devergie's work supported the prevailing norms of science of the Paris school, or so the report claimed, whereas Donné's challenged them.

Clearly the committee framed its investigation and report within the norms of science of the Paris school and the Academy of Medicine. Although in France the Academy of Sciences and the Academy of Medicine were both political creations, academic rules required that extrascientific factors should not influence scientific judgements – even though everyone knew that they did. While the norms of science inculcated by the academicians were not just 'mere rhetoric', scientific judgements could be, and often were, political. In the case of Devergie and Donné, while the evidence suggests that the committee was right in citing Devergie as the better scientist, he was also the Establishment scientist by virtue of his positions within the Parisian medical community. Donné, for his part, was not without good scientific credentials, and he was in favour at the Court. But political intrigue as well as questionable science in all likelihood played a major role in the Academy of Medicine's decision.

Microscopy also provided opportunities for professional advancement within Paris Medicine for Lebert, who learned to use the microscope from Schönlein while in medical school in Zurich. Later, while working as a cantonal physician in Switzerland, he began to do research with Swiss microscopist and embryologist Jean-Louis Prévost. Lebert was torn between two career goals: clinical medicine and scientific research. First in Switzerland, then Berlin, and finally, in Paris, he tried to combine both. His early career exemplified the integrationist approach he preached with regard to microscopy and clinical medicine.[52]

Lebert settled permanently in Paris in 1846 and quickly became the pre-eminent microscopist in the city, in great part due to the publication of his *Physiologie pathologique* (1845) which secured his reputation among the Parisian medical elite. Lebert's reputation rested in part on his theory of the specific cancer cell which he introduced in his book. According to Lebert, the cancer cell was a distinctive cell, observable under the microscope, which indicated the presence of cancer in the organism. Conversely, Lebert argued that unless the cancer cell could be observed, no cancer was present.[53] This theory and his book broadened and intensified the ongoing debate over tumours. Just a year earlier the Royal Academy of Medicine had been the site of a three-month-long debate on breast tumours (January–March 1844).[54]

Lebert sought professional acceptance by establishing his credentials as a clinician and researcher. For him, as for Donné earlier, microscopy was a point of entry to the 'Paris hospital'. He built up a successful private practice, opened his own laboratory where he taught microscopy to four of the most promising young medical students: Paul Broca, Charles Robin, François Follin, and Aristide Verneuil.[55] He got leading surgeons and clinicians to assist him by providing specimens for microscopical examination. His association with Andral, Louis, Velpeau, Cruveilhier, and others lent respectability and authority to his work, since by their cooperation they acknowledged the legitimacy of his research. Lebert, realizing the importance of institutionalizing his microscopical endeavours, was one of the founders of the *Société de biologie* (1848), an organization devoted to research in medicine and natural science, with a hard core of microscope users and promoters as members.[56] More than the other microscopists, Lebert developed and publicized an integrated approach which allowed microscopy to be incorporated into the existing clinical and pathological anatomical framework. Such an integration was Lebert's strategy for securing a place in the 'Paris hospital'.

Lebert used microscopy to gain access to the Parisian medical elite. But, in the end, he remained on the periphery in spite of much widely hailed, although controversial research, an international reputation, and a thriving practice. Microscopical success was not enough to acquire a position at the Faculty of Medicine, a hospital position, or entry into the Academy of Sciences or the Academy of Medicine. Lebert left Paris in 1852 to accept a clinical post in Zurich. He was nominated to the Academy of Medicine in 1854, but his candidacy was unsuccessful. Only after his later clinical success in Switzerland and Germany, and with increasing acceptance of microscopy and cell theory among his French colleagues, was he successful in being elected a corresponding member of the Academy in 1866.[57] A major problem for Lebert was that microscopy had become controversial at about the same time he had settled in Paris, and part of the controversy was due to his own theory of the specific cancer cell, over which there was serious dispute among European microscopists. The majority of Parisian physicians, surgeons, and foreign microscopists such as Virchow, Paget, Rokitansky, Remak, Mandl, and Delafond rejected it (Lebert's 'school' and Strasbourg physicians Sédillot and Küss accepted it).[58] Indeed many of the Parisian medical elite did not accept the cell theory. Lebert's German origin also retarded his professional advancement, since those clinicians who questioned the utility of microscopy associated the instrument with German medicine, which to them meant inferior, or non-French medicine.

Seeing microscopy as opportunity, Lebert went to Paris to make his reputation. In a sense, he did. But his espousal of an unpopular and controversial theory and the debate surrounding the microscope in the late 1840s and early 1850s contributed to his own perceived failure to reach the pinnacle of French medicine and science. Contemporaries did not necessarily agree with Lebert's assessment of his position. Writing in the 1860s, historian of medicine Charles Daremberg elevated Lebert to the highest position within Paris medicine:

> Lebert ... was in France ... one of the first and most eminent propagators of doctrines from across the Rhine.... with Lebert the clarity, neatness of the French method are unified with the erudition and the philosophical tendencies of the German schools...[59]

And Jean Cruveilhier, who had worked side by side with Lebert on the microscopical examination of tumour sections, ranked him the best of the medical microscopists: 'Among the medical micrographers ... Lebert ranks in first place'.[60]

Success could clearly be measured in other ways than institutional affiliation. It also meant recognition by peers, or election to the Academy of Medicine or the Academy of Sciences or both. To achieve that, Lebert had to return to his native Germany and establish his reputation as a clinician as well as a microscopist. Only then did the French allow him the institutional entrée he sought, when they elected him to the Academy of Medicine as a corresponding member in 1866.[61]

Both Donné and Lebert realized some success in using microscopy to carve out a niche within the Parisian medical elite. Lebert achieved a more central position than Donné in that he was more highly regarded by contemporaries and later chroniclers. It would seem that being German was less of a handicap than being a royalist. Donné became politically unacceptable because of his royalist leanings and never acquired the reputation of Lebert. The latter emerged as the leader of the Paris microscopy school, working closely with leading surgeons and physicians. It is true that being a German hurt him, if we are to believe what contemporaries said. Nevertheless, microscopy did secure him a professional reputation within the Paris school.

The Era of Uncertainty: The Microscope on Trial

The problem introduced by the microscope into the study of tumours – an area pursued in the late 1840s and 1850s by Lebert, Mandl, Broca, Follin, Velpeau, and others – involved their classification. Were tumours to be classified according to gross and microscopical structure or clinical observations? Some clinicians claimed there was no parallel between the structure of tumours and their properties – or between their anatomical and clinical characteristics – and that microscopical findings were illusory in any case. According to Broca, many clinicians took this point of view, setting up a conflict between clinical and scientific-laboratory medicine. Broca accounted for this disagreement over classification in two ways. First, the new doctrine, according to which tumours were classified based on structural and microscopical characteristics, complicated diagnosis and prognosis. Secondly, with its new language, the new doctrine required the use of an instrument difficult to handle and imposed on surgeons the necessity of a special education – as long as it was tiring. Of the microscope, Broca commented: 'Disrupting thus all habits, it could not count on the welcome that is ordinarily accorded to new views, in a profession where progressive men are in the majority.'[62] Lebert had proposed a classification based on microscopical pathological anatomy, a method which he saw as merely continuing and enlarging upon the work of traditional gross pathological anatomy. Some physicians and surgeons, however, felt threatened by this approach. They believed that accepting microscopical anatomy meant abandoning gross pathological anatomy for a new method, as yet unproven. Broca recounts that:

> The argument was pressing, and to respond to it there were only two expedients: one could doubt that part of anatomy studied with the microscope, and say the only essential characteristics are those that can be seen with the naked eye; or, resign oneself to a painful sacrifice, and make pathological anatomy descend completely from the high position that it had held up to then.[63]

Broca explained that the first response – doubting all microscopical observation – could only have a temporary success. He asserted, however, that although microscopical observations could lead to contradictory interpretations, all the observational sciences were like that. The difference was that, more than for any other observational science, the study of microscopical elements was an invitation to hypothesizing. He claimed that, because the elements are only accessible to one of our senses, they can only be studied in one way, and we can only know part of their character. Our curiosity, ever more excited because we think we are closer to 'lifting the last veil', is not satisfied. Thus:

> The science of microscopical elements is studded with more or less philosophical hypotheses, more or less transcendent theories: objects of belief for some, of negation for others, of doubt for many, and of discussion for all. In hearing for the first time, the echo of these innumerable debates, persons unfamiliar with microscopy could believe for an instant that everything was uncertain and illusory in this science, and that one could, from then on, without examination, distance oneself from the study of discoveries of the notion furnished by histology and pathology, that one could at least do that until all the microscopists were in agreement, that is to say, until the end of time.[64]

Thus Broca argued that disagreement was a central feature of an immature science, that competing ideas were the engine that drove scientific progress. But, Broca continued, in the case of microscopy this disagreement was shortlived. When the new science acquired a certain constancy of results so that many gained a superficial knowledge of it, physicians had to recognize that histology was divided into two parts – one transcendent and conjectural, the other purely descriptive – whose certainty was equal to ordinary anatomy, and that microscopical characterizations of tissues were as fixed and certain as those visible to the naked eye. Microscopical and naked-eye observations verified each other.[65]

Broca, an integrationist like his teacher Lebert, emphasized that the new method of studying and classifying tumours was not a departure from or a challenge to Paris clinical medicine. In fact, Lebert, Broca, and Rudolf Virchow – probably following Lebert – asserted that microscopy was only valid as a way of studying tumours if grounded in pathological anatomy and clinical observation. Without such verification, Lebert and Broca found microscopical investigation wanting. Thus, from their perspective, for critics to set up a dichotomy between clinicians and laboratory physicians was completely erroneous. For integrationists, the microscope carried pathological anatomy to another level – that of elemental structure – but microscopical findings had to be verified in the clinic.[66]

Dichotomy or Integration?

Broca commented extensively on the surgeons' response to the integrationist approach of Lebert, claiming that the publication of Lebert's *Physiologie pathologique* brought on a deep division between surgeons who were willing to take pathological anatomy to the microscopical level and those who were not:

> As long as microscopy remained a speculative science, the surgeons welcomed it with a benevolent curiosity.... But when they were confronted with the practical application, when they saw that it was necessary to distinguish two types [of tumour] at the bedside, when they saw diagnosis weakened daily by the findings of the microscope, then resistance began.
>
> At first they wanted to contest the exactitude of microscopical observations. You heard eminent professors ... pretend that the microscope was a misleading instrument, and that with a little imagination you could see whatever you wanted to see. I was even obliged to devote part of my M.D. thesis (1849) to the refutation of this singular nonsense. Soon, however, it was necessary to change the language. They wanted to recognize that microscopical observation was exact, but they added that it was useless; that pathological tumours were characterized by their colour, their consistency, their exterior structure, in short, by characteristics confirmed by naked-eye observation, and not at all by the molecular appearance of atoms that the microscope showed.[67]

Broca argued that these objections were valid, but maintained that naked-eye observation typically coincided with elementary differences revealed by the microscope. He made this point in a work submitted to the Academy of Medicine essay contest for which he received the Prix Portal in 1850.[68] In that work, Broca, following in Lebert's footsteps, placed microscopy squarely within the tradition of pathological anatomy, with the intention of smoothing out difficulties and satisfying the malcontents. His hopes were not realized. Suspicion toward the microscope did not dissipate; instead, the argument widened. Part of the reason for increased scepticism was no doubt that usage became more widespread among Parisian physicians and surgeons. Velpeau dated 1847 as the beginning of the era when use of the microscope became general among the Parisian medical elite. From that date he submitted all the tumours he removed to microscopical examination.[69]

Similar doubts about the application of the microscope to pathology also began to surface in England and Germany. By 1847,

Dichotomy or Integration?

Rudolf Virchow, Lebert's friend and collaborator, reported that, after a decade of enthusiasm, doubts about the utility of the microscope in pathology had begun to appear among German physicians.[70] British physiologist and microscopist William Carpenter noted that, in spite of the early acceptance of microscopy in Britain, by the 1850s the instrument and its practitioners were under attack by many physicians:

> The instrument fell under a temporary cloud ..., for having been applied by Anatomists and Physiologists to the determination of the elementary structure of the animal body, their results were found to be so discordant, as to give rise to a general suspicion of a want of trustworthiness in the Microscope, and in everything announced upon its authority. Thus both the instrument and its advocates were brought into more or less discredit.[71]

Yet, at about the same time, doubts about the microscope in some areas of medical research began to dissipate. By the early 1850s most Parisian physicians and surgeons acknowledged the importance of microscopy for diagnosing skin diseases – mites carrying scabies, plant parasites that caused ringworm and thrush – as well as knowledge acquired by examining body fluids. What was still hotly contested was the usefulness of the microscope for diagnosing cancerous tumours, a dispute which came to a head in the Academy of Medicine debate in 1854–5.[72] The debate was a major turning point in the history of early medical microscopy in Paris, after which the integrationist position came to prevail as medical microscopy became incorporated into Paris clinical medicine. This debate can also serve as a key to understanding the historiography of Paris Medicine, because it was a debate as much over differing perceptions of Paris Medicine as over microscopy. Microscopy was a way of bringing into focus two differing constructions of Paris Medicine at mid-century.

Microscopy and Paris Clinical Medicine: The Debate of 1854–5

Two questions were proposed for debate at the Academy of Medicine: first, was the microscope useful for diagnosing cancer, and second, was cancer curable? Although the latter question generated considerable discussion, the most heated and controversial part of the debate focused on the microscope and microscopists and their role in Paris Medicine. The academicians constructed the debate by pitting one adversary against another and by dividing the speakers up informally into those who were pro-microscopy and those who were anti-microscopy. Dividing the Parisian medical elite into two opposing camps exemplified the military rhetoric in which the debate was framed,[73] but did not reflect the reality of the controversy or of Paris Medicine. In actuality, no one came forth as an opponent of the microscope. Quite the opposite was the case. The rhetoric used suggests that by the mid-1850s, it was important within the scientifically minded progressive Parisian medical elite for all to declare themselves pro-microscope. One might argue that this was merely a rhetorical strategy to establish intellectual assent before attacking the opposition. But I think it shows that it was no longer acceptable to appear to be an enemy of scientific medicine, which by then had come to mean the incorporation of laboratory methods into clinical medicine. Both Velpeau and Bouillaud, who emerged as the principal critics of some aspects of the practice and theory of microscopy, took great pains to present their microscopy credentials dating from the 1830s.[74] Perhaps as a rhetorical flourish, a disclaimer to take opponents offguard, Bouillaud, exhibiting great oratorical skills and expressing his faith in the instrument, declared himself 'un ami du microscope', and invented his own terminology: he was, he claimed, a 'microscophile'.[75] The first area of disagreement over the instrument was practical. While clinicians and surgeons present at the debate readily acknowledged most applications of the microscope, in serious dispute was the use of the instrument to diagnose cancer. And underlying this dispute was a fundamental disagreement over the existence of Lebert's specific cancer cell. But behind it all was the question of authority and which model of Paris Medicine would prevail.

The principal actors were Velpeau, the head surgeon of the Charité hospital, a specialist in tumours of the breast, Robert, who emerged as the self-styled defender of the microscope, the surgeon Malgaigne, and Bouillaud, pathological anatomist, specialist in diseases of the heart and brain. Although Bouillaud billed Velpeau as the leading opponent of the microscope, the latter clearly was not.[76] But he did represent the clinical as opposed to the microscopical point of view on the question of cancer diagnosis. Curiously, as Hippolyte Larrey pointed out, there were no microscopists present to defend themselves, because none was a member of the Academy.[77] Of the first generation of microscopists, both Donné and Lebert had left Paris by this time. Gruby had abandoned microscopy research and teaching to devote himself full-time to private practice. Mandl was the only one of the four who had any involvement with the debate and then only from the outside. During the debate he wrote a letter to the Academy clarifying his position on the specific cancer cell.[78] (Although Mandl was one of the earliest proponents of the cancer cell, he had come to reject it, because he found that the theory was not supported by his own observational evidence.) The second generation of microscopists was too young to have been elected to the Academy: Charles Robin, Paul Broca, François Follin, and Aristide Verneuil. The only participant in the debate with strong microscopic credentials was Delafond, who had been engaged in microscopic research since 1839.[79]

Broca, Follin, and Verneuil attended the debates, however, as reporters for the *Moniteur des hôpitaux* (Broca), the *Archives générales de médecine* (Follin), and *Gazette hebdomadaire de médecine et de chirurgie* (Verneuil).[80] Broca emerged as the self-appointed spokesman for the 'Young Paris School', the name given by Velpeau to the younger generation of clinicians and the second generation of microscopists.[81] However, Broca's voice cannot be seen as representative of the microscopy community in general. As it came out in the debate, Lebert and his school, who accepted the notion of a specific cancer cell, were in the minority, with most other French, British, and German microscopists in opposition. Indeed, Lebert's postulation of a specific cancer cell, along with his re-classification of tumours, became the main focus of attacks by Bouillaud and Velpeau. Lebert had previously defended his position and had been one of the major actors in a similar debate in 1852–3 before the Surgical Society of Paris, but, in the Academy debate, he was not present to defend himself.[82]

Velpeau presented the principal arguments against the use of the microscope in diagnosing cancer. In the early days of medical microscopy, he recalled, surgeons had hoped that cancer might be identified by a microscopical analysis of the blood, making a pre-surgical diagnosis possible. These hopes had not been realized. Diagnosis was still impossible for internal cancers, and whether the tumour was cancerous or not could only be decided post-mortem. At that point microscopical examination was useful for pathology, but not for diagnosis. For external tumours, such as breast cancer and skin cancer, tumours could be examined microscopically and a diagnosis made. But Velpeau argued that diagnoses founded upon clinical examination, that is, naked-eye observation, were superior to those based on microscopical examination.[83] Furthermore, Velpeau, who had for fifteen years worked closely with Lebert and his students by furnishing them with specimens, levelled a more serious charge, arguing that microscopists had consistently made diagnostic errors and regularly disagreed with each other. In some cases, by using the microscope, they had failed to recognize cancerous tumours and, conversely, had found cancerous some benign tumours. Thus, based on his own experience, Velpeau maintained he had no reason to trust microscopical analysis of tumour sections or to think the microscope had any practical value for surgeons.[84]

The second part of the dispute was at a more philosophical level. Lebert's postulation of and strict adherence to the specific cancer cell, his elevation of the cancer cell to an overarching system, along with his reclassification of tumours based on microscopical anatomy, became the main focus of attacks by both Bouillaud and Velpeau. This disagreement was methodological and epistemological: how was scientific knowledge to be acquired? Velpeau and Bouillaud argued for an empirical approach, contending that theories had to be derived from and confirmed by observation. If the observations did not support the theory, then the theory was no good. They accused defenders of Lebert's theory of the specific cancer cell of deducing observations from theory.[85]

The crux of the problem, Velpeau contended, was that Lebert had created yet another system. Like Claude Bernard some ten years later, and like many of his colleagues, Velpeau feared medical systems.[86] The observational, empirical approach of Paris clinical medicine, he believed, had freed medicine from philosophical systems which were negatively associated with, first, eighteenth-century medicine; second, German medicine; and third, the recent memories of Broussais's 'physiological medicine', which had divided the Parisian medical community for a decade. For Parisian clinicians philosophical medicine was seen as the antithesis of Paris Medicine; it was associated with either German or Montpellier medicine.[87] One way of defining Paris Medicine was to state clearly what it was not, and this was the strategy employed. Now Lebert had created a new system, supported by a new classification. In doing this, Velpeau argued that Lebert challenged the authority not only of individual physicians like himself but of the whole Paris clinical tradition. Importing a German philosophical approach, people like Lebert threatened to undermine the authority of Paris Medicine.

Velpeau saw Lebert and his school as a threat. Even though he worked closely with Lebert, Velpeau found him arrogant about the microscope, and Velpeau considered the microscopists upstarts. As he, with his thirty years of clinical experience, explained, clinicians were diagnosing cancer long before microscopists began examining tumour fragments.[88] He recounted that he told Lebert that his theory of the specific cancer cell was not supported by clinical observations, but Lebert held fast, in spite of all evidence to the contrary. Velpeau accused Lebert and his 'school' of being disdainful of the tradition of Paris Medicine, that is, of wanting to replace clinical with an unproved laboratory medicine.[89] In fact, Lebert wanted no such thing. He wanted to be accepted by the Parisian medical elite, to be regarded as a clinician who practised microscopy, not as a mere 'micrographer'. In his appearance before the Surgical Society of Paris in 1852–3, as a participant in that debate over cancer and microscopy, Lebert had protested against the use of the term 'micrographer'. The gist of his complaint was that he and his microscopist colleagues were not technicians, but clinicians and pathologists above all.[90]

Yet Velpeau, having had his say, in a final rhetorical burst, concluded the debate on a conciliatory note. In a spirit of *noblesse oblige* he wanted to welcome the enemy into the camp, that is, welcome the errant and arrogant microscopists into the clinic: "In the end, however, I am not so opposed to the micrographers as I have perhaps seemed, if they want to make reasonable concessions that the clinic requires of them, we will soon be in agreement." Sounding like Lebert himself, he conceded that microscopy did not have to be at odds with clinical medicine. Both clinical and microscopical observations should confirm each other. Microscopy belonged in the clinic to be practised by clinicians.[91] It was important for all concerned at the end of the debate that the solidarity of the entity of Paris Medicine be affirmed. Velpeau had called the debate in the first place as a vindication of the Paris Clinical School and the clinical viewpoint as he understood them. Paris Medicine could be held together by opposing forces. The integrity could be maintained by dichotomy. A desirable synthesis could be reached.

In concluding his report on the Academy debate for the *Moniteur des hôpitaux*, Broca constructed the debate on his own terms to vindicate the integrationist position. Thus he declared that microscopy had carried the day, that great progress had been made, that the microscope was now accepted within the Parisian medical community. As he put it: 'It's a whole revolution!'[92]

Broca redefined the central question of the debate to fit the agenda of the integrationists. The question posed was: is the microscope useful for the diagnosis of cancer? The consensus among the surgeons present at the debate was 'no'. But if the question was re-stated as 'is the microscope useful for pathology?', then the answer was 'yes'. With Broca, the utility of the instrument was assured, at least in the laboratory, if not in the clinic. As Malgaigne had suggested, by forcing a distinction between science and practice, the microscope was not yet very useful in medical practice, but it was useful in medical science, by which he meant medical research.[93]

Broca not only wanted to declare that the microscope had triumphed; he also wanted to heal the breach that he believed had been created by the debate. It was important to him to portray the debate in a positive light, to recast the criticisms of Velpeau and Bouillaud. Broca suggested that any innovation of importance, like the microscope, threatened to displace entrenched interests and arouse resistance. But, Broca maintained, this was all to the good, for this was the way science worked.[94] Broca used the controversy over the microscope and over two views of Paris Medicine to illustrate what he regarded as the broader features of the practice of science. Such resistance moderated scientific revolutions and set up a healthy dialectic, which was, he believed, the key to scientific progress. Broca believed that dichotomy was a necessary precursor to integration.

In the end, the distinction between microscopists and clinicians was forced and artificial. The debate could more accurately be characterized as a dispute over two approaches to Paris Medicine. Those who were labelled 'microscopists' represented 'the young Paris school'.[95] In no case did these young clinicians want to subordinate clinical to laboratory medicine. Like Virchow and Lebert, the young clinicians believed that the microscope had to be used in conjunction with pathological anatomy and clinical medicine. But the older generation, challenging the microscope's diagnostic utility, interpreted microscopists' willingness to rely on an instrument for diagnosis as a challenge to the experience and judgement of clinicians like themselves. It was seen as an attack on what they regarded as the ideals and practices which characterized and were the strength of Paris Medicine. These were the ideals of patient observation, rooted in sensualism, naked-eye observation of gross pathology, observations of patients in hospital clinics, and an emphasis on the centrality of the judgement of the clinician in interpreting data.

Discussion: Dichotomy or Integration?

In his preface to *Medicine at the Paris Hospital*, Ackerknecht justified his decision to exclude any detailed discussion of 'the work of physiologists, microscopists, chemists, or other French scientists of

Dichotomy or Integration?

the period' by explaining that he was writing a *medical history* [italics mine]. He argued that since 'the philosophy or the prejudices of the Paris clinicians effectively prevented their incorporating the discoveries of other branches of science into medicine', he was following their model. Since the Parisian clinicians had excluded science, or the so-called accessory sciences, so would he. Thus, in conceiving of this work, Ackerknecht perpetuated the dichotomy which some clinicians tried to establish between clinical medicine and laboratory science, between practice and research.[96] Just as Foucault took Bichat as his guide and wrote about the birth of the clinic by applying Bichat's approach to disease to his own analysis, so Ackerknecht found in the clinical perspective of the Paris school support for his own clinical point of view.[97]

But Ackerknecht could not maintain the dichotomy he set up. Like the Parisian clinicians about whom he was writing, he could not in the end take the science out of clinical medicine. Several examples illustrate this point: first, to show the disdain of clinicians for scientists, at a couple of places in his book he points out the important scientific-medical men who never had chairs at the Faculty of Medicine, such as Pierre Louis and François Magendie. Here his attempt was to circumscribe clinical medicine within the Faculty of Medicine. This effort was self-defeating, for one of the main points of the book was to put forward the notion of the 'Paris hospital', the full battery of institutions, organizations, disciplines, and specialists that made Paris medicine what it was. And the 'Paris hospital' had to include the physiologists, microscopists, chemists, and clinicians, all those outside the Faculty, all who contributed to the reputation of Paris Medicine.

Second, in his discussion of eclecticism, 'the fourth and last episode in the supremacy of Paris medicine', Ackerknecht calls it 'the richest and most brilliant period of them all'.[98] And it was the eclectics who in the 1830s began to incorporate new approaches like microscopy and medical statistics into clinical medicine and pathological anatomy. The problem with dichotomizing science and the clinic is clearly exemplified in Ackerknecht's discussion of Pierre Louis, whom he calls 'this true clinical scientist'.[99] What in fact did the clinicians of the 1830s and 1840s do if not move in the direction of developing clinical science? And what did the microscopists mean by their integrationist approach if not clinical science? They argued that not only was clinical medicine a science, but that in order to become more scientific, clinical medicine had to incorporate the accessory sciences. To do so was to continue the tradition of Paris Medicine, not to subvert it. Paris Medicine as constructed by eclectics such as Bouillaud was scientific medicine.[100]

John Lesch's work on physiology and my own on medical microscopy suggest that Ackerknecht's demarcations do not adequately reflect the reality of Paris Medicine. Physiology, including animal experimentation, microscopy, medical chemistry, and the numerical method had become key features of Paris Medicine by the late 1830s and the 1840s.[101]

Two approaches dominated in the relationship of medical microscopy to the Paris clinical school. Among the Parisian medical elite there was a need to make distinctions clear, in part because Paris Medicine was and had always been an umbrella entity containing a variety of constructions of disease and medicine and in part because of the rhetorical rules of debate: us and them, pro and con. Thus the debaters divided the Paris medical community into two camps: the microscopists and the clinicians; into two schools: the Paris School and the Young Paris School; into two approaches to microscopy: the German approach and the French approach; and even two kinds of medicine: medical science versus the practice of medicine, laboratory versus clinical, German versus French.

The rules of academic debate required a certain rhetorical argumentation. This was the rhetoric. And the rhetoric was central to the construction of the entity of Paris Medicine by its practitioners. The reality behind the rhetoric was more complex and less dramatic. Individual clinicians and surgeons took different points of view, making it impossible to articulate then or now a common viewpoint toward the microscope. Velpeau had used the microscope for over twenty years, even while denying its superiority to naked-eye observation in the case of tumours. Malgaigne declared the microscope useful for research, but not for practice. His was probably the dominant point of view within the Paris school. Andral and Rayer used the microscope regularly, had incorporated it into their research and practice, but felt no need for grand statements regarding the instrument. For them the microscope – as well as the entity of Paris Medicine – was non-problematic.

Some physicians, such as Lebert, were accused of making microscopy into a system, of making overarching claims for the instrument. Microscopists took different approaches: Donné made large claims for the instrument and staked his reputation on microscopy. But he worked in areas that were less controversial than cancer research. For clinicians and surgeons, cancer was a much more compelling problem: it was a disease that was always with them; they were confronted with patients suffering and dying. This provided a kind of reality check against unsubstantiated claims for the instrument.

The microscope became a symbol, an icon. For those who feared changes in medicine, the microscope symbolized all they feared: the changing face of medicine, reductionism, the objectification of the patient, the fear of new technology and the accompanying new skills it required. Once again the symbolic power of the microscope to frighten must be recognized. The microscope stood for ideas some clinicians feared: large claims, a monistic approach, yet another medical system, the connection with cell theory which many did not embrace, and German medicine. For proponents of scientific medicine, the microscope stood for progress, improved diagnostic capabilities. According to positivist historians the microscope was the wave of the future. For Charles Daremberg, for example, it was the consummate instrument of positivism.[102] Looking back, we see the microscope as forward-looking. But this was not clear to the clinicians and surgeons of the 1840s and 1850s. What did the instrument really offer them? A false hope? Another system? More speculation and philosophizing? They took a guardedly sceptical position, as good scientists.

The symbolic power of the microscope was greater than its actual utility. What could physicians in fact use it for? They could detect a few skin diseases, analyze blood and urine, identify a few parasites. By this time milk studies had become a dead end. And its use in pathology was uncertain. Thus a certain ambivalence prevailed. Was the microscope the wave of the future or an instrument which could not live up to its expectations?

When we try to understand the reality behind the rhetoric of the debate, when we try to articulate a clear-cut clinical and a microscopic point of view, the dichotomies become unclear. What we are left with are various individuals' points of view with general agreement only on the issues involved. Differing perceptions of clinical medicine and microscopy prevailed. Some clinicians constructed clinical medicine to suit their professional needs, to defend their interests. Hence they resisted the microscopical intrusion. Others felt no compelling need to embrace the instrument. The daily reality check of sick and dying patients meant that misdiagnosis could be crucial. They wanted to avoid any overarching claims regarding the microscope.

Thus in the debate microscopy was a 'way in', a way to force the articulation of national styles of science and medicine, to articulate what Paris Medicine was and what it was not. In calling the debate, Velpeau used the microscope and microscopists as a way to force a

Dichotomy or Integration?

discussion and formal articulation of two constructions of the Paris Clinical School. The clinical microscopists saw the integrationist approach as a way of reinvigorating clinical medicine, a way of moving clinical medicine to a new level. What the clinicians feared, the microscopists embraced. The clinicians believed that the microscope challenged the authority of physicians by bringing into question their expertise and judgement, by suggesting that they could not diagnose without the instrument. Some clinicians saw this as a personal and professional affront. The microscopists for their part claimed that the authority of the clinician was as great as ever, they just needed to incorporate new data.

In this mid-century debate two competing visions of Paris Medicine were articulated. It was not clear which would prevail or if they would co-exist. In the final analysis, Broca was probably right when he enthusiastically claimed that a revolution in microscopy had occurred.[103] But for the participants in the debate, for Parisian clinicians and surgeons, it was not clear which direction Paris Medicine would take.

Notes

1. Erwin Ackerknecht, *Medicine at the Paris Hospital, 1794-1848* (Baltimore: Johns Hopkins Press, 1967), 121-7. Quotes: 123, 125.
2. Ackerknecht, *Paris Hospital*, 125. For my own study of the Parisian microscopy community, see Ann La Berge, 'Medical Microscopy in Paris, 1830-1855', in Ann La Berge and Mordechai Feingold (eds), *French Medical Culture in the Nineteenth Century* (Amsterdam and Atlanta: Rodopi, 1994), 296-326.
3. Cited in Elizabeth Haigh, *Xavier Bichat and the Medical Theory of the Eighteenth Century* (London: Wellcome Institute, 1984), 97. The quotation is from Xavier Bichat, *Anatomie générale appliquée à la physiologie et la médecine*, 4 vols (Paris: Brosson and Gabon, 1801), 2: 576. On the philosophy of Ideology, see the classic article by George Rosen, 'The Philosophy of Ideology and the Emergence of Modern Medicine in France', *Bull. Hist. Med.* 20 (1946), 328-39.
4. Stanley Reiser, *Medicine and the Reign of Technology* (Cambridge and New York: Cambridge University Press, 1978), 75.
5. *Ibid.*; Brian Bracegirdle, *A History of Microtechnique* (Ithaca: Cornell University Press, 1978), 9; Haigh, *Xavier Bichat*, 96-9.
6. Reiser, *Reign of Technology*, 76; Charles Chevalier, *Des microscopes et de leur usage* (Paris: Crochard, 1839), 79-105; John Quekett, *A Practical Treatise on the Use of the Microscope*, 2nd edn (London: Baillière, 1852), 25-39.

7. Dora Weiner, *Raspail: Scientist and Reformer* (New York: Columbia University Press, 1964), 78-111; Bracegirdle, *History of Microtechnique*, 24-5; Chevalier, *Des microscopes*, 187-90.
8. Brian Ford, *The Leeuwenhoek Legacy* (London and Bristol: Biopress and Farrand Press, 1991), 175-6. On the cost and design of early microscopes, see James Cassedy, 'The Microscope in American Medical Science, 1840–1860', *Isis* 67 (1976), 82-3.
9. On pathological anatomy and Paris medicine, see Russell C. Maulitz, *Morbid Appearances: The Anatomy of Pathology in the Early Nineteenth Century* (Cambridge and New York: Cambridge University Press, 1987).
10. Donné's work is summarized in his *Cours de microscopie complémentaire des études médicales* (Paris: Baillière, 1844); François Magendie, *Les phénomènes physiques de la vie*, 4 vols. (Paris: Baillière, 1842), 3: 34-377. On Rayer, Bouillaud, Andral and Gavarret, see Ackerknecht, *Paris Hospital*, 101-13. On Gluge, see Paul Broca, *Traité des tumeurs* (Paris: Asselin, 1866), 30-1. For Gluge's communiqué on pathological tumours to the Royal Academy of Sciences, see 'Recherches microscopiques sur le fluide contenu dans les cancers encéphaloïdes', *Comptes-rendus de l'Académie des Sciences*, 2 January 1837, 20. On Magendie's use of the microscope in teaching physiology, see La Berge, 'Medical Microscopy in Paris', 305-7.
11. La Berge, 'Medical Microscopy in Paris'.
12. *Bulletin de l'Académie de Médecine* 9 (1843-4), 330-653.
13. Hermann Lebert, *Physiologie pathologique* (Paris: Baillière, 1845).
14. *Bulletin de l'Académie de Médecine* (1854-5), 7-447.
15. On the teaching of pathological anatomy, see Maulitz, *Morbid Appearances*, 60; Ackerknecht, *Paris Hospital*, 167; Pierre Huard and Marie-José Imbault-Huart, 'La vie et l'oeuvre de Jean Cruveilhier, anatomiste et clinicien', *Episteme* 8 (1974), 46-57.
16. Ackerknecht, *Paris Hospital*, 101-13. On medical eclecticism, see Eugène Bouchut, *Histoire de la médecine et des doctrines médicales*, 2 vols (Paris: Germer-Baillière, 1873), 2: 585-7. Bouchut attributed the origins of medical eclecticism in France to the publication by Jules Guérin of an 1831 essay: *Eclectisme en médecine* (2: 586). Physicians borrowed and adapted the idea of eclecticism from the philosophical eclecticism of Victor Cousin (2: 585).
17. Neither the introduction of animal experimentation nor of medical chemistry as far as I know has been the subject of a major investigation by medical historians. On the debate over the numerical method and the introduction of medical statistics into Paris

medicine, see Terence Murphy, 'Medical Knowledge and Statistics Methods in Early Nineteenth-Century France', *Medical History* 25 (1981), 301-19. See also John Rosser Matthews, *Quantification and the Quest for Medical Certainty* (Princeton, New Jersey: Princeton University Press, 1995), ch. 2; Theodore M. Porter, *The Rise of Statistical Thinking, 1820-1900* (Princeton, New Jersey: Princeton University Press, 1986), 151-62; I am currently working on a book on medical statistics, medical microscopy, and the clinical tradition in nineteenth-century France.

18. For biographical material on Donné, see Camille Dreyfus, 'Alfred Donné (1801-1878): Un précurseur en hématologie', *Nouvelle revue d'hématologie* 2 (1961), 241-55; A. Lennox Thorburn, 'Alfred François Donné, 1801-1878, discoverer of *Trichomonas vaginalis* and of leukaemia', *British Journal of Venereal Diseases* 50 (1974), 377-80; La Berge, 'Medical Microscopy'.

19. Alfred Donné, *Recherches physiologiques et chimico-microscopiques sur les globules du sang, du pus, du mucus, et de ceux des humeurs de l'oeil* (Paris: Didot le jeune, 1831), 5.

20. *Ibid.*, 6.

21. *Ibid.*, 7.

22. Donné, *Cours de microscopie complémentaire des études médicales*, 32.

23. Gabriel Andral, *Pathological Hematology: An Essay on the Blood in Disease*, trans. J. F. Meigs and Alfred Stillé (Philadelphia: Lea and Blanchard, 1844), 16-18, 26-9, 32-7, 46-7, 83-7, etc. Pierre Rayer, *Traité des maladies des reins et des altérations de la sécrétion urinaire*, 2 vols (Paris: Baillière, 1839), 1: viii-ix, 92-3, 114-23, etc.

24. Thorburn, 'Alfred François Donné'.

25. Dreyfus, 'Alfred Donné'; Thorburn, 'Alfred François Donné'. There is no agreement on priority. Maxwell Wintrobe credits John Hughes Bennett and Rudolf Virchow with the first description of the new disease, leukaemia. See Maxwell Wintrobe, *Hematology: The Blossoming of a Science* (Philadelphia: Lea and Febiger, 1985), 12-16. For Donné's work on this, see Donné, 'Sur la constitution microscopique du sang', *Comptes-rendus de l'Académie des Sciences* 6 (1838), 17-18 and *Cours de microscopie*, 135-6.

26. V. Kruta, 'David Gruby', in *Dictionary of Scientific Biography*, 5: 565-6; Raphael Blanchard, 'Notices biographiques. III. David Gruby, 1810-1898', *Archives de parasitologie* 2 (1899), 48-59.

27. Alfred-Armand Velpeau, *Traité des maladies du sein* (Paris: Masson, 1854), VI-XVI, 481-505. Velpeau had consistently maintained this position since the 1840s.

28. Paul Broca, *Traité des tumeurs* (Paris: Asselin, 1866), vi-vii.

29. Paul Broca, 'La microscopie pathologique est-elle utile?', *Moniteur des hôpitaux*, 17 Oct. 1854, 985, and 2 Dec. 1854, 1156.
30. On Gruby, see Kruta, 'David Gruby'; and Blanchard, 'David Gruby', 43-74; Jean Théodoridès, 'L'oeuvre scientifique du Dr. Gruby', *Revue d'histoire de médecine hébraïque* 27 (1954), 27-38.
31. These proto-dermatologists were referred to as and called themselves specialists in 'maladies de la peau'. On nascent specialities in French medicine, see George Weisz, 'The Development of Medical Specialization in Nineteenth-Century Paris', in La Berge and Feingold (eds), *French Medical Culture*, 149-87 and Ackerknecht, *Paris Hospital*, 163-80.
32. Blanchard, 'David Gruby', 55-6. Bazin, Devergie and others were receptive, but Cazenave was still resisting.
33. Louis Mandl, 'De la structure intime des tumeurs ou des productions pathologiques', *Archives générales de médecine* 8 (1840), 313-29; 'Histogenèse', in *Anatomie microscopique*, 2 vols (Paris: Baillière, 1838-47), 2: 339-70; Leland Rather, *The Genesis of Cancer* (Baltimore: Johns Hopkins University Press, 1978), 109. On Mandl's microscopy course, see La Berge, 'Medical Microscopy in Paris'. Louis Mandl, *Traité pratique du microscope* (Paris: Baillière, 1839); Chevalier, *Des microscopes et de leur usage*; Félix Dujardin, *Nouveau manuel complet de l'observateur au microscope* (Paris: Roret, 1843).
34. See Lebert's own account in Hermann Lebert, *Biographische Notizen* (Breslau: Korn, 1869), and Francis Schiller, *Paul Broca: Founder of French Anthropology, Explorer of the Brain* (Berkeley: University of California Press, 1979), 59-76. For more on Lebert, see La Berge, 'Medical Microscopy in Paris'.
35. Andral, *Pathological Hematology*; Rayer, *Traité des maladies des reins*.
36. Lebert, *Physiologie pathologique*, viii, ix.
37. *Ibid.*
38. *Ibid.*
39. George Sussman, 'The Glut of Doctors in Mid-Nineteenth-Century France', *Comparative Studies in Society and History* 19 (1977), 293-303; Ian Dowbiggin, *Inheriting Madness: Professionalization and Psychiatric Knowledge in 19th-Century France* (Los Angeles: University of California Press, 1991), 13.
40. For details on public and private microscopy courses see La Berge, 'Medical Microscopy in Paris'.
41. Donné, *Cours de microscopie*, 8-9. Although this article does not address it, legal medicine specialists were among the first physicians to adopt the microscope. See, for example, Henri Bayard, 'De l'examen des tâches diverses qui peuvent être l'objet de recherches

médico-légales dans les expertises judiciaires', *Annales d'hygiène publique et de médecine légale* 29 (1843): 162-84.

42. The Société de biologie included leading microscopists like Lebert among its founders. E. Gley, 'La Société de biologie et l'évolution des sciences biologiques en France de 1849 à 1900', in E. Gley, *Essais de philosophie et l'histoire* (Paris: Masson, 1900), 168-9, 175, 272-4. For more on Lebert and the Société de biologie, see La Berge, 'Medical Microscopy in Paris'.

43. On Donné's milk studies and his work in proto-paediatrics, see Ann La Berge, 'Alfred Donné and the Medicalization of Child Care in Nineteenth-Century France', *J. Hist. Med.* 48 (1991), 20-43. For full citation, see Harvey's note 5, this volume.

44. *Comptes-rendus de l'Académie des Sciences* 9 (1839), 485-6. See also Alfred Donné, 'Procédés de gravure des images photogéniques sur plaques d'argent', *Comptes-rendus de l'Académie des Sciences* 10 (1840), 933-4.

45. Thorburn, 'Alfred Donné'.

46. In the debate on microscopy in *Bulletin de l'Académie de Médecine* (1854-5), 43-4. Hereafter referred to simply as Microscopy debate with the page reference. '... my reproach is addressed, not to the instrument itself, but to those who use it.' (p. 45). See Bouillaud's similar comment on p. 312.

47. On Pinel as clinician, see Philippe Pinel, *The Clinical Training of Doctors*, ed. Dora Weiner (Baltimore: Johns Hopkins University Press, 1980); on the conflicting values that beset Laennec's medical practice and research, see Jacalyn Duffin, 'Private Practice and Public Research: The Patients of R. T. H. Laennec', in La Berge and Feingold (eds), *French Medical Culture*, 118-48.

48. See 'Correspondance', in *Comptes-rendus des l'Académie des Sciences* 17 (1843), 815-7; and 'Falsification du lait', in 'Académie des Sciences', 20 Feb. 1843, *Gazette médicale de Paris* 11 (1843), 128.

49. Alphonse Devergie, 'Sur la valeur de l'examen microscopique du lait dans le choix d'une nourrice', *Mémoires de l'Académie Royale de Médecine* 10 (1843), 206-22.

50. *Bulletin de l'Académie de Médecine* 7 (1841-2), 197-210.

51. *Ibid.*

52. Lebert, *Biographische Notizen*.

53. The best discussion of Lebert's theory of the specific cancer cell is Michel, 'Du Microscope, des ses applications à l'anatomie pathologique, au diagnostic et au traitement des maladies', *Mémoires de l'Académie de Médecine* 21 (1856), 315-30.

54. *Bulletin de l'Académie de Médecine* 9 (1843-4), 330-653; Rather, *The*

Genesis of Cancer, 109-10. For a good short summary of the debate, see Jean Cruveilhier, *Traité d'anatomie pathologique générale*, 5 vols (Paris: Baillière, 1849-64), 3 (1856): 710-11.
55. On Lebert as microscopy teacher and the Lebert 'school', see La Berge, 'Medical Microscopy in Paris'.
56. On the Société de biologie, see above, note 42.
57. Lebert, *Biographische Notizen*, 32-3.
58. Michel, 'Du microscope', 322.
59. Charles Daremberg, *La Médecine: Histoire et doctrines* (Paris: Didier et Baillière, 1865), 290-304. Quote, 290-1.
60. Cruveilhier, *Traité d'anatomie pathologique*, 3 (1856), 713, 736. Quote: 713. 'Parmi les médecins micrographes … se place en première ligne M. Lebert… .'
61. Lebert, *Biographischen Notizen*, 32-3.
62. Broca, *Traité des tumeurs*, x-xi.
63. *Ibid.*, vii.
64. *Ibid.*, viii.
65. *Ibid.*
66. *Ibid.*, xi.
67. *Ibid.*, 40.
68. Paul Broca, 'Anatomie pathologique du cancer', *Mémoires de l'Académie de Médecine* 16 (1852), 453-824.
69. Microscopy debate, 30.
70. Erwin Ackerknecht, *Rudolf Virchow, 1843-1901: Doctor, Statesman, Anthropologist* (New York: Arno Press, 1981, reprint of original 1953 edition), 54.
71. William Carpenter, *The Microscope and its Revelations* (Philadelphia: Blanchard and Lea, 1856), 39.
72. *Bulletin de l'Académie de Médecine* 4 Oct. 1854-16 Jan. 1855, (1854-5), 7-447.
73. *Ibid.*, 279-80. To set the stage for this debate framed by military rhetoric, see Robert A. Nye, *Masculinity and Male Codes of Honor in Modern France* (New York: Oxford University Press, 1993). On debates at the Paris Academy of Medicine, see George Weisz, *The Medical Mandarins: The French Academy of Medicine in the Nineteenth and Early Twentieth Centuries* (New York: Oxford University Press, 1995), 73-83, 159-88.
74. *Bulletin de l'Académie de Médecine* (1854-55), 26-44.
75. *Ibid.*, 282, 284.
76. *Ibid.*, 202, 205.
77. *Ibid.*, 120-3.
78. *Ibid.*, 194-8.

79. *Ibid.*, 242-66; 382-405.
80. 'Séance de l'Académie de Médecine', *Moniteur des hôpitaux*, 5 Oct. 1854-23 Jan. 1855.
81. Microscopy debate, 445.
82. *Bulletin de la Société de Chirurgie de Paris* 3 (1852-3), 232-356; Microscopy debate, 41-4, 159-60, 307, 312, 436-47.
83. Microscopy debate, 28.
84. *Ibid.*, 34-41. See also L. S. Jacyna, 'The Laboratory and the Clinic: The Impact of Pathology on Surgical Diagnosis in the Glasgow Western Infirmary', *Bull. Hist. Med.* 62 (1988): 384-406.
85. *Ibid.*, 41-4, 159-60, 307, 312, 436-47.
86. Claude Bernard, *Introduction to the Study of Experimental Medicine*, trans. Henry C. Greene (New York: Dover, 1957).
87. On Broussais, see Ackerknecht, *Paris Hospital*, 61-80, and Ackerknecht, 'Broussais or a Forgotten Medical Revolution', *Bull. Hist. Med.* 27 (1953): 320-43; see also Michel Foucault, *The Birth of the Clinic: An Archaeology of Medical Perception* (New York: Vintage Books, 1965; originally published in French in 1963), 174-92.
88. Microscopy debate, 39-44.
89. *Ibid.*, 158-66, 436-43.
90. *Bulletin de la Société de Chirurgie*, 310-11, 314.
91. Microscopy debate, 446-7. Quote: 446.
92. Broca, *Moniteur des hôpitaux*, 23 Jan. 1855, 73.
93. Microscopy debate, 131-46.
94. See above, note 29. See also Paul Broca, 'Des tumeurs fibroplastiques', *Moniteur des hôpitaux*, 2 Dec. 1854, 1156.
95. Microscopy debate, 445.
96. Ackerknecht, *Paris Hospital*.
97. Foucault, *Birth of the Clinic*.
98. Ackerknecht, *Paris Hospital*, 101.
99. *Ibid.*, 102.
100. For Bouillaud's construction of Paris Medicine, see Jean-Baptiste Bouillaud, *Essai sur la philosophie médicale et sur les généralités de la clinique médicale* (Paris: Rouvier and le Bouvier, 1836) and the introductory essay in this volume.
101. John E. Lesch, *Science and Medicine in France: The Emergence of Experimental Physiology, 1790-1855* (Cambridge, Mass.: Harvard University Press, 1984); La Berge, 'Medical Microscopy'.
102. Daremberg, *La Médecine: Histoire et doctrines*, 297-9.
103. For support for the idea of a microscopical revolution, see Cruveilhier, *Traité d'anatomie pathologique*, 3 (1856): *passim*.

8

'Faithful to its old traditions'?
Paris Clinical Medicine from the Second Empire to the Third Republic (1848–1872)

Joy Harvey

A definition of clinical medicine written in the 1870s, in Dechambre's *Dictionnaire de Médecine*, might almost be read as an anticipation of both Erwin Ackerknecht's classic study on the Paris hospitals and Michel Foucault on the development of the clinic.[1] Louis Hecht, the author of this short article, emphasized the French use of the term 'clinic' in a double sense. The first sense was as a designation of 'that branch of medical science which incorporates all others in a practical aim to study a sick organism in order to return it to its normal state or at least to alleviate and prolong its existence'. In the second sense, it referred to 'a hospital service in which the patients, while receiving medical care, serve at the same time to instruct those who study medicine'.[2] The double aspect of practical medicine taking place at the bed of the patient echoed the definition made by the physician, Jean Baptiste Bouillaud, later quoted by Michel Foucault to such good effect.[3]

This chapter seeks to enquire to what degree French clinical medicine can be said to have flourished during the Second Empire and in the first years of the Third Republic.

Searching for information concerning how Paris clinics actually functioned in the decades between 1848 and 1872, one can turn to two kinds of primary sources. The first is provided by descriptions and case reports printed in the multiplying hospital gazettes of that period. The second is provided by regular reports as detailed in the letters of two unusual young doctors who shared with their families the experience of studying and practising in the Paris hospitals. Covering most of this period of thirty years is the correspondence of Paul Broca over the years from 1841 to 1857 and that of Mary Corinna Putnam (Jacobi) from 1866 to 1871. Both sets of letters offer extensive and vivid word pictures about clinical procedures and instruction while describing the physicians and fellow students encountered. Between the two of them, they cover medical and surgical services in most of the Paris hospitals.[4] These sources display the public face of clinical medicine described in the medical press and the private face shown in the letters, each supplementing and highlighting the other.

In the early 1840s when medical journals first began to proliferate, a satirical article appeared on 'Le Médecin', describing methods of self-advancement which could make one noticed in the medical community. The aspiring doctor could 'affect the periodical press'. If he manages to found a journal of 'medical or chirurgical sciences, medico-surgical or surgical-medical', he's done it, 'he has put down a foundation for his unlimited renown. This will be his Archimedes lever. Science won't be able to take a step without his permission; no malady will exist which has not appeared in his gazette. Young doctors will search out his approval, the old ones will humour him, everyone will fear him. He will succeed in giving a fever to the Faculty itself!'[5]

The periodical fever struck almost every well-known physician in the Paris clinics in the period between 1820 and 1860. After that period, although the physicians continued to contribute, professional medical editors took over major control. There had been combined medical-surgical journals since the original Medico-Chirurgical Society was founded in Paris in 1805, to be followed within a few years by a London society by the same name.[6] Societies and journals imitating these societies sprang up in the provinces and around the world.[7] In the 1820s and the 1830s, as medical journals proliferated, a few journals bore not only the title 'medico-chirurgical' but added the word 'clinic' to the title.[8]

An interesting development of the medical periodical press in the period was the appearance not just of the medical journal devoted to a medical society or general medical reviews, but also of true gazettes, devoted to the hospital clinics and medical news. The hospital gazettes give some indication of how Paris clinics functioned. They open a window on not only the medical educational system which they served in the decades between 1840 and 1870, but the wider hospital system. Judging by the medical press, French clinical medicine was gaining institutional strength and positions in clinical research through the end of the 1860s, revitalized with the addition of medical laboratories in the early 1870s.

The hospital gazettes provide a rich, almost untapped source about clinical medicine in the mid-nineteenth century. They differ

'Faithful to its old traditions'?

from the medical society journals, which reflected presentations by a select group of prestigious physicians. Admittedly, reports of the medical societies featured in every medical gazette, including the latest debates in the Académie de Médecine. Like the periodical press intended for the general reader, the medical gazettes appeared weekly or even more often. They presented information about both national and foreign medical news, reprinted materials from lectures and reports, and gave updated summaries of current clinical observations. Excluding from consideration medical speciality journals, medical society journals, or academy bulletins, there were about six medical gazettes by mid-century which covered general clinical subjects. As a sign of the vitality of clinical medicine after 1847, four were founded between 1847 and 1853, only two in the earlier clinical period: *Gazette des Hôpitaux civils et militaires* (1828–1925) edited by François Fabre; *Gazette Médicale de Paris* (1830–1916) edited by Jules Guérin; *L'Union Médicale* (1847–1926) edited by Amédée Latour; *Revue Médico-Chirurgicale de Paris* (1847–1855) edited by Joseph-François Malgaigne; *Gazette Hebdomadaire de Médecine et Chirurgie* (1853–1902) edited by Amédée Dechambre which was soon after its formation sponsored by the Ministry of Public Instruction; and *Moniteur des Hôpitaux* (1853–1862) edited by Henri de Castelnau with some unacknowledged help from Louis Joseph Fleury and Paul Broca. Additional clinical journals sprang up in the period which followed, most notably *Tribune Médicale* (1867–1933) and *Progrès Médicale* (1873–20th century). The clinical osteologist, Jules Guérin, who edited *Gazette Médicale de Paris*, has been hailed by one of his later competitors as the real father of the medical periodical.[9] The Paris hospital gazettes soon increased their appearance from weekly to as often as three times a week by the mid-1840s, when *L'Union Médicale* was first published.

The medical press received a second boost around 1867 when journals accepted advertising for the first time. A few editors-in-chief tried to hold out against this and finally conceded after the advertisements were screened, but still prohibited advertising from their front pages.[10] Earlier the practice had been frowned upon by editors. Some gazettes, seeking advertising to sustain the publication, temporarily acquired an unsavoury reputation. François Fabre's *Gazette des Hôpitaux*, in 1841, solicited advertising from the makers of various unguents, lotions and medical apparatuses. The editor, requiring regular contributions to the journal about the clinics from aspiring *internes*, used the unorthodox method of including tickets to variety shows in the wrappers of free copies delivered to the *salle de garde*, where the hospital residents stayed. One young *externe*, Paul Broca, an upright young Protestant, was shocked. He wrote satirical songs about the gazette, leading a successful boycott against it, and forcing it to change its method of solicitation.[11] Later, he almost became a professional medical editor when he flirted for a short period with the possibility of taking over Malgaigne's journal, *Revue Médico-Chirurgicale de Paris*.[12] Since the hospital gazettes depended to a large extent on the accounts of clinics and reports of the lectures of the medical faculty by the *internes*, their support was a major factor in survival for the gazettes.

Most gazettes that lasted over many decades had close ties to particular prestigious hospital physicians and major medical societies. One such gazette was *L'Union Médicale*, established in 1847 by Amédée Latour. The visibility of this gazette was probably due primarily to its link to the prominent physician and clinician Armand Trousseau through whose influence it reported upon and published papers given at the Société des Hôpitaux. Since this hospital society, in turn, owed its power to Gabriel Andral, also a powerful member of the Faculté de Médecine, the gazette could claim at least two major sources of medical power. While not himself of major importance in the medical clinics, since he never taught in the faculty, Latour acquired a sufficient reputation from his medical journal to become an associate – but never a full member – of the Académie de Médecine.[13]

Like the earlier gazettes, *L'Union Médicale* reported on hospital clinical cases. The review of a case or group of cases would be made by an aspiring young *interne*, who routinely recorded the observations, methods, and innovations of his clinical chief. Since these were signed articles, this form of publication offered a common road for advancement for an *interne* who wished to establish his own name and enhance the reputation of his *chef de service* and patron. Sometimes the focus was on a wide range of cases as these were diagnosed and treated on a particular medical or surgical service, sometimes the reports were organized around a specialized topic. The gazette included formal clinical lectures by physicians *agrégés* in the Faculté de Médecine, on specific topics forming part of medical education. It included reports of discussions held in the Académie de Médecine, as did all the gazettes, and occasionally included debates before the Académie des Sciences when these were relevant to medicine.

The hospital gazette also included statistics on epidemics and national public health issues, like vaccination and puerperal fever. Occasionally it reported professional news about the position of physicians and surgeons or discussed the changes in personnel of medical and surgical clinics and hospitals. No gazette focused on a single hospital as was common in England or America (for example *Guy's Hospital Reports* in England or *Mount Sinai Hospital Reports* in New York), but instead surveyed the full range of Paris hospitals under the control of both the Faculty of Medicine and the Assistance Publique, including the military hospitals, with occasional provincial hospital reports. It is difficult to indicate the wide range or to do justice to the richness of these journals in a brief summary.

Although Paris clinics have been accused, with some justice, of stressing diagnosis and pathology, they never ignored discussions of therapies or techniques that might offer relief to the patient. In the first issue of *L'Union Médicale* in 1847, Jean Baptiste Bouillaud's method for typhoid fever diagnosis was described as well as his treatment by bleeding. Admittedly, other reports from his clinics stressed diagnosis of unusual cases such as an anomalous double aorta resulting in aneurysm. The early issues included a report from Pierre Briquet's clinic at the Hôpital de la Charité suggesting a different treatment of typhoid by purgatives along with descriptions of cases of paralysis and hysteria. The surgical clinic of Antoine Joseph Jobert de Lamballe at Saint Louis reported on various indications for amputation of the lower jaw while Auguste François Chomel's clinic at the Hôtel-Dieu was represented by cases on liver tumours and pleurisy with a review of possible treatments for each condition. All of these regular reports, as well as those from the Hôpital de la Pitié and the Hôpital de la Ville depended on analyses written, as indicated above, by clinical or surgical *internes*.[14] In contrast the formal clinical lectures had a more structured form, although again they were often summaries provided by an *interne*. For example, François Leuret's lectures at the Bicêtre covering diagnosis of general paralysis of the insane were reported upon in sequential issues of the same gazette along with summaries of Charles Daremberg's lectures on the history of medicine.[15] On the whole, *L'Union Médicale* reflected a more conservative opinion than one associates with medicine in the later decades of the century. The anti-clerical physicians of the Third Republic later rather naughtily referred to this journal as the only hospital paper which regularly invoked the name of God.[16]

Although much of the hospital gazette was self-reflective of the French system, new methods or techniques developed in English and other European hospitals were regularly discussed, especially where new techniques in surgery or new therapies were concerned. The results of English sanitary commissions were detailed with marked interest. Reports on new styles of practice were examined also throughout the Paris system. For example, in the early issues of *L'Union Médicale*, sixteen different reports on the efficacy of chloroform were presented from a variety of doctors and surgeons. Methods or techniques developed in English and other European hospitals were also discussed especially in the case of surgery, or radically new therapies, or the important topic of English sanitary reform.[17] In later volumes there were more complete reviews of both the British and German medical press. However, the primary focus remained the Paris hospitals.

Important features consistently available in all the journals were medical examination results and consequent placement of *externes* and *internes* in the hospitals, and the movement of major professors from hospital to hospital as various clinical positions opened up.[18] At certain politically significant moments, the editor of the gazette presented a problem he considered to be of major importance: sometimes a professional debate about the teaching or practice of medicine, sometimes a discussion of an issue concerning the health of the population at large.

In 1853 the *Moniteur des Hôpitaux*, a new style of hospital gazette, was founded by Henri de Castelnau, a self-proclaimed positivist and a good friend of Paul Broca. Castelnau had originally worked on one of the other hospital gazettes and was charged by that gazette of taking lists of subscribers when he left in order to build up his own journal. The attack may have been motivated partly because Castelnau and his friends, who had supported the Second Republic, challenged the conservative establishment, particularly those physicians like Pierre Adolphe Piorry and Paul Dubois favoured by the Second Empire. The journal reflected the new 'positivist' medicine that the recently created Société de Biologie had insisted upon. It incorporated a more confrontational editorial style on professional issues and regularly printed medical satires attacking thinly disguised members of the Paris faculty. Regardless of his attacks on powerful medical figures, neither Castelnau nor his associates challenged the fundamental structure of Paris clinical medicine.

In the early issues of the *Moniteur des Hôpitaux*, long articles appeared on the inordinately high death rate of women in childbirth at the Maternité, an issue being argued before the Académie de

Médecine. The *Moniteur* took a polemical stance which it sustained over the next three years, depending primarily on comparative studies done by a clinical physician, Alexandre Thierry.[19] Castelnau's report in December 1856 detailed Alfred-Armand Velpeau's response in the Académie de Médecine to the defensive positions of Armand Trousseau and Paul Dubois. Velpeau's statistics showed that while the Hôtel-Dieu had been condemned for its unsanitary condition, only 1 in 38 women died in childbirth in that hospital in contrast to 1 in 19 at the Maternité. At Saint Louis, a specialist hospital for the treatment of skin diseases, only 1 woman in 216 had died in labour. Velpeau had cited the British 'contagionist' James Simpson who had identified one careless midwife (in a group of twelve) as the source of 20 maternal deaths, as she carried contagion from woman to woman. The suggestion had been made that the administration should either reduce the number of women giving birth in the hospitals or eliminate the great maternity hospitals completely. A resolution had been presented by Alexandre Thierry, originating from the Paris municipal government, advocating that the *maternités* be closed since they served as 'centres of infection'. Dubois, an obstetrician favoured by Napoleon III, whose son Dubois later delivered, argued that this was difficult and expensive to do, and would destroy clinical teaching on this subject.[20] Trousseau, who believed in the existence of post-operative fever but not puerperal fever, according to Castelnau, supported Dubois against the obstetrical judgement of Velpeau. In his editorial response, Castelnau, referring to Dubois with thinly disguised contempt as 'M. le Baron', agreed that closure of the hospitals would affect clinical teaching but added: 'It was necessary first to serve humanity, then science, and only finally the needs of the profession.'[21] In spite of the overwhelming evidence brought against the maternity hospitals, the Assistance Publique simply took the measure under advisement, refusing to act, much to the dismay of the editor.

One might add parenthetically that Armand Husson, then director of the Assistance Publique, which controlled hospital administration, argued six years later that the death figures at the maternity hospitals were unjustifiably inflated by neonatal deaths and stillbirths added to the total hospital maternal death rates. He argued, with what justification we do not know, that this was a practice not followed in England. The inadequacy of Husson's self-justifying response is shown by the enormous difference Velpeau had shown in maternal death rates between hospitals.[22] Husson had further justified the high death rate in all wards of the Paris hospitals by arguing that unlike the London hospitals, there was no selection of patients. All the sick poor of Paris had to be accommodated.[23]

An English reviewer, Blanchard Jerrold, took up the theme of the Paris hospitals at the end of the 1860s, publishing a series of articles on the Paris hospitals entitled 'The Sick Poor of Paris'. He compared the hospitals of Paris and London to the definite disadvantage of the English hospitals. Admiringly, he described the centralized stores and the experience of the patient from initial diagnosis at the central bureau of the Assistance Publique, through the acute or chronic wards of the hospital.[24] As was often true of the medical journals of both countries, praise for foreign medicine occurred primarily when journalists were pushing for reform within their own system.

The hospital journals offered a chance for young physicians to make their names known outside the clinics where they studied. Castelnau's new journal had provided a forum for young physicians like Paul Broca and his friends who had submitted reports to prestigious medical societies but whose discussions might not be fully recorded in the bulletins of those societies. When Broca, for example, wished to respond to the Académie de Médecine he was hampered from replying in the journal of the Academy because he was not a member. Broca used the hospital journal as a forum for his interpretation of cancer and his advocacy of microscopy in pathology in opposition to the views of established physicians. He became involved in a heated fight in the early 1850s with the distinguished clinician Velpeau about the movement of metastastic cancer through the blood, using the *Moniteur des Hôpitaux* to publish his replies to Velpeau's attacks in the Académie de Médecine.[25]

The *Moniteur des Hôpitaux* followed the unusual practice of featuring satirical pieces as a running column underneath the main news stories, beginning with the first page of the paper. While some of the satirical pieces were simply jokes, illustrating for example comical misapplications of the clinical method, others attacked well-known figures.[26] One of the most sustained satires involved a humorous rendering of Trousseau's rather casual clinical lecturing style (which contrasted to his magnificent writing style). This satire began as a dialogue between an 'auditor' 'who believes in common sense' (possibly Pierre Adolphe Piorry who endorsed the concept of 'bon sens' in medicine) and a satin 'toque' (symbol of the successful *agrégé* professor) as a demonstration of the 'art' of clinical lecturing.

The 'toque' imitated Trousseau's clinical presentation which, through continual asides, moves further and further away from the case at hand.[27] Paul Broca also contributed to the satirical poems and dialogues which were a feature of the journal. Broca had learned not to sign his satires after a parody of one of Piorry's religious poems had been recognized under the anagram Bap. Lacour.[28]

The comparatively short life of the *Moniteur des Hôpitaux*, in spite of its support for what Ackerknecht has termed the 'young Paris school' (the new wave of medical men including Paul Broca), may have been doomed by its challenge to established physicians who controlled many of the rival gazettes. By 1859, the journal had gone into decline, becoming little more than a review journal, eliminating both the humour and the controversial editorials which had been a feature of its first six years. This may have been due to the lessened interest of Broca and his colleagues who, along with Castelnau, founded the Société d'Anthropologie de Paris in that year with its own journals, and moved into established positions.[29] The other medical gazettes, however, continued to develop and expand their clinical commentary. By 1873 it was possible for a young medical student or visiting clinician to consult a new gazette, *Le Progrès Medical*, for information about the location of interesting clinical cases throughout the Paris hospital system. The type of case, hospital, service, and even bed number were helpfully provided.[30]

The correspondence of Paul Broca with his parents, which sadly exists only between 1841 and 1857, extends our image of the range of clinical experience available to young students. He passed through an extensive sequence of hospital clinics during the fifteen-year process that took him from beginning student, to *externe*, to *interne*, finally winning, through examination, his place as *agrégé* professor at the medical school.[31] As a young medical student, Broca attended clinics given by Chomel, Roux, and Cloquet at the Hôtel-Dieu; Rostan, Dubois, and Fougieur at the Pitié. He dismissed the formal medical lectures given by Piorry on therapeutics as a waste of time, since he believed the physician simply pushed his favourite diagnostic and therapeutic methods regardless of success. He regarded surgical lectures by Pierre Nicolas Gerdy and Gabriel Andral with great respect, later editing and publishing Gerdy's lectures. When he passed the *internat*, Broca was placed in the service of François Leuret at Bicêtre. Although Leuret practised clinical psychiatry, he was in the process of preparing his great text on neuroanatomy, introducing Broca to that field. Broca went on to serve as an *interne* to Pierre Nicolas Gerdy in surgery at the Charité, under Stanislas Laugier at Hôpital Beaujon, under Joseph François Malgaigne at Saint Louis, moving to the Hôtel-Dieu, where he finished the rest of his internship during the revolutionary year of 1848. Later, as an *agrégé* professor, he taught clinics and ran services throughout the Paris hospital system supplementing surgical teaching with both lectures and clinics for major professors who were ill or on vacation through the late 1850s and early 1860s. In 1867, Broca was made a professor of external pathology at the Charité, moving to a chair in clinical surgery in 1868. With the usual shift of teaching chairs as individuals died or moved on, Broca became professor of clinical surgery at Hôpital des Cliniques in 1872, although he continued to make his greatest scientific reputation in neuroanatomy and biological anthropology.[32]

The interesting feature of Paris medicine throughout this period was the wide range of experience available to the medical student and the ease with which many physicians trained in this school passed from clinical observation to experimental research. Paul Broca, although trained as a surgeon and neuroanatomist, was proficient in microscopy and did research on cancer using this instrument, as Ann La Berge has discussed in this volume and elsewhere.[33] Broca won a prize from the Académie de Médecine on this work. He published a monograph on aneurysms, and his *agrégé* thesis had been on hernias! In the 1860s, as he began to be more interested in brain pathology, he extended the work of one of his professors, Jean Baptiste Bouillaud, on brain localization with so much success that he is still cited for his anatomical and clinical investigation of the speech area of the brain. As the founder of the Société d'Anthropologie he wrote many articles on race, craniology and evolution. While still teaching clinical surgery, he began a twenty-year work on comparative brain anatomy, tracing the limbic lobe in a large number of primate species.[34]

The broad training offered by mid-century Paris clinics is shown by the careers not only of Paul Broca but also of many of his friends. His contemporary and friend Jules Gavarret studied the physics of blood flow and later became Professor of Medical Physics. Another close friend, the neurosurgeon Charles Edouard Brown-Séquard, had already begun to make his name by investigating clinical manifestations of spinal cord (and later claimed inheritance of experimentally produced damage to the spinal cord) while publishing an internationally recognized journal of anatomy and physiology. Eventually Brown-Séquard would succeed to Claude Bernard's chair at the Collège de France.[35]

Scientific experiment and observation were encouraged through the growing number of scientific societies. Paul Broca described his week, hour by hour, as a young *agrégé* professor of medicine in 1855 to his parents. After completing his medical rounds, every afternoon he participated in a different medical society: the Société de Chirurgie, the Société Pathologique, the Société Anatomique and the Société de Biologie. Although not yet a member of the Académie de Médecine, he attended its meetings, following the debates avidly in order to write reviews of the discussions and to prepare later submissions to that body. So closely linked were these societies to the medical school and its faculty, that the history of the school written in the 1890s listed these and other medical societies as an important aspect of Paris medicine and a source of encouragement for the development of medical specialities. Although a detailed discussion of these societies lies outside the scope of this paper, it is important to add that they were vital to the development of French scientific medicine through the encouragement of basic research and the encouragement of public discussion of results.[36] More than one medical speciality had gained from both the development of a medical society and its associated journal.

If clinical teaching was still vital in the 1850s, its continuation in Paris in the late 1860s can be demonstrated through the letters and publications of Mary Putnam, later married to the paediatrician Abraham Jacobi.[37] These cover the period both before and after she was admitted to the Ecole de Médecine. She had come to Paris in 1866, already armed with two degrees: one from the New York College of Pharmacy and a medical degree from the Woman's Medical College of Pennsylvania. Like Broca, her accounts of the Paris clinics and clinical debates come not only from her letters to family but also from her regular reports on Paris medicine for a journal, the *New York Medical Record*, as the anonymous Paris correspondent.[38]

By 1867, soon after she came to France, Putnam Jacobi had obtained permission to attend general and specialized clinics in a number of hospitals. She also heard clinical lectures given in the hospital amphitheatres and attended an anatomical class. She described the manner in which medical clinics served as practical classes on diagnosis. Although the only woman physician in the first clinics she attended, she was listened to with respect by the attending physicians.

Putnam Jacobi's account of the almost deserted clinics of the cardiologist and neurologist Jean Baptiste Bouillaud made her aware of the political nature of medical rejection. Putnam found him sympathetic to her situation as a young woman physician in a period when her presence in the clinics was unique. She told her parents of his personal kindness, describing him as 'heroic' with a sense of fellow feeling towards her as someone fighting a rather different although equally unpopular cause. Bouillaud had defended Broca's studies of brain localization as proof of the truth of phrenology before the Académie de Médecine.[39] Although no other evidence of a connection between this young woman and Paul Broca exists, Putnam Jacobi, while on Bouillaud's service, reported to the *Medical Record* on a case of a brain cyst which appeared to provide clinical support for Broca's speech area in the frontal lobe.[40]

Putnam Jacobi's formal admission to the Paris school at the very end of 1867 meant she began to attend regular medical lectures and the official clinics. She reported to the *New York Medical Record* about the surgical clinics at the Charité, 'one of the official clinics held by a professor of the Faculty', Léon Gosselin, whose clinical teaching method impressed her. She had been introduced to Gosselin by Bouillaud and perhaps for that reason, although the clinic was very crowded, both the *interne* and the other students yielded her a place near the professor.[41]

Among her clinical reports on Paris medicine, she included accounts of debates of the Académie de Médecine, following the custom of the hospital gazettes. She drew other material directly from the gazettes, reporting on the heated arguments over use of tracheotomy in cases of child croup, which had a number of fatal results in France. She also incorporated some of the medical humour of the gazettes. In one case she repeated a humorous tale about the constant linking of the names of Edmé Félix Vulpian and Jean Martin Charcot, who regularly published together. Charcot's newborn son was attributed to their joint production.[42] Another story gave the account of a fight between two orderlies, reported in *L'Union Médicale*, who came to blows over the validity of treatment of typhoid fever by bleeding, as advocated by their respective chiefs.[43] She continued to be surprised and amused at the belligerency between physicians who attended the dermatology clinics of Saint Louis hospital. These were so exaggerated that she wondered nervously about the consequences should the opposing chiefs encounter one another on the narrow staircase of the hospital.[44]

Putnam Jacobi praised the French system for opening to the young doctor an opportunity to attend medical debates presented by senior physicians in the medical societies. She emphasized the importance of well-organized clinical rounds for clinical instruction which gave each student an opportunity to present his (or her) observations and recommendations. She singled out the advantages of competitive hospital placements for medical students as eliminating the personal patronage by established medical men required in England and America. The range of clinical experience Putnam Jacobi received provided her with a solid background for her later teaching and research career in New York. On her return to New York she tried to incorporate Parisian-style clinical teaching in her courses for the New York Woman's Medical School, finding this difficult in a situation where no hospitals outside of the New York Infirmary and a few out-patient clinics were open to women.[45]

One of the weaknesses of the French clinical system acknowledged by Putnam Jacobi was the lack of laboratory space for students, since she had hoped to do laboratory work in chemistry. As this began to seem unlikely, she had sought permission to attend the histology course given by Charles Robin while she waited for admission to the Ecole de Médecine. She also studied microscopy in the private laboratory course run by Victor Cornil and Louis Antoine Ranvier, later significant names in French scientific medicine. She finished her study in Paris in 1871 with an award-winning thesis on fats and fatty acids in clinical disorders, probably inspired by Cornil's studies of disorders of the kidney which had shortly preceded hers.[46]

Laboratories in chemistry and physics within the medical school had existed from 1847, when, following the report of Dumas, they were created by the Minister of Public Instruction. This did not ensure that students had routine access to these laboratories. They initially were research laboratories, sometimes available for medical demonstrations. Although private laboratories existed as adjuncts to clinical teaching, they were not firmly established within the medical curriculum. Charles Rayer, head of the Société de Biologie, during the period when he was dean of the medical faculty had used his influence to create a laboratory of comparative medicine. Like Robin's laboratory of histology in the 1860s, this was part of the Ecole Pratique des Hautes Etudes organized by Victor Duruy during his administration of the Ministry of Public Instruction. Broca's laboratory of anthropology, which taught both medical men and other interested professionals methods of craniology and other anthropometric measurements, was created at the same time as part of this school.[47]

Although many medical men pursued basic research through the Société de Biologie and other scientific societies, the lack of laboratories for clinical teaching and scientific research within the medical school began to trouble a number of the professors even before the Franco-Prussian war. A special investigation of clinical laboratories in other European countries was undertaken by Paul Lorain in 1868. His report, requesting new clinical laboratories as part of medical reform, was endorsed by Adolphe Wurtz, then dean of the Faculté de Médecine who soon left this position to take the chair of medical chemistry. Husson, the director of Assistance Publique under the Second Empire, had opposed the formation of new research and teaching laboratories. The far more liberal Municipal Council of Paris (which later took it on itself to partially fund Broca's School of Anthropology in the 1870s and a chair of evolution at the Sorbonne in the 1880s) advanced a credit to the Medical School to create two laboratories, one in microscopy and one for comparative pathology.[48]

Under the Third Republic, the newly appointed director of the Assistance Publique, Michel Möring, strongly supported the creation of clinical laboratories. In 1872, the National Assembly endorsed the decree of Jules Simon, Minister of Public Instruction, which detailed that: 'in each of the hospitals of Paris there should be a laboratory of clinical teaching'. (In practice this meant that laboratories were established in the major teaching hospitals, the Hôtel-Dieu, Charité, Pitié, Hôpital des Cliniques.) Twelve additional laboratories for teaching, experimentation and research were created by 1874. These laboratories in surgery and medicine were 'instituted for doing microscopic, chemical, physiological, and physical research necessary for clinical teaching'.[49] Cornil, who had privately taught microscopy to Putnam Jacobi, obtained one of these official clinical laboratories in the 1870s, located in the Charité Hospital, that carried professorial rank, and Ranvier later ran the laboratory of histology at the Collège de France. French medicine, with a growing awareness of the need for scientific laboratories, was finally attempting to make good that lack.

If clinical medicine was flourishing in the period that followed 1848, why have these years been neglected even by French historians of medicine? Not only a revolution (1848) but the period of both the Second Republic and the Second Empire begin and end during those twenty years. One explanation is that the definition of the 'era' of Paris clinical medicine is considered to be the period highlighted by Erwin Ackerknecht's great study, 1794–1848, although Ackerknecht has chosen an arbitrary year in which to end this period.[50] Many of the physicians he discusses reached the apex of their careers by the

'Faithful to its old traditions'?

end of 1848 but continued to teach and publish twenty and in some cases thirty years beyond this date, as Ackerknecht himself demonstrates in both the text and the bibliography of his book. The great clinicians of the second generation whom Ackerknecht discusses as 'eclectics' – Gabriel Andral, Armand Trousseau, and Armand Velpeau – lived until the end of the 1860s. Trousseau's great clinical lectures were published only in 1861, while Jean Baptiste Bouillaud was actively practising medicine still in the 1880s, although he was a bit of a fossil by then.[51]

The next generation which had been taught by these men forms Ackerknecht's 'young Paris School': Paul Broca, Charles Edouard Brown-Séquard, Edmé Félix Vulpian, Jean Martin Charcot, all flourished from the late 1850s to the 1880s and, in a few cases, well beyond. It is likely that the French historians of medicine have been unusually silent partly because they have followed the lead of republican physicians who, from the start of the Third Republic, had little wish to glorify the medical world of the Second Empire. Instead they preferred to celebrate the previous generation as the medical historian, Charles Daremberg, for example, glorified the world of Laennec.

While it has become almost a truism that English, German and American clinical medicine took over the lead from the 1850s to the end of the century, the combination of clinical research and clinical teaching that comfortably passed from bedside to the laboratory and back to bedside continued to develop in French clinical medicine in the post-1848 period. Ackerknecht indirectly has made the same argument by including references from the 1850s to 1870s in his bibliography and giving some space to the younger physicians in his book.

American historians of medicine have been influenced by another historical accident. Young American physicians who so enthusiastically gathered around Louis in the 1830s did not find the clinicians and clinical teaching in the great Paris hospitals of the mid-century as welcoming to them in the 1850s and 1860s, as John Harley Warner details in this volume.[52] While Paul Broca mentioned that he regularly taught American and English physicians in surgical courses in the 1850s, he did so in private courses intended to supplement medical clinical lecturing. Few English-speaking physicians followed the medical clinics on a daily basis. An exception to this general experience of Paris medicine by Americans in the late 1860s and early 1870s was that of Putnam Jacobi discussed above.[53]

Michel Foucault has commented on the double definition of the medical clinic as both a science and a method of medical instruction which Bouillaud presented as a banality even in his own time. Foucault adopted this definition to emphasize his contention that the 'matrimonial' doctor–patient couple codified a situation in which 'two living individuals are trapped in a common but non-reciprocal situation'.[54] In Foucault's view, the patient becomes collapsed to his disease in order to provide clinical objectivity which 'forces the disease to speak' in a visible and later three-dimensional manner which can be understood by the clinician. As this new discourse is developed, Foucault described medical instruments as serving to distance the physician from his former partner, the patient. This uncoupling of doctor and patient forms a core of Foucault's analysis.

The question remains to what degree the image the medical couple presents is an accurate description of Paris medicine at mid-century. The hierarchical structure of the Paris hospitals, with its nursing nuns administering in the wards, lower-class male and female nurses, medical students, *externes,*' *internes*, had been for many years ranged in rows between Foucault's couple, each pushing in front of the other to observe and participate in what had always resembled a piece of public theatre rather than a private physician–patient interaction. In the face of this public performance, we can only ask how many physicians insisted to their students that the young doctor must never forget that he was dealing with an individual patient whose concerns were his first obligation, as Putnam Jacobi recorded Gosselin as insisting to his students. Ackerknecht has described Trousseau as having 'condemned experimentation on the sick and preached respect for the poor: two rules apparently not always obeyed'.[55] Nevertheless, Louis Hecht in his description of *la clinique*, accused German, not French, medicine of this collapsing together of the disease and the patient. Hecht described German medicine in these words:

> Fascinated by the mathematical exactitude with which instruments for physical examination and chemical reagents permit them to understand morbid lesions, too preoccupied on the other hand by the kind of material alterations which pathological anatomy has taught them is incurable, certain clinicians [from the outer Rhine]... seem to have forgotten, let us say, that they have not just illnesses to study and to classify, but sick organisms to cure and to care for.[56]

We cannot ignore Foucault's underlying concern that we need to attend to the patient's point of view. Few accounts in the medical literature give us a sense of what it is like to be on the receiving side of the clinical apparatus. An exception is Maxime du Camp's description of the Paris Hospitals in the *Revue des Deux Mondes* in 1870. He wrote about hospitals and patients in a similar spirit with which he described other Paris institutions of the nineteenth century (the banking system and the justice system) for the same journal. Du Camp expressed awe at the importance of the famous physicians who considered it an honour to treat the sick poor. But he also described the experience of the individual trying to enter the hospital, by the ready admission during emergencies, free consultations for poor patients by the elite of the medical or surgical world. He described the poor, sometimes not seriously ill, desirous of admission because of the opportunity to be fed and clothed. The sick man or woman with no fixed abode was admitted more readily than the poor man who had a home. Once admitted, the patient was undoubtedly overwhelmed as du Camp described himself, with a sense of awe before the vast spaces, large windows, billowing curtains, waxed floors, the beds with 'all their necessary utensils'. He pictured the chart with its necessary medical information at the end of the bed, the food that was well prepared and eagerly eaten, the vast cellars, the administrative nuns 'gliding like beneficent shadows'. But du Camp also described little telling details like the standard costumes for male and female patients that included not only robes but head coverings. The young women at the venereal hospital, he observed, had found a way to make even the plain blue caps they were issued very fetching indeed.[57] Perhaps this was an overly romantic view of the hospital whose final stop was often the morgue or the dissecting table.

Was the French clinic as Hecht claimed 'faithful to its old traditions'? Practical medicine took place at the bed of the patient and in doing so, he insisted, Paris medicine considered the illness 'without losing sight of the patient'. 'The clinic on the contrary does not study the maladies but sick organisms, it appreciates the modifications that individual conditions of age, sex, race, temperament, constitution, idiosyncrasy etc. produce that are inherent in each organism'.[58] While all of medical science aimed at the cure and alleviation from pain and disease, '*la clinique* is the crowning achievement'.[59] The degree to which the French clinic could be said to wear that crown during the 1860s and 1870s is still in the process of reinterpretation.

'Faithful to its old traditions'?

Notes

1. Erwin H. Ackerknecht, *Medicine at the Paris Hospital* (Baltimore: Johns Hopkins Press, 1967); Michel Foucault, *The Birth of the Clinic: An Archaeology of Medical Perception* (1963), translated from the French by A.M. Sheridan Smith (New York: Random House-Vintage, 1973).
2. L. Hecht, 'Clinique', in Amédée Dechambre and Raige-Delorme, *Dictionnaire Encyclopédique des Sciences Médicales* (Paris: Asselin and V. Masson, 1864-89), 18 (1876): 126-32.
3. Foucault, *Birth of the Clinic*, 115.
4. Paul Broca, *Correspondence*, 2 vols (Paris: Schmidt, 1886); Mary Putnam Jacobi, *Life and Letters of Mary Putnam Jacobi*, edited by Ruth Putnam (New York: G. P. Putnam's Sons, 1927) and its companion volume, Women's Medical Association of New York, *Mary Putnam Jacobi, A Pathfinder in Medicine* (New York: G. P. Putnam's Sons, 1925). The second of these contains her reports to the *Medical Record*. For a more detailed look at her experiences in the Paris clinics than is offered here, see Joy Harvey, '"La Visite": Mary Putnam Jacobi and the Paris Medical Clinics', in Ann La Berge and Mordechai Feingold (eds), *French Medical Culture in the Nineteenth Century* (Amsterdam/Atlanta: Rodopi, 1994), 350-71.
5. L. Roux, 'Le Médecin' (1841), from the *Encyclopédie Morale du XIXe Siècle*, ed. Jules Janin. Reproduced in *Les Gens de Médecine* (Paris: Les Editions Errance, 1982), n.p. He continues, 'One could use the microscope to prove there were organisms in the milk of wet-nurses', a reference to the work of Donné's microscopical studies of human milk, discussed by Ann La Berge in 'Medical microscopy in Paris 1830-1855', in La Berge and Feingold (eds), *French Medical Culture*, 296-326.
6. *Medico-Chirurgical Transactions of the Royal Medical and Chirurgical Society of London* (1809-1907), vols 1-90.
7. For example, the Medico-Chirurgical Society of Edinburgh which began in 1821 and the Medico-Chirurgical Society of Parma which began in 1806.
8. This was *Répertoire annuel de clinique médico-chirurgicale* (1833-6) which became *Revue annuelle et universelle de clinique médico-chirurgicale, Paris* by 1837.
9. The biographical article on Jules Guérin that makes this claim, was written by a later collaborator of Amédée Dechambre, in *La Grande Encyclopédie*. When Thomas Wakley started his feature 'Mirror of the Practice of Medicine and Surgery in the Hospitals of London' in his

330

journal the *Lancet* in the late 1840s, he was following clinical reporting in the style of these gazettes. Later in 1856 he would claim he was the originator of the 'Mirror', the weekly hospital report, and was being imitated by the French.
10. Jacques Léonard, *La Médecine entre les pouvoirs et les savoirs* (Paris: Aubier, 1981), 171.
11. This occurred at the very beginning of Paul Broca's medical career in 1841. See *Correspondence* 1: 25. This is also cited in Francis Schiller, *Paul Broca: Founder of French Anthropology, Explorer of the Brain* (Berkeley: University of California Press, 1979), 39-40.
12. Broca, *Correspondence*, vol. 2.
13. Gabriel Andral, who taught medical pathology, is supposed to have said of himself that he had studied medicine three times: pathological anatomy, physical diagnosis and then haemopathology, working with the medical physicist, Jules Gavarret, on studies of the blood. See Ackerknecht, *Paris Hospital*, 105-7. Gavarret, a good friend of Broca, was far more liberal both politically and socially than Andral.
14. This is evident throughout the first volume of *L'Union Médicale*, Jan.-Dec. 1847.
15. *L'Union Médicale* 1: 410-12, 17 August 1847.
16. See Harry Marks, 'Attitudes of French Physicians towards Women (1840-1900)', M.A. thesis, University of Wisconsin, 1972. The first issue of the new series of *L'Union Médicale* in 1859 included an editorial by Latour in which he emphasized that his gazette would never be used to 'propagate (religious) doubt'. 'Editorial', *L'Union Médicale* (1859), vol. 1, n.p.
17. See *L'Union Médicale*, 31 July 1847, for example, on English sanitary reform. This includes an interesting comparison with the English system: 'England is the mother country of associations: no one knows better than an inhabitant of Great Britain how much isolation creates embarrassments and difficulties for executing the most modest projects, no one appreciates better the part which one can derive from a unified view and shared efforts. [The sanitary and health associations] include, doctors, important men (from the nobility for example) ... [Also there are] more general "meetings" in which the public participates, in which men of the highest class demonstrate the advantages of improvement of sanitation for working classes.'
18. Harry Marks in 'Attitudes of French Physicians' discussed the political attitudes of the medical press to detail controversies over the admission of women to the Paris Medical School and later over their right to take examinations for the *externat* and *internat*. See also Jacques Léonard's chapter on the medical press in his interesting

study of French medicine. Léonard, 'L'emprise de la presse', *Pouvoirs et savoirs*, 195-200.

19. Alexandre Thierry, *Statistique comparée de la mortalité des femmes en couche dans les hôpitaux de Paris et dans ceux d'Allemagne et d'Angleterre* (Paris: P. Dupont, 1856). This book consisted of articles that first appeared in the *Moniteur*.

20. *Moniteur des Hôpitaux*, 4 (1856): 490-1.

21. The final discussion of this debate appeared in *Moniteur des Hôpitaux*, December 1856. Dubois is described with great dislike in Broca's letters to his parents between 1854 and 1856. His delivery of the Emperor's son, satirically referred to as 'Napoleon the fourth' , resulted in a bad bruise on the infant's forehead following the inept use of forceps, delighting Dubois' enemies. Attacks on Dubois, common in the early years of the *Moniteur*, must have been rather unwise since Dubois was dean of the Faculté de Médecine from 1852 to 1862.

22. Armand Husson, *Etude sur les Hôpitaux de l'Assistance Publique* (Paris: Paul Dupont, 1862). This contains a great deal of information, including plans of the hospitals. Husson's point might be answered by Michel Möring's later collection of documents of the Assistance Publique, Administration générale de l'Assistance publique à Paris, *Collection de documents pour servir à l'histoire des Hôpitaux de Paris commencée sous les auspices de Michel Möring continuée par Charles Quentin*, 5 vols (Paris: Imprimerie nationale, 1881-87).

23. Husson cited T. Holmes in the *British and Foreign Medical Chirurgical Journal* 14: 225 on the greater number of poor in the French hospitals.

24. Blanchard Jerrold, 'The Sick Poor of Paris', *Lancet* 2 (1869). This was reprinted in the New York edition of this journal: *London Lancet* (N.Y.) I (1869): 282-8; III (1869) 396-8; V (1869) 499-503; VI (1869) 566-8. The article was accompanied by an editorial in the New York journal, 'The French and English hospital systems', III (1869): 392-4.

25. See, for example, the discussion by Broca of the importance of microscopy in pathology, presented in opposition to Velpeau. *Moniteur des Hôpitaux*, 16 October 1854. This debate is discussed by Ann La Berge in her essay in this volume and by Schiller, *Paul Broca*, 71-4. Ann La Berge has also discussed Broca's microscopic studies of cancer in 'Medical Microscopy in Paris, 1830-1855' in La Berge and Feingold (eds), *French Medical Culture*, 296-326.

26. The joke on the clinical method involves a man who, having observed a mason recovering from a fever and stomach ailment after

(against medical advice) consuming a dish of herrings in oil, prescribes the same dish to a second patient, a carpenter, who then dies. He writes up his clinical conclusions, basing the difference of survival on the difference in profession. 'In cases of fevers and stomach disorders: prescription: herrings in oil: good for masons, bad for carpenters.'

27. Piorry's concept of 'bon sens' in medicine had been earlier satirized by Broca in earlier articles in the *Moniteur*. Another satire concerned a court case in which a merchant of dubious medications and the woman who runs the store are supported by a 'well-known' Gascon 'doctor', whose name begins with G who runs a clinic for venereal disease. (The identity was obvious to the contemporary readers, not so obvious to the modern reader.)

28. This had appeared in Dechambre's *Gazette Hebdomadaire* in 1855. Broca had discussed this in *Correspondence* (vol. 2) and it is analyzed by Schiller, *Paul Broca*, 59-76. Léonard attributes the humour of some of the medical journals (specifically Fabre's *Gazette des Hôpitaux*) to a 'more plebeian, pseudo-democratic and satiric style current in the writings of Béranger and Daumier'. Léonard, *Pouvoirs et savoirs*, 199. Or does it derive, rather, from the well-known satirical tradition of the *internes* in the *salle de garde*?

29. Broca's colleagues – Eugène Dally, Charles Edouard Brown-Séquard, Charles Robin, Louis-Adolphe Bertillon who had all contributed to Castelnau's journal – were founding or early members of the Société. Castelnau was also a founding member.

30. This journal was edited by Désiré-Magloire Bourneville, former editor of another journal, *Movement médicale*. A free-thinker, he later became very active as a politician as well as a physician in the Municipal Council of Paris and later in the Chamber of Deputies. He pushed first for the opening of secular nursing schools and later for the secularization of hospital administration. See Léonard, *Pouvoirs et savoirs*, 288.

31. Broca, *Correspondence*.

32. For Broca's biography and his detailed movement through the Paris hospitals, see Schiller, *Paul Broca*, although Schiller does not detail all the hospital services and clinics that are to be found in the Broca correspondence cited above.

33. Ann La Berge, 'Medical Microscopy in Paris, 1830-1855'.

34. See Schiller, *Paul Broca*, for Broca's wide range of contributions to medicine. See also my own thesis on the Société d'Anthropologie, *Races Specified, Evolution Transformed: The Société d'Anthropologie de Paris as a Forum for Debate 1859-1902*, Ph.D. thesis, Harvard

University, 1983, in which many of Broca's contributions to politics, evolution, and the human sciences are discussed. His work on craniology helped establish this field and his discussion of evolution was crucial in a period when Darwin was being offhandedly dismissed in France.

35. 'Jules Gavarret', *La Grande Encyclopédie*. Gavarret had trained in both the Ecole Polytechnique and the Faculté de Médecine. He studied the physics of blood flow, publishing a major clinical and pathological study with Andral in 1844, while still a young doctor. Later he developed the field of medical physics and emphasized heat exchange as a professor in charge of the laboratory of medical physics. The best-known biography of C. E. Brown-Séquard is that of J. M. D. Olmsted, *Charles Edouard Brown-Séquard: A Nineteenth Century Neurologist and Endocrinologist* (Baltimore: Johns Hopkins Press, 1946).

36. A. Corlieu, *Centenaire de la Faculté de Médecine de Paris (1794-1894)* (Paris: Imprimerie nationale, 1896). On the importance of the Société de Biologie to French medicine, see John E. Lesch, *Science and Medicine in France, The Emergence of Experimental Physiology 1780-1855* (Cambridge, Mass.: Harvard University Press, 1984), 222–4.

37. See for a more detailed discussion, Harvey, "'La Visite'".

38. In these contributions, she followed the style and content of the Paris hospital gazettes, signing the articles with her initials in reverse order 'P.C.M'. Even the occasional medical joke she relates refers to members of the medical faculty under whom she worked. These are included in the collection of her papers, Putnam Jacobi, 'Letters from Paris to the Medical Record', in *Pathfinder*, 1-170.

39. Mary Putnam to V[ictorine].H[aven].P[utnam], 27 December 1867, *Life and Letters of Mary Putnam Jacobi*, 160.

40. This was a case reported in the St-Antoine hospital under the service of M. Jaccaud in which a brain cyst produced temporary aphasia, with the reappearance of speech once the cyst broke. Putnam Jacobi, 'Letters to the Medical Record', *Pathfinder*, 2-3.

41. *Ibid.*

42. Putnam Jacobi, [July, 1867], *Pathfinder*, 19.

43. *Ibid.*, 11.

44. Putnam Jacobi, *Pathfinder*, 115. August 21 [1868].

45. Harvey, "'La Visite'".

46. *Life, Letters, Putnam Jacobi*, 286–9. The title of her thesis, awarded a bronze medal, was 'De la graisse neutre et des acides gras'. She discussed some of the background material, including Cornil 's *agrégé* thesis in a number of her 1869 letters to the *Medical Record* in Putnam Jacobi, *Pathfinder*, 143-70.

47. For details of the creation of laboratories as part of the French system of medical education, see A. Corlieu, *Centenaire de la Faculté de Médecine de Paris (1794-1894)* (Paris: Imprimerie nationale, 1896).
48. Corlieu, *Centenaire*, cites the study of Paul Joseph Lorain, 'De la réforme des études médicales par les laboratoires' (Paris, 1868), 45 pp. The Municipal Council gave a credit of 14,695 francs for the two labs.
49. Corlieu, *Centenaire*, 151. There was a limit of twenty students allowed in a lab. They had to apply and have the request signed by the dean of the faculty and the chief of the hospital.
50. Ackerknecht, *Paris Hospital*.
51. Ackerknecht, *Paris Hospital*, 109. If we look at the publication date of Armand Trousseau's great clinical lectures, cited by Ackerknecht in his bibliography, we note that the first edition was published only in 1861. See also Ackerknecht, *Paris Hospital*, 105-7.
52. See John Harley Warner's essay in this volume: 'Paradigm Lost or Paradise Declining? American Physicians and the "Dead End" of the Paris Clinical School'.
53. Harvey, '"La Visite"'.
54. See Foucault, *Birth of the Clinic*.
55. Ackerknecht, *Paris Hospital*, 188.
56. Hecht, 'Clinique', *Dictionnaire Encyclopédique,* 130.
57. Maxime Du Camp, 'Les Hôpitaux à Paris', *Revue des Deux Mondes* 88 (1870): 513-47.
58. Hecht, 'Clinique', *Dictionnaire Encyclopédique*, 127.
59. Hecht, 'Clinique', *Dictionnaire Encyclopédique*, 130.

9

Paradigm Lost or Paradise Declining?
American Physicians and the 'Dead End'
of the Paris Clinical School

John Harley Warner

By the middle of the nineteenth century, Erwin Ackerknecht asserted in *Medicine at the Paris Hospital, 1794–1848* (1967), '*French medicine had maneuvered itself into a dead end*, as all empiricisms had done so far in medical history'.[1] Somewhere in the course of drafting his text Ackerknecht adjusted the date of that event from 1850 to 1848, bringing his medical story into line with a political narrative.[2] 'By 1848, Paris "hospital medicine" had come to a dead end, its momentum spent'; the Paris School, the dust jacket put it more luridly, was 'swept away by the Revolution of 1848'.[3] In more recent years, both his depiction of the Paris School and the discontinuity implied by its putative dead end have been drawn into question. Our emerging image of the Parisian medical world of the first half of the nineteenth century is more complex than Ackerknecht's bold portrait – far less monolithic in its consecration to radical clinical empiricism and exclusion of the basic sciences, for example – while the notion that exhaustion of the empiricist programme brought the whole thing to a dead end has begun to appear overstated and simplistic.

It is surprising, therefore, that what Ackerknecht invoked as the most powerful testimony to a dead end – the massive shift in the stream of foreign medical students that once flowed into Paris toward German cities instead – has remained little questioned. The imposing influx of German, British, and American medical practitioners into Paris after the peace of 1815, according to Ackerknecht's interpretation, offers unambiguous evidence of the intellectual vibrancy of the Paris Clinical School. Equally, the redirection of students after mid-century from France to Germany – that is, to both the states that later would form a unified Germany and other

German-speaking centres in Austria-Hungary such as Vienna – is a clear indication that the vigour of the Parisian medical model had been spent. 'French medicine paid for its practicalism, clinicism, and conservatism by losing its superiority to Germany', Ackerknecht asserted, a loss of supremacy the shift in migration betokened.[4] With the creative promise of the Parisian empiricist programme lost, those abroad in search of medical science at its cutting edge duly abandoned Paris in favour of the next ascendant centres in Germany, where the laboratory-based medical sciences ostracized by the Paris clinicians were vigorously cultivated. Others have shared this interpretation. Historians of American medicine, for example, charting the transformation from its 'Paris period' to the German period that followed, have seen the shift in itinerary of American physicians abroad both as evidence of the shifting balance of intellectual power in medicine and as among its inevitable consequences.[5]

The shift in destination of American physicians was real enough, but its interpretation is rather more problematic. Ackerknecht assumed, without analyzing, the motivations that lay behind the migration of American doctors. In particular, he assumed that French superiority in medical science, so celebrated by the Americans, was what attracted them in such large numbers to Paris, just as the supplanting of French by German medical leadership was what redirected their travels to Vienna and Berlin. As the French medical model brought Paris to its dead end, the power of the Paris School to attract students waned, while at the same time the ascendancy of the German medical model made Vienna and Berlin natural destinations for American physicians pursuing study in Europe. It is the underlying assumption that what attracted students to one centre rather than another was the prospect of studying at the cutting edge of Western medicine that gives migration its utility as an index of the rise and fall of the Paris School.

My objective here is to begin to reassess these assumptions – and thereby the conclusions based on them – by looking closely at the experiences and perceptions of the American medical migrants to Paris. My starting premise is that the reasons why Americans journeyed to Paris cannot be equated with the stories they later told about its significance or the meaning they came to attach to their studies there. We must look instead at what they actually did, at what they most valued in Paris, and at the process of decision-making that informed their choices, recognizing that they were selective reporters who sometimes misunderstood the French system and its workings. To comprehend why they travelled in such numbers to Paris and why they later began to bypass France on their way to Germany and Austria, we need to investigate what drew them to Paris in the first place, their valorization of the experiences Paris afforded, and what came to persuade them that Germany offered a more promising destination. This is a preliminary and suggestive exploration, and any fuller appraisal of shifts in medical student migration and their meaning will have to go beyond American perceptions to look closely at the intellectual and pedagogical realities that governed educational experience in the lecture halls, dissecting rooms, pathoanatomical museums, and wards of Paris.

Why Paris?

Why would an American physician go to Paris? Much of the answer seems obvious. Out of the reorganization of medical thought and institutions in the wake of the French Revolution, Paris emerged as the most vibrant centre of Western medicine. Parisian clinicians created new canons of medical science, represented by such technical and conceptual innovations as the stethoscope and physical examination, tissue pathology, systematic correlation of clinical with autopsical findings, and clinical statistics. After Waterloo and peace, Paris became a mecca for foreign medical practitioners, who were duly impressed by the new tools for investigating disease and by the vigour with which the Parisian clinicians applied them. As Anson Colman wrote from Paris in 1833 to his wife in Rochester, New York, 'I shall have gathered such hints, and shall bring back with me such aids to study and investigation, as will, I hope, render the few months that I am now spending abroad the most important to me in my whole life'.[6] Like Colman, many American physicians wrote home extolling the new vision of medicine they encountered in France and returned to proselytize the lessons of the Paris School.[7]

Of these, none loomed larger than the ideal of empiricism. In American portraits, the Paris School stood above all else for a strident, sceptical empiricism set against the rationalism that dominated medicine through the early nineteenth century. Americans were pointing to the sensual empiricist legacy of the medical *idéologues*, but ordinarily they expressed it in simple terms: what was most significant about French medicine was its allegiance to empirical fact, to truth, to knowledge attained and verified by direct observation and analysis of nature. They praised French superiority in medical science, but attributed that success to the epistemological stance they regarded as its most notable feature. There was nothing inevitable about this depiction, as I have argued elsewhere, and while the Americans tended to stress French epistemology – its empiricism and antirationalism – English medical visitors to Paris explaining the French achievement tended instead to stress French medical polity.[8] For the Americans, an ideal of empiricism both emblemized what was most admirable about the French medical model and offered a key to the social and intellectual transformation of medicine in their own country.

Yet by and large, what Americans depicted as being most important about the Paris School after their return was not what drew them across the Atlantic. What they remembered and told about medical Paris and its significance, that is, was not necessarily the same as what they hoped to gain when they set off for Paris; and it is critical not to equate later perceptions and story-telling with earlier motivations and expectations. American physicians were attracted to Paris for a wide variety of reasons, reflecting the diversity of those who made the journey. But, as I want to suggest here, overwhelmingly it was the promise of practical experience at the bedside and dissecting table that drew them to Paris, not its intellectual vigour or the chance to witness the cutting edge of medical science. Once in Paris, many Americans would be recruited to French ideals, and after their return would energetically proselytize the French example as a way of propelling the campaign 'against the spirit of system' they believed would bring a thoroughgoing reformation of American medicine.[9] But what principally drew them to France was the promise of acquiring experiential knowledge.

An inventory of the reasons American doctors gave for making the trip to Paris is easy to compile from the abundant accounts they left of their deliberations before departing and reflections once they arrived. As they endlessly recounted, they went to enjoy medical facilities far more expansive than anything found at home. They went to attend clinical rounds of physicians whose medical writings they had read, to witness operations performed by the famous surgeons, and to listen to lectures on wider-ranging realms of natural history. They went to observe patients gathered together in the great hospitals, pathological specimens collected in the museums, and natural history specimens assembled at the Jardin des Plantes. They went to observe the natural history of disease in the wards through its outward signs and symptoms and on the autopsy table through the internal lesions it left; to practise surgical techniques on the dead body; and to gain experience in anatomical dissection. At the same time, they went because time spent abroad was a source of professional distinction in a society committed to egalitarianism. And they went for myriad idiosyncratic personal and professional reasons: to acquire specimens for the museum or books for the library of an American medical school; to give professional legitimacy to an established physician's sabbatical from the burdens of practice, or to a young doctor's escape from the United States while neighbours' recollections of his misdeeds at home had a chance to fade; or to have the heady exhilaration of functioning at the intellectual centre of their profession before resigning themselves to a routine life of practice on the periphery.

Such a list, however, describes why Americans went to Paris between the mid-1810s and 1850s without explaining why they went *there* rather than elsewhere. One way of isolating what was *singular* about the attraction of Paris is to turn the problem on its head and ask why American doctors elected to go to Paris in greater numbers and for longer stays than to the other cities they commonly visited, such as Edinburgh, Dublin, London, Heidelberg, Berlin, Vienna, Florence, and Rome. Why, in particular, Paris rather than London? On the face of it, London would seem an especially appealing place for Americans to study medicine. There, they did not have to learn a foreign language or endure the frustrations of stumbling along with only a little French. Moreover, American observers nearly all agreed that the English were superior to the French as healers. And even the most ardent American disciples of Parisian medicine acknowledged that in many respects English values were more congenial than French values to Americans, including morality, religious sentiment, and practicality. A sizeable proportion of the American doctors who studied in France visited London as well, if sometimes only for tourism or as a pilgrim's act of filial piety, and after Paris it was the most common stop on their medical tours of Europe. Nevertheless, they went to Paris in greater numbers than to London and ordinarily for much longer stays.[10]

Reports by American doctors on medical London included most of the major elements that appeared in their accounts of Paris. They were charmed by the great physicians and surgeons, men whose names were as prominent in the American medical literature as those of the Parisian stars. Americans walked the wards with them, attended their lectures, and witnessed their surgical operations. London medical institutions were also imposing, and the sheer size of hospitals like Guy's, St Bartholomew's, and St Thomas's sometimes elicited admiration every bit as awed as that elicited by La Pitié, La Charité, or the Hôtel-Dieu. London medical museums even seemed unsurpassed to their American viewers. What is more, Americans often felt that the great medical figures of London were more responsive than their French counterparts to letters of introduction brought from home. American visitors were guided about the hospitals, dissecting rooms, and museums; taken to medical and scientific society meetings where papers were read in their native tongue; and sometimes introduced into polite society. The richness of London's medical institutions and medical minds, as portrayed in American accounts, should have made that city a serious rival to Paris. Still, Leonidas M. Lawson could write from London in 1845:

> Very few American physicians visit London; indeed, I am not aware of any one being here at this time except myself. I cannot but conclude that the advantages offered by London are greatly overlooked by our countrymen who go abroad.[11]

The single element most prominently and consistently missing from accounts of London that pervades accounts of Paris is enthusiasm about free access to facilities for medical study. 'Here I am in Paris in accordance with a desire which possessed me for years', Ashbel Smith, echoing the tone of many medical Americans in France, wrote in 1832 to a friend in North Carolina. 'When in America I sighed as you know after opportunities for improvement; here on the contrary I have only to regret that I can avail myself of but few comparatively of the almost innumerable facilities which this metropolis affords. Yet science displays its cabinet and Instruction opens its halls *gratuitously* to all who ask knowledge[.] I have not time in the 24 hours'.[12] Comparable outpourings of enthusiasm written by Americans in London are vanishingly rare.

American travellers in the aggregate had more praise for French medical science – pathological anatomy, the natural history of disease, and techniques of clinical investigation – than for that of the English; but this difference was only one of degree. All but a tiny hard-core of American disciples of the Paris School admired English medical science, and, indeed, by and large had higher esteem than later historians for the scientific merits of the London clinicians. They spoke with delight about the extensive facilities for the scientific study of disease they found in London, but not (as in Paris) about the ease and freedom with which the prospective student could gain eyes-, ears-, and hands-on use of these facilities.

Paradigm Lost or Paradise Declining?

With a few exceptions, Americans were remarkably consistent in their failure to enthuse over access to practical experience in London, a marked contrast to the way they reported on Paris.

What the absence of awed and excited rhetoric about free access in London contrasted with its central prominence in accounts of Paris suggests is that access more than scientific brilliance was the most important distinction between London and Paris that directed American doctors to the French capital. But this is indicated by more than negative evidence alone. In their letters from Europe, Americans routinely noted that restrictions on access in London made it a less appealing place for study than Paris. 'The American physician who arrives in London for the purpose of observing what pertains to his profession', Carleton B. Chapman warned after visiting both cities, 'may be greatly disappointed. ... The hospitals of London are well calculated to answer the end for which they were created, *viz.*, to afford a temporary home with medical and other attendants for the sick poor, *and to get a great name* for the favored ones who have charge of them'.[13] James Jackson, Jr, complained that the English hospitals were simply not arranged to facilitate clinical study. 'I suppose I shall of course follow Elliotson's Clinique', he wrote sulkily while *en route* to London after Paris. 'Altho' I presume the student may be admitted at all hours & other days yet fr. what I have seen of & heard fr. the English medical students in Paris, I doubt much whether one will be allowed to study *disease*, comme il faut'.[14]

Even if medical London had facilities that in some ways rivalled those of Paris, English medical polity, as Americans viewed it, fostered a closed rather than open system. In American accounts, contrasts between the access to experiential knowledge in London and in Paris often were explicit and invidious. The Parisian hospitals were controlled by the government, which employed clinicians to attend patients and to teach, and fostered the access of instructors and students to the bodies of living patients and their remains after death. By contrast, the London hospitals were private charitable institutions with lay boards of governors that vested medical control in a small number of socially elite physicians and surgeons. The latter tended to see the hospitals as their private domains, guarding their privileged access to patients for research as a source of professional eminence and for teaching as a source of income. 'Without the personal interest of somebody it is impossible to see anything in this country', the young Oliver Wendell Holmes complained from London in 1834.[15] Jackson, Jr, succinctly expressed a widely shared perception when he reminded his father that 'at Paris I am to study under the influence of men whose aim is science – at London, *gain*'.[16]

On the other hand, American enthusiasm for the openness of the Paris School was routine and persistent over time. 'If I were to tell you how much I am delighted with the opportunities I found here, I should go into raptures', Abel Lawrence Peirson wrote from Paris to his wife in Massachusetts. 'God be thanked for the opportunities with wh. I am surrounded'.[17] 'What a feast is here presented', a Virginia student echoed, 'and yet all this is *gratis*'.[18] William Gibson, in a published account of his visit to Europe in 1839, reported:

> Of the advantages of a residence in Paris for medical purposes, beyond most other cities, I was well apprised, but the real amount and value of such advantages I certainly had no adequate conception of until they were presented to my view, nor could I fully understand why pupils, after having completed their studies in this country, and sailed for Europe in quest of additional information, should, almost to a man, take up their quarters, exclusively, in the French metropolis, and never think, afterwards of attending the lectures and walking the rounds of the English, Scotch, and Irish colleges and hospitals. But I had not been a week in Paris before I understood, perfectly, the nature of the case, by finding that there were hundreds, nay thousands of individuals, employed in demonstrating, teaching, and unravelling, in every possible way, the most intricate subjects, in every branch of our science and art, and for a compensation so exceedingly small, and, oftentimes, without any compensation at all, as to be within the limits of the poorest and most destitute student. ... Above all, I found that the regular lectures in the different hospitals and institutions, by men of the first eminence, were paid for by government, and *gratuitous*, as respected the pupil.

Paris, he concluded, was a place 'where the student revels from dawn to sunset, and, if he please, throughout the night, among lectures, dissections, demonstrations and preparations, until he is stuffed and crammed, and saturated with knowledge to such extent, as to leave no room for additional supply'.[19] F. Campbell Stewart summed up 'that in no part of the world can the same practical experience be acquired by the attentive student as in the French capital'.[20]

The scientific supremacy of the Paris School would be one leading message in reports by Americans, certainly, but it was not this that principally drew them to the French capital in such large numbers in the years between the mid-1810s and the 1850s. Even Pierre Louis, who came to represent to his American disciples the chief achievement of French medical science, its empiricist departure, was sought by Americans in the first instance as a conduit to practical experience in the clinic, not as a sage mentor working at the cutting edge. The migration of American physicians to France was testimony above all, not to the intellectual vigour of Paris medicine, but to the singular access to practical experience that the Paris School afforded.

'The Paradise of Parisian Life'

'The capital of France is now-a-days regarded as the medical emporium of the world', an American professor of surgery just returned from Paris told students at the 1838 commencement of the Louisville Medical Institute. 'Her School of Medicine, with its score of Professors – her ample facilities for the pursuit of practical anatomy – her spacious hospitals, thrown open, with the most commendable liberality, to all who seek instruction – her copious medical literature, in a language which has well nigh supplanted the Latin as the "communis lingua doctorum" – conspire to give to Paris a position in regard to external equipments for the prosecution of medical studies, unequalled by any other city'.[21] In the American medical literature from the 1820s through the 1850s, such catalogues of the facilities for medical instruction in Paris were commonplace. The usefulness of these facilities was enhanced by the '*cheapness*, or rather *the non importance of human life*!!' as one American put it in a letter home, trying to capture the widespread perception that the human body was treated in the Paris hospitals as a mere object for scientific scrutiny. As he explained, 'This gives every opportunity for investigating diseases; of experimenting; of operating; of examining them in their minute details every morbid condition to which life is incident; and finally when the poor devils make their final exit, are, as matter of course the property of the Hospitals in which they died for the purpose of dissections'.[22] All this tallied up to what Oliver Wendell Holmes, contrasting England with France, called in 1833 'the paradise of Parisian life'.[23]

Ackerknecht's study, like nineteenth-century American accounts, abounds with such inventories of Parisian facilities. Indeed, in characteristically Westernunionesque fashion, he overwhelms the reader with lists of what the medical student in Paris found on offer, and goes on to conclude that 'a review of the teaching resources of Paris in the first half of the nineteenth century makes it easy to understand why, for several decades, it became the Mecca of medical students from all over the world'.[24] But in fact, real understanding is not quite so easy. Ackerknecht never closely investigated the nature of clinical experience – that of French much less foreign students – that was at the core of Parisian teaching and learning. Yet it is not enough to catalogue the resources that were available; to begin to understand the educational 'paradise' that the Paris School represented to American students, we must look at how these resources were actually used. What can we learn from the letters they wrote home about which, out of all the imposing opportunities that confronted them, they most elected to cultivate during their limited time abroad? How did Americans decide what to focus on and what to gloss over? What was the actual nature of clinical instruction, as they experienced it?

Didactic instruction was never foremost in their attention, save for the very small number of Americans (mainly French Creoles from Louisiana) who studied in Paris for their medical doctorate.[25] As one American noted, after hospital rounds in the morning 'those who are studying the rudiments of medicine go to the school; but this institution is very little frequented by the Americans, who generally devote themselves to clinical studies'.[26] Most Americans wanted to return able to say that they had seen the famous professors and took advantage of the fact that lectures at the Ecole de Médecine were free to make them part of their sightseeing rounds, and some regularly followed lectures elsewhere in other branches of natural history. But, as one American, explaining why he had elected to spend little of his time in the lecture rooms, wrote to his father, 'I came to Paris not to study theories for I could study those as well or better at home – nor yet to study practice for the French practice is entirely opposed to the English and American Schools – But to study disease as it exists in the living and in the dead body'.[27]

On the other hand, nearly all American physicians who passed any time at all in Paris spent some of it at the dissecting table, and some few came to regard this as the core of their Parisian studies. Their letters home recounted the government policies that ensured a steady supply of bodies from the hospitals to the anatomy rooms, and they widely shared the conclusion voiced by Frank H. Hamilton that 'it is this enlightened policy which renders Paris the greatest school of anatomy in the world'.[28] So too, they routinely described the facilities at the Clamart or the Ecole Pratique, and reported on the modest fees demanded for access to anatomical experience. 'There is a delightful dissecting Establishment at the Clamart, for the summer, on a most extensive scale. There is room (& material) for two hundred upwards, tho there is but a few at present there', John Young Bassett wrote in 1836 to his wife in Alabama. 'There is not the [illegible] prejudice existing here against dissections & even the patients themselves do [not] seem to mind it, tho' they are aware of their fate, for more than two-thirds of the dead are carried to the Ecole Practique, or *Clamart*'.[29] Nowhere in the United States were bodies for dissection available in such reliable supply or the facilities for systematic dissection so extensive. Nevertheless, unlike the English, who often travelled to Paris principally for access to experience at anatomical dissection that was exorbitantly expensive at home, Americans relished the convenience and economy of extensive dissecting experience in France without regarding it as something all but unobtainable in their native land.[30]

Access to clinical instruction, however, was a different matter. Hospitals of any substantial size existed in only a few of America's largest cities, and even in these, patient populations were tiny compared with those of the great hospitals of Paris. Moreover, student access to patients in most American hospitals was meagre, and even though some American physicians returned from France determined to re-create courses of clinical instruction modelled after what they had enjoyed in Paris (courses almost invariably termed 'clinique' at American medical schools), opportunities for extensive clinical instruction remained slim.[31] It was a persistent source of wonderment to visiting American physicians that they needed only to show their diploma or passport in order to have the vast programme of clinical instruction in the Paris hospitals open up freely to them. 'Of the opportunities for studying diseases of every nature you will be able to form an opinion when informed that during the course of a year eighty thousand persons are admitted to the Hospitals', one American recently arrived in Paris wrote home describing the system in 1853. 'To obtain a ticket it is merely required to show one's passport. Each Hospital has medical and Surgical wards, attended by the most prominent Physicians and Surgeons. Each of these have an Amphitheater attached to his position, and is required to lecture on the cases under his treatment to the students who attend them whilst prescribing, a certain number of times a week. In the Amphitheatres also all the operations are performed'.[32]

And yet, as a vehicle for acquiring the kinds of clinical knowledge and experience that Americans most sought, there were serious limitations to this official system of clinical instruction.

Many Americans complained that the instruction offered at the bedside was superficial. 'As the physicians go to the hospitals every day, they do not say much about a patient except the first time of visiting him', Robert P. Harrison wrote from Paris to an American medical journal, 'and as the examinations are made in the consultation room before the patient enters, the students have but little opportunity of studying what is to them very important, the commencing examination and treatment of the cases'.[33] Thus Samuel Brown lamented to his diary in 1824, 'This morning I attended the Hotel Dieu but did not profit much by my visit owing … to my attending a Physician who was in much haste to go his rounds'.[34] More than this, because all of the professors made their rounds at the same hour, Americans found they had to choose only one to follow each day. 'My greatest difficulty in employing my time is the selection of courses', one recently arrived American explained. 'There is so much offered & so much that I would like to undertake that until now I have been skipping from place to place, unable to give the preference to any one. The only chance of doing any thing, I find, is to undertake one or at most two courses at a time'.[35] Such arrangements greatly diminished the actual value to the student of the clinical lectures given in the Paris hospitals.

Language posed another problem. Many Americans arrived with little knowledge of French and even less experience trying to understand the spoken language. Most engaged a language tutor shortly after their arrival, but comprehending French lecturers often remained a daunting task. Thus, after his first day visiting the Hôtel-Dieu, Henry Willard Williams confessed to his wife that 'one professor I listened to for an hour today without understanding a single sentence', explaining that he had resolved to attend the rounds of the professors he was best able to understand. 'I hope, however, to become familiarized to the sound of the language and able to catch the sense as well as from a book in reading', he wrote optimistically.[36] This lack of ability in understanding French lecturers encouraged Americans to concentrate on the clinical information they could actually see or otherwise directly experience. 'Though knowing little of the language upon my arrival', a Charleston physician wrote to the editor of that city's medical journal, 'I was nevertheless determined to take in whatever information I could through my eyes, notwithstanding that but little could be forced through my ears'.[37]

Seeing, however, much less touching, was not easy, for the ward visits that were so freely open were also notoriously crowded. Abel Lawrence Peirson, witnessing Dupuytren's morning visit for the first time, wrote to his wife: '"Two hundred pupils follow him to bed side of each patient. How much they must learn!"'[38] Just how much his irony was intentional is unclear, but others were explicit about the difficulty even of seeing the patient under such circumstances. Competing for space with French students, at the bedside and in the lecture hall, was a routine cause for complaint. 'There was jamming, kicking, bullying, cursing, and, what is so common among French students, *blackguarding* as we style it', one American typically grumbled.[39] What the American student wanted most from the Paris clinic was, as one of them noted, the chance to 'auscult, and percuss, and *touch* for himself', yet the realities of the official ward visits and lectures afforded little opportunity for such an education of the senses.[40]

Despite such impediments, most Americans did devote many of their mornings to the regular clinical rounds and lectures. Seeing the great hospitals, following the famous physicians and hearing them teach, witnessing the famous surgeons operate – it was all part of the heady experience of being at the very centre of things. The rhetoric Americans used in describing such clinical instruction commonly included vividly detailed attention to the physical staging of the room, how the orator's voice sounded, how he dressed, and the character his physical presence conveyed. Such reports betrayed an underlying sense of clinical instruction as spectacle, a relished sense of the theatricality of seeing the medical lions perform. Americans took such clinical teaching seriously as one way of gaining knowledge, more so in surgery than in internal medicine. But, like the visits Americans made to the renowned professional sites and figures of London, attending the hospital instruction of the professors was also medical tourism. 'A great number of the lectures we attend but a few times – merely as a matter of curiosity and to see the professors', Elisha Bartlett explained to his sister in 1826.[41] The visiting American, Austin Flint told a Kentucky medical class, 'may gratify his curiosity by visiting, on different days, different hospitals, or different wards of the same hospital, but there is little advantage in this beyond the mere gratification of curiosity'.[42] Yet as Flint had noted earlier, while still in Paris, 'Curiosity, of course, leads the medical visitor in Paris to see most of them'.[43]

There was, however, another form of clinical instruction – private lessons – that obviated many of the problems Americans encountered in the regular course of hospital teaching by the professors. Arrangements varied considerably, but typically a group of four or five students would arrange with an *interne* to admit them to his wards at hours when they were otherwise shut to students. In return for a fee, the *interne* would point out interesting cases, allow the students to examine the patients, and answer questions. 'Though the lectures are given publicly & the hospitals open in the morning during the visits of the attending physicians, they are not attended by the students during other parts of the day, except under these circumstances', James Lawrence Cabell wrote to his uncle. 'The *Internes* or medical assistants who reside in the Hospital & prescribe for the sick in the absence of the Professors, generally make an evening visit through their wards giving clinical instruction to a small class, these numbering generally limited to 4 or 5, on the payment of 30 francs a month from each'.[44] Such an arrangement gave students access to the bedside in a way impossible during ordinary morning clinical rounds. 'If one wishes to visit and examine patients at other times than during the regular hour of service for the clinical professor', Flint, then in Paris, commented in 1854, 'he must make an arrangement with an *interne*, who for a moderate fee, will at a different hour attend at the bedside, give any information that may be desired respecting the history, treatment, etc., of the cases, and at these visits any reasonable amount of examination of the cases is allowable. In this way special diseases may be studied to any extent'.[45]

Such private instruction got around many of the obstacles that spoiled the usefulness to Americans of the regular course of clinical instruction. It compensated for their imperfect command of French, for instead of gaining knowledge mediated by the remarks of the clinical professor, they could learn largely through their own sensual experience and from the patient guidance of an *interne* they employed. 'Bedside instruction in Paris is the most profitable and fortunately the most easily understood by the student', commented one American who found French lecturers very difficult to follow, yet one could learn directly from the patient only if access to the bedside was not blocked by a large crowd of students.[46] By avoiding the large clinical visits, a Massachusetts physician explained to his father, 'you are able to make the visit all most alone few if any medical students going the rounds – You are thereby enabled to experience each patient as much as you please'.[47] As another American described it, 'Form a class of four, or even two, and offer an *interne* five dollars per month each, and the doors of the hospital turn noiselessly on their hinges, ... the patients are your own, to be examined at your leisure, and the *interne* at your side to assist, direct and instruct you'.[48] Such arrangements permitted a full exercise of the senses – made it possible to stand at the bedside and systematically look, listen, and touch. Courses of private instruction became for the majority of Americans the most valued core of their studies in Paris, and this pattern persisted from the 1820s through the 1850s.

Actually there were at least two quite different types of proprietary instruction, often conflated as 'private classes' in the minds and reports of visiting Americans. On the one hand, as F. Peyre Porcher reported in 1853, 'Each Interne or Chief of the Cliniques of any note, has his private class of four or five at the Hospitals, who, for twenty-five to fifty francs per month, enjoy the privilege of making visits and examinations, and of studying auscultation and percussion with him during the evening'.[49] James L. Cabell explained in 1837, 'During the visit of the attending physician in the morning, there being generally a large crowd, it is just possible to see the patient & to hear the remarks of the physician, but hardly ever practicable for the student to examine for himself. For this reason the *Internes*, who are graduates of two, three, four or five years, limit their classes to so small a number. Most american students are in the habit of taking thus a course at one hospital on diseases of the Heart, another on those of the lungs, another of the eyes & another of the skin, while some add to these a course on surgery & midwifery &c'.[50] Such an arrangement became an established, albeit informal, institution, and nearly two decades later Carleton B. Chapman could describe a nearly identical system.[51]

The other kind of private class had a more formal structure and defined focus, most often but not always clinical. Private, for-fee classes, often given by *agrégés* of the faculty, were offered on such topics as diseases of the lungs, skin, or eyes; diseases of children; the use of the stethoscope or microscope; physiology; legal medicine; pathological and surgical anatomy; and 'touching' in midwifery. 'Paris abounds in private teachers', one American physician reported in 1848. 'Private instruction can be obtained on any subject. Magendie's assistant delivers lectures on Physiology; Blandin's assistant on Operative Surgery; Paul Dubois' assistant on the *Toucher*; the keeper of Dupuytren's Museum on Pathological Anatomy. The price of these tickets varies from six to ten dollars. Then there are Sichel's, and Desmarre's, and Tavignot's clinics on diseases of the eye, a clinic on diseases of the ear, etc. etc'.[52] Lists of such courses appeared in the guidebooks to medical Paris published for students, and, as one American noted, were posted at the Ecole Pratique and in the vicinity of the Ecole de Médecine.[53]

Just as arrangements with *internes* provided special access to the body in the clinic, so in other private courses – on normal, pathological, and surgical anatomy – Americans were able to combine the expertise of Parisian instructors with the special access to cadavers that French policies afforded. Especially popular was a private course, offered at various times both at the Ecole Pratique and at Clamart, that gave the student the opportunity to perform surgical operations on the dead body. Ashbel Smith, for example, wrote home enthusiastically in 1822 to describe the extensive surgical experience he was gaining from such a course, for which he paid five dollars.[54] 'It is true the courses are all public but they are crowded', John Young Bassett, like so many of his compatriots, reported on the official programme of instruction in 1836; therefore, 'I have found much advantage in employing private instructors & paying them'. He went on to describe the private course he had arranged: 'Six of [us] engaged *Mons. Chassaignac* – he is ajuge [*sic*] to the Faculty – and one of the best anatomists in France – to give us private instruction in Surgery. We perform all the operations two or more times ourselves under his eye'. Bassett added, 'I have also entered another private class of six with *Mons. Robecchi* for anatomical instruction; these gentlemen are both aiming at Professorships & *Mons. Chassaignac* aspiring at present for the Chair of Anatomy, & consequently they spare no pains'.[55] In this way, he explained, 'I have an opportunity of performing all the surgical operations myself two or three times over during the course (but I pay for it)'.[56]

However much Americans relished seeing the famous professors in action, then, and however much they revelled in the free access they had to their hospital rounds and lectures, they did not believe such official instruction was what best rewarded their limited time abroad. Most Americans made both kinds of private course central parts of their Parisian studies, taking advantage of clinical instruction and what one described as 'a legion of Lecturers, public and private, who occupy almost every hour of the twenty-four at the Ecole Pratique, and in private rooms in the neighbourhood'.[57] Though they often rose early to follow the eminent clinicians on their candle-lit rounds, and often stayed for their lectures, operations, and autopsies, most devoted the balance of the day to work at the dissecting table and to courses of private clinical instruction. 'Many of the irregular students – and nearly all of the American and many of the foreign students come under this class – pay but little attention to the lectures delivered at the School, with the exception of those upon Chemistry', one American explained. 'These, after visiting the hospital, will probably attend to dissections, Operative Surgery, or attend a private course on Midwifery, Bandaging, Diseases of the Eye, Auscultation and Percussion, Skin Diseases, Diseases of Children, or some other subject to which they wish to pay particular attention'.[58]

Americans were well aware that their experience of the Paris School was different from that of its French students. As a footnote to a letter from Paris published in an American medical journal, which described the array of private courses, an American editor noted in 1854, 'It is a fact well known here, that much the larger proportion of the amount of fees paid for the private courses, and to *internes* for clinical instruction at the hospitals, comes from foreigners, and especially from the American students and practitioners who visit Paris for medical improvement'.[59] The cost of such courses was one factor, for, as one American in Paris observed, 'these are tolerably expensive, and hence are not enjoyed but rarely by others than the English and Americans', though he added that 'this is the very best clinical instruction that one can acquire'.[60] More than this, for Americans, who sought most in Paris what was least available at home, time spent attending the official course of lectures, despite the fact that admission to them was gratuitous, was uneconomical. As one noted, 'The skilful and intelligent instructors, who have what are called "private courses", are mainly paid by Americans, whose generally short stay prevents their attending to the courses given by the faculty, as they are extended through too great a length of time'.[61] Consequently, as Austin Flint noted, 'The private courses of lectures and demonstrations, constituting the most valuable portion of the educational advantages which Paris offers, are in a great measure sustained by the foreigners resorting to Paris for professional improvement'.[62]

Private clinical instruction embodied what Americans most expected from the Paris School. It was what they told those at home to anticipate from a journey to France and what those who made the trip in turn relied upon. Already in place by the early 1820s, this pattern of expectation and behaviour was remarkably durable, and, with some fluctuations, paid private tutelage was what most powerfully attracted American doctors to Paris through the 1850s. From a professional point of view, it represented 'the paradise of Parisian life' to two generations of American medical migrants. Throughout that period, an ideal of empiricism stood in American depictions as what was most important about the French medical model. But it was not necessary to make the voyage across the Atlantic to adopt such an ideal. Instead, sensual experience, gained at the dissecting table and most especially at the bedside in the kind of context that private instruction alone readily made possible, was what most attracted American doctors to Paris and what seemed to assure that their migration there would continue.

Dead End?

If the Paris School reached a dead end in 1848, there was no indication of it either in American reports on medical Paris or in patterns of migration there by American doctors. Indeed, through the 1850s the number of Americans annually making the journey grew markedly. 'Scarcely a day passes without the arrival of new members of the medical profession from America', one observer in Paris noted in 1854, 'and probably every steamer carries home some who have just completed their tour of observation and study here'.[63] So large was the influx that in 1851 the American Medical Society in Paris was founded with the aim 'of aiding American students to hear and see whatever is worthy of their consideration', and by 1853 the society was reported to be larger than either the Anglo-Parisian Medical Society (f. 1837) or the Verein deutscher Aerzte in Paris (f. 1844), its English and German counterparts.[64]

At the same time, what the American disciples of the Paris School had made it stand for in their own country – an ideal of empirical truth – retained its symbolic power in the American context. Even though the crusade 'against the spirit of system' they had launched in its name appeared decreasingly French as it was assimilated into the American mainstream, reformers continued to use the lessons of their Parisian experience to rail against the dangers of rationalism and speculative medical theory. During the 1840s and 1850s, essays lambasting rationalistic systems were common among the M.D. theses submitted at American medical schools; and in such works, 'the gush of speculation' that the empiricist message of the Paris School promised to stem continued to be held responsible for many of the profession's social, intellectual, and economic ills.[65] The cultural power of empiricism in antebellum American medicine, in other words, was far from spent.

What did change, gradually, was the significance attached to a trip to Paris. Still unusual enough to be a source of considerable professional distinction during the 1820s and 1830s, by the 1850s study in France had come to be an expected step in the career-building of any American physician with ambition and means. Thus in 1845, a Harvard College student sketching a plan for his future could include study in Paris as an assumed stage in his medical training. 'My way is clear for at least 6 years if my health and prosperity continue', he wrote to a friend. '3 years here and a degree of M.D. – and then two years in Paris and Europe – After that I may begin to look after a wife'.[66] As more and more Americans journeyed to Paris, the utility of that experience in setting the traveller apart from the masses of an overcrowded and competitive profession diminished. And as study in Paris became less and less a source of distinction and special identity, the meaning of a trip to France changed in turn.

During the decades when Paris stood unrivalled as a magnet for American doctors abroad, many of them did of course include British, Italian, and German cities on their itineraries as well. Those who visited Vienna through the 1850s often did so as tourists, though ordinarily they included medical institutions and figures in their sightseeing. After a year and a half studying medicine in Paris, for example, Charles T. Jackson explained that 'I resolved to lay aside the scalpel & stethoscope for a while & take a tour through the most interesting portions of Europe'. When he visited Vienna in 1831 it was as part of a leisurely grand tour, and only when cholera appeared in that city six days after his arrival did he decide to take advantage of the occasion to study at the Allgemeine Krankenhaus, later recalling, 'I lost no opportunity of instructing myself in the nature of the terrible disease & I had my hands full'.[67] Around the same time his kinsman, James Jackson, Jr, considered taking a short break from study in Paris to see what he could learn in Germany, but his father, a medical professor at Harvard, persuaded him that there was too little going on in German medicine to warrant the trip.[68] Levin S. Joynes wanted to spend six months exploring German medicine in 1841 before returning home from France. 'But to one who does not know the language, it would be folly to go to Germany to study, unless he has at least four months to throw away in acquiring it', he wrote to his father in Virginia, explaining that he had resolved to visit England instead; 'I abandoned all ideas of going to Germany, and why should I regret it after all? – for there is no *Paris* in Germany. To exchange one for the other would be "paying dearly for a whistle."'[69]

The reports of those who did include Germany in their European tours, combined with translations and summaries of German works that increasingly appeared in the American medical press, meant that American physicians were generally aware of the medical facilities and activities in Vienna and Berlin. But through the 1850s, most elected to study in Paris instead. There, private instruction remained paramount, but the late 1840s and early 1850s did witness some shift in the kinds of courses most prominent in American reports, particularly a greater emphasis on medical specialities.

In antebellum America, medical specialism remained illegitimate – a hallmark of the charlatan – and at least through the 1840s to a large extent Americans believed the French shared this view. 'All specialists as they are called that is men who confine their attention to one particular thing as diseases of the eyes &c are looked upon [in] Paris as quacks', one American wrote from Paris in 1844, 'for there is no doubt that the more a man confines his mind to one subject the more dogmatic narrowminded he will become – It is bad enough to be obliged to separate the profession into the three great branches without subdividing them into eye doctor ear doctor nose doctor and belly doctor'.[70] Nevertheless, American students felt comfortable concentrating on one or a few branches of medicine, so long as they did not declare any intention of becoming a specialist. 'On account of such numbers of sick being congregated at so many points in Paris, students from all countries flock hither. The specialities too, or places where only one disease is treated, cannot be otherwise than very instructive', one noted in 1851.[71] Studying diseases of the skin at the Hôpital St Louis had long been a favourite focus of Americans, while by the early 1850s, Americans avidly attended the clinic of the Vienna-trained Julius Sichel on diseases of the eyes.[72] Thus, when Augustus Kinsley Gardner noted in 1848 that 'my great object in visiting Paris' was to study midwifery, especially in the clinic of Paul Dubois, his admission was not unusual, and enthusiastic descriptions of private 'touching' courses in midwifery abounded.[73] Americans generally spoke of studying diseases of the skin or diseases of the eyes – not dermatology or ophthalmology – but the specialized focus of their work was nonetheless apparent.

Courses on experimental physiology and microscopy also became more prominent in American accounts. In fact, Americans claimed that in both fields, they were more ardent students than their French counterparts. Not only did many Americans frequent Claude Bernard's lectures, but one could assert in 1854 that 'in the class which attended the Spring Course of Lectures on Physiology by Bernard, and which was quite a numerous one, there were only two who were not Americans'.[74] In the same year, another American could write from Paris that 'among the most notable defects of French teaching, may be noticed the neglect of general pathology and the use of the microscope. Robin is nearly the only teacher of the microscope, and his class is generally confined to a small number of American students. Nachet, one of the principal manufacturers of microscopes, told me that his best customers were from America, and that nearly all his most expensive instruments were sent there'.[75] Robin's courses won a devoted American following. 'He gives two courses, one theoretical, in which he gives description of the histological tissues; the second one is practical in which he shows them all under the micro[sco]pe in addition to all morbid and malignant growths', John A. Murphy, who, along with a compatriot, had just taken both of Robin's courses, wrote from Paris in 1854. Embracing what he saw as the coming importance of the microscope, Murphy predicted that 'the results of investigations now going on with it, joined to the philosophical researches of M. Bernard, will produce a great change ere long, in the treatment of disease, as well as in pathological anatomy'.[76]

Indeed, by the early 1850s some older Americans committed to French medicine could be heard complaining that the Paris School was slipping precisely because it was departing from a strict focus on their kind of clinical medicine. Thus Alfred Stillé wrote in 1851 to George Cheyne Shattuck, both of them devout students of Pierre Louis who had made their experience in Paris during the 1830s a central part of their professional identity, that a contemporary who had recently revisited Paris and judged it declining might have a point. 'I do not wonder Swett should have felt that there was a falling off in the scientific status of the present generation of physicians in Paris', Stillé admitted to Shattuck. 'Yet', he continued, perceptively, 'the change is perhaps less in them than in himself. When a man has devoted himself as he, and you, and many of our associates did, in Paris, to a certain field of investigation, it is not easy to enter upon a new one with the same interest, or estimate so highly those who cultivate it'. Stillé went on to reflect that 'I begin to find it no longer a matter of wonder that men who have become accustomed to practice with a certain degree of knowledge should have so much difficulty in being persuaded that there is still more to learn'. Nevertheless, writing from Vienna after revisiting Paris himself, Stillé confessed that 'I am sensible of being quite behind the age in several matters, and especially in all that relates to the application of chemistry to morbid processes; and at the same time I feel something of that want of appreciation of the methods of diagnosis at present employed which I blamed in my Seniors when I was studying auscultation & percussion'. Stillé went on to say that if he knew German and his health were better, he would be tempted to remain in Vienna and join the other six or seven American students then engaged in medical study there.[77]

Grumblings that Paris was not what it once was generally remained muted, tentative, and very qualified. Nevertheless, early in the 1850s some Americans did begin to suggest that perhaps the kinds of instruction they most valued in Paris might be equally obtainable in Vienna. Comparing the advantages of Paris, Berlin, and Vienna for studying diseases of the eye, George Doane, back in Burlington, Vermont, after a study tour of Europe, asserted in 1853,

> Nothing can be conceived more admirable than the arrangements at Vienna for instruction, in this, and other branches of medical, and surgical knowledge. Having for a short period experienced them, I regard it almost as a duty to call to them the attention of those who have in view a visit to Europe, after the completion of their studies here. There were only five Americans in Vienna last winter, while Paris could boast of between three and four hundred.* These latter crowded every private lecture-room, and clinique of the 'Quartier Latin' to their own discomfort, and that of the teachers; while in Vienna the same, and in many cases, greater facilities exist, unknown and unimproved. The latter city has but one hospital for general practice, but it is the largest in the world.[78]

Austin Flint, addressing medical students at the University of Louisville in 1854, typically told them that 'Paris has been generally considered to possess greater facilities for pursuits connected with medical science, than any other city in the world. Students and medical men from widely separated quarters of the globe, have been attracted thither in greater numbers than at any other point'. Yet, he went on to note, 'of late there has been some diversion in favor of other places, such as Berlin, Vienna, Giessen and Dublin', but he nonetheless concluded that 'the supremacy of Paris is still maintained'.[79]

At the same time, some Americans did begin to assert that the medical faculty of Paris was not being kept up to its earlier standards. In part, the clinicians of earlier decades Americans had so identified with the Paris School showed their advancing age and, as one American put it in 1847, seemed 'to belong to the by gone generation'.[80] More than this, some American observers maintained that the changing political climate had lowered the scientific standards for making medical appointments. Those in Paris in

Paradigm Lost or Paradise Declining?

1848 witnessed the political turmoil and duly noted it in their journals, but by and large it did not interfere with their medical studies.[81] Some, however, believed that its aftermath was more intrusive. Stillé, writing to Shattuck after revisiting Paris in 1851, noted that 'the political state of the French capital is unfavorable to scientific progress, & the peers of our old masters do not at present exist there'.[82] After his return to Philadelphia, Stillé reflected that while in Paris, 'I did not visit any of the hospitals, but was told that very little was doing in medicine; politics are undermining & belittling science as they have done here'.[83] Similarly, another American physician reported from Philadelphia in 1854 that 'to the stranger who was familiar with the Institutions in 1840, it does not appear, on a return at present, that much progress has been made, either in the means of teaching the doctrines taught, or the qualifications of the Professors'. In particular, 'It will be seen that in the Faculty, the gain scarcely compensates for the loss, and if the reputation of the School of Paris depended upon that alone, it might well be supposed to be upon the decline'. And yet, he concluded that 'such is not the case', dismissing the notion of decline by pointing out that what American physicians most valued – not teaching by the faculty but private instruction by less eminent clinicians – remained intact. 'The able corps of hospital physicians and surgeons, with the agrégés[,] chefs de clinique, *internes*, etc, keep up the public and private course to their former standard of excellence'.[84]

In 1855, however, this changed dramatically. On the first of January of that year, Americans then in Paris reported, a new edict issued by the Dean of the Faculty went into effect that suppressed all teaching by *internes* of private clinical courses. As Robert A. Kinloch reported from Paris less than two weeks later in a letter to a South Carolina medical journal,

> The Bureau of administration of the hospitals, has seen fit to put a stop to all private instruction by the '*internes*'. This is greatly to be regretted, since most of our young men have derived what practical knowledge they obtained in Paris, by the freedom they have heretofore enjoyed of entering the hospitals, and examining the patients more closely with the intelligent '*internes*', than they could possibly do when following the physician or surgeon in his daily visit.[85]

Kinloch went on to say that 'many explanations have been offered, but I believe none of them sufficient to account for the procedure'. He noted that 'amongst other reasons, the '*internes*' sometimes tell

Americans that they believe our country-woman, Mrs. Clarke, ... to have been the cause of the change, from her *close scrutiny* of the male patients'.[86] In a letter written two months earlier he had offered a detailed account of 'Miss or Mrs. Clarke', an 'American female M.D'. who 'is always accompanied by her brother who is said to be a Homeopathic physician'. As he reported, 'I have encountered her several times in the wards of M. Dubois, where she seems to be attentively and courageously observing the diseases of the parturient state. Her attention though, seems not to be of an exclusive kind, as I have heard of her in the surgical amphitheatres of some hospitals, witnessing bloody operations'.[87] Kinloch dismissed the rumour as 'only a "*funny*" explanation, and no doubt a scandal upon the good lady'.[88] Another American also reported on the Dean's action that 'the cause of this change did not seem to be well understood', but noted that 'it was said to be owing to an abuse of the privilege formerly allowed to the *internes*, and which it was thought had resulted in injury to the patient'.[89]

Other observers agreed with Kinloch that this new move boded ill for the prospects of medical study in Paris by Americans. In the spring of 1855, Henry Smith, a Philadelphia professor of surgery who had studied in Paris sixteen years earlier, revisited that city to collect pathological specimens for the University of Pennsylvania. Though saddened to find that 'my old preceptors, Lisfranc, Roux, Marjolin, and Breschet, were numbered with the dead', it was the recent edict of the Dean that forced his conclusion that 'in comparing the present position of Paris, as a residence for the young American student, with that which it held in 1839, I am sorry to say that its advantages appeared to me to have diminished'. He recognized that 'its anatomical theatres, with the facilities for the practice of operative surgery, seem, it is true, unchanged', but lamented that 'its private clinical courses have been much impaired by a decision of the Dean, which has forbidden the formation of private classes under the charge of the hospital *internes*'. As he explained to Philadelphia medical students after his return,

> Formerly it was the custom for four or five young Americans to unite in a class, and under the direction of the house-physician to visit, at a private hour, the new patients who each day entered the wards, examine them carefully, and express an opinion of the nature of the complaint, this opinion being subsequently verified or disproved by the future visit of the clinical professor on the next morning. Such facilities furnished opportunities for practical

instruction and experience in diagnosis, which rendered Paris the great centre of medical attraction, and caused hundreds to seek its hospitals after the completion of their preliminary courses elsewhere; but now it is forbidden, and the student is limited to the public visit of each morning in connection with the crowds who follow the rounds of the surgeon.

As Smith concluded, 'Owing to the changes which, as stated, have been recently made in the arrangement of the courses of instruction in the Parisian hospitals, it cannot be denied that Paris does not now present the attractions which it once offered to the medical student'. Smith predicted that just as Paris had superseded Edinburgh as the favoured destination for American medical students abroad, Vienna might well supplant Paris as 'the great centre of medical attraction'.[90]

The edict of the Dean was not unprecedented, and earlier proscriptions on private courses seem always to have been temporary. Extolling the extensive opportunities for private clinical instruction that he had taken advantage of in Paris, for example, one American wrote in 1845, after his return to Philadelphia, 'Unfortunately all this is at an end. Last January, Orfila, the Dean of the Faculty, and the managers of the hospitals, put a stop to these private courses. The reason assigned for this was, that such repeated examination was injurious and cruel to the patients. But those *internes* who were engaged in the business said that the real opposition was on the part of their fellow internes, and arose from their jealousy'.[91] Yet private arrangements continued. As another American explained in 1848, 'Some years ago private clinical instruction in the hospitals was sanctioned by the administration, but being carried by the *internes* to too great an extent, the patients made such loud complaint that it became necessary to prohibit it'. He noted, however, that 'under the present system private clinical teaching is conducted *sub rosa*', and suggested that 'the laws of a hundred faculties and administrations would be little heeded by the *internes*, when pecuniary reward was in question'.[92] Still, when Orfila had abolished private classes in 1845, a move 'much to the regret of all the foreigners', it had led one American to predict that 'if this privilege be not again granted, Paris has in my opinion lost its great charm for the American student'.[93]

Even if the Dean's action of 1855 was temporary as well, its timing assured that it would have serious, far-reaching consequences for Americans. A decade earlier, when the 1845 action had been taken, the Paris School reigned as unquestionably the leading place for professional improvement by the American physician abroad. Not only its status as the uncontested centre of medical science, but also (and more important for Americans) its reputation as a clinical school unparalleled in the access students could gain to the bedside, for modest fees, had been secure. In 1855, however, the singularity of Paris seemed less self-evident. Some observers had been voicing their concern, qualified as it usually was, that the standards of the Paris School were slipping. Equally, occasional reports from American physicians in Vienna were newly enthusiastic about the potential of the German clinic as a place for medical study. At the same time, American society as a whole was starting to pay increased attention to German culture, and at least one American medical student in Paris could write home in 1854 that he wanted to spend time in either Berlin or Vienna before returning, partly to study medicine but mainly to master German, for, as he explained, 'fortune may bring me in contact with the German emigrants of whom such vast numbers pour into our country every year'.[94] Above all, in 1855 there was a growing awareness that if anything threatened to impede the free access to private clinical instruction that was what Americans chiefly valued in Paris, there might be attractive alternatives elsewhere.

During the second half of the 1850s, quite abruptly, invidious comparisons of Paris with Vienna began to proliferate in the American medical literature. Henry K. Oliver, Jr, for example, one of the earliest American disciples of the Vienna School, wrote in 1857 from Vienna to the *Boston Medical and Surgical Journal* enthusiastically describing arrangements in that city for clinical instruction:

> The clinics are distributed throughout the entire day, so that one may go from the medical wards into the midwifery wards, and from there into the surgical, &c. Not to speak of other advantages, this single arrangement enables one to pick up as much medical knowledge in Vienna in six months, as in a year or more at Paris, where all the clinics take place at the same hour in the morning. Each student who wishes, is charged with the care of a patient, whom he visits at least twice a day. On the first day of the patient's entrance, the student examines him and writes out the result and the history of the case generally. In this he is guided by the *chef de clinique*, who points out the main features of the case, teaches him to percuss, auscult, &c. The following day, the student reads the account of the case, as written off, to the professor at the bedside,

who then examines the patient himself, and afterward questions the student, laying especial stress upon the means of arriving at the diagnosis. The advantage of this mode of lecturing, instead of just examining the patient and retiring to the lecture-room to enlarge upon the case, as in Paris and with us, can hardly be questioned.

The editor of the journal, J. Mason Warren, prefaced Oliver's letter by noting that 'the superior advantages of the Vienna hospitals, for students, over those of Paris, have of late years attracted much attention. The great facilities afforded for both medical and surgical study and observation, have quite turned the tide in favor of the German institutions; and much more time is now spent in them by some of our young medical men, than in those of the French capital'.[95]

Into the 1860s, comparisons of Paris with Vienna that found the former wanting became commonplace, most especially after 1865, when peace renewed the flow of American doctors to Europe that the American Civil War temporarily had slowed. Tellingly, what Americans most often celebrated about Vienna as a place for study was access, for a fee, to practical clinical instruction, what they had always valued most in Paris, but which had become hard to come by in the French capital. 'Little can be done in the application of the theory, in Paris, except by comparatively few, because of so little being done in private classes', H. Z. Gill wrote in 1868, 'while at the German cities every facility is afforded to strangers, at very low fees'. Having just returned from two years of study in Austria, Prussia, France, and England, he concluded that 'private instruction in the general branches can be obtained in Germany more thoroughly and at less expense, perhaps, than in any other country'. Gill urged, for example, that 'in Vienna, Prague and Berlin are offered the greatest advantages for personal examination of patients by members of the class in all diseases of the chest. Especially is this true at the two former cities, where much attention is given to teaching practical diagnosis, as well from physical signs as from chemical and microscopical means; and at the same time, due attention is given to pathology and post-mortem examinations'. He added that 'the remarks already made in reference to private classes in the general branches apply, in an eminent degree, in nearly all the special subjects', and noted that 'for studying *venerial diseases*, as well as for *cutaneous affections*, Vienna affords the greatest facilities for the foreign students'.[96] Thus an Ohio physician could write from Vienna in 1868, 'There are some thirty American Students here and I think if the others in Europe only knew of the advantages here they would not waste their time in Paris & other Cities'.[97]

Instruction in the clinical specialities loomed especially large in rhetoric extolling Vienna. From the 1850s onward through the 1870s, of course, Americans also increasingly emphasized the opportunities for studying the medical specialities in Paris. 'The great attention given to specialities will strike the foreigner impressively, especially if he comes from a section where the condition of society and the circumstances of the profession have not favoured specialities of practice', a North Carolina physician wrote from Paris a few months after his arrival in 1861, noting in particular the opportunity to study the use of the ophthalmoscope in a private course. He applauded the fact that 'for a moderate sum you can also receive daily lessons at the Hospitals on any branch you choose, from the assistants of the Hospital surgeons and physicians. These assistants are generally young men of talent and are well qualified, and being anxious for distinction, they carry on these private courses with great benefit to their classes'.[98] In reporting on their Parisian studies, Americans underscored their work in, for example, diseases of the eyes. Yet, as one recalled his experience there in 1860, 'There was an abundance of material, but it was not as profitable as I hoped. They were far behind the clinics of Berlin under Graefe, or of Vienna under Arlt and Jaeger. They were but an exhibition rather than instructive. But for private instruction from Galezowsky and Cusco I should not have learned much'.[99] In the same year, a Boston editor prefaced a letter sent to his journal by an American physician in Vienna, on courses of study in diseases of the eye, noting, 'It certainly well illustrates, at least in one respect, the advantages claimed for that over other European cities, as the place for American students to complete their studies'.[100] Similar comparisons in other specialities, such as obstetrics, abounded.[101] As David F. Lincoln, writing from Vienna in 1871, summed up, 'For us foreigners, Vienna is a school for *specialities*'.[102]

In all their discussions about the advantages of Vienna over Paris, though, Americans made it clear that what they valued most was precisely what they had valued most in Paris – that is, not teaching by the great professors so much as ready access to practical instruction at the bedside. Just as Americans in Paris were eager to return home able to say that they had followed Louis's ward rounds or seen Dupuytren operate, so in Vienna they wanted to see Rokitansky, Oppolzer, and Skoda in action. But, as one American wrote bluntly from Vienna in 1871, it was not the professors but the assistants, who for a fee taught special courses to small groups in the clinic, that were of the greatest value to the American student. 'Those who are the most prominent before the medical profession at large, those who have acquired a world-wide reputation already, perhaps, and who might be supposed to be the real foundation of Vienna's popularity, have practically little to do with it'. As he explained, 'Their lectures are fashioned for students who are learning the elements, and who are required to study for years before graduating here, rather than for the graduate who has learned the elements already, and who wishes to acquire special advanced information in relation to particular parts'.[103] The quality of the professors of the Vienna School was not the key issue.

The American physicians who travelled to Vienna, in other words, went for much the same reasons that had drawn their predecessors to Paris. Thus, in 1874, Frederick Shattuck could write from Vienna to his father, the eminent Boston disciple of the Paris School, George Cheyne Shattuck, Jr, that even though 'the regular work of the Professors has really stopped', that would not interfere with the routine of his studies, for 'the private courses with the assistants which I take will nearly all run on during the vacation'.[104] As another Boston physician in Vienna noted in 1871, 'The idea may still linger in the minds of some, that a student comes to Vienna to hear Rokitansky, Skoda and Oppolzer – or their respective successors. This can hardly be said to be the case'. Instead, 'the real glory of the school at present consists in the fact that one can learn anything, quickly and thoroughly'.[105]

Certainly the attraction of Vienna had nothing to do with the notion that its clinicians might be better at therapeutics or at patient care in general than their Parisian counterparts. Just as Americans had long insisted that the Americans and the English were better healers than the French, whatever the excellence of Parisian pathology and diagnosis, those who travelled to Vienna and Berlin were equally strident in asserting Anglo-American superiority to the Germans in medical treatment. 'In the Hospitals they study to know what is the matter; then they stop', Joseph Webb wrote home to his mother from Berlin in 1866. 'In *"Diagnosis"*, they excel; but in *Treatment* we excel'.[106] More than this, as William Williams Keen wrote in 1865 from Vienna, 'I thought that in Paris the patients were made subservient enough to the instruction & Enlightenment of the Students but here they are nothing but animals trotted out for the gaping crowds'. Like most American observers he insisted proudly that public opinion would never allow in American hospitals the kind of treatment of patients he witnessed in the

Paradigm Lost or Paradise Declining?

Allgemeine Krankenhaus; 'but it is certainly jolly for the Students. It's a magnificent place to learn & in many respects is far superior to Paris'.[107] Indeed, it was partly for this reason that Webb, visiting France after his studies in Germany, could observe in 1867 that 'there are many reasons, why one should give Vienna the preference for studying medicine, over all other Cities'. As he wrote from Paris, 'There is much to learn here; but I am satisfied that Vienna, is all things considered the best – you get more at the patient in Vienna, than here'.[108] Whatever ambivalence Americans retained about Viennese attitudes toward patient care, and toward what they saw as an objectification of the patient more extreme even than in Paris, they recognized that it enhanced free access to the bedside, what as students they most valued.

Some Americans who travelled to Paris continued to celebrate what it offered them, impressed by facilities for instruction far beyond anything they could find at home. 'I have already seen enough to justify me in expressing the belief that the medical advantages of Paris, are greater than those of any city in the world', one American wrote confidently from Paris in 1861. 'Paris has, at no former time, been so justly entitled to this distinction as now'.[109] So too, a young New Haven physician wrote home in 1867 that 'the lectures at the "Jardin des Plantes", at the Sorbonne and at the "École de Médecine", together with my exercise in the Laboratory, Hospitals and museum, certainly affords mental exercise sufficient, to keep in activity all my powers'. In Europe to study not only medicine but comparative anatomy, he wrote that 'the unequalled opportunities, which one finds for study in Paris, impresses me more and more every day .... It is not strange, then, that this Mecca attracts from every quarter of the globe, pilgrims, who searching after truths, regard distance and separation as nothing'.[110]

By the 1870s, however, in the American medical journal literature, in professional addresses, and in private correspondence, assessments of the advantages for study that different European centres offered the American physician were less likely to compare Vienna with Paris than Vienna with Berlin. 'Now that you have been longer in Berlin, and already know Vienna so well, I shall very gladly read a few more lines from you on their comparative merit and defects', a young American physician in Vienna wrote in 1872 to a compatriot studying in Berlin. 'Dr Knight says that indeed there is a quantity of *material* here which Berlin cannot offer, but for scientific & thorough methods of investigation and instruction Berlin has a great advantage, not to mention Virchow.

– and he advised me if I had two winters to spend in Europe, to study in Berlin during the whole of one'. As he concluded, 'I *suppose* I ought to secure a winter in Berlin for sake of pathology i.e., to go there next October, but I should leave Vienna so with some grudging'.[111] By 1880, an American physician in Vienna could write to a Cincinnati medical journal, reflecting that 'medical centres have their day like the states and empires of which they are so often the capitals, and if Vienna now holds out attractions, which at one time Paris possessed in the first degree, what is more conceivable than that Berlin in its turn may assume first rank?'[112]

Growing from concerns in the 1850s that the access to experiential knowledge that for decades had attracted them to the Paris School was diminishing, American physicians abroad increasingly concluded that Vienna afforded them greater advantages for medical study. What most of them sought in German-speaking lands was neither any new epistemological departure – any fresh approach to medical knowledge – nor the scientific brilliance of the German teachers. To be sure, some found the extent to which the Vienna School cultivated specialism in medicine appealing, as they did its stress on newer chemical and microscopical diagnostic techniques. And some – a minuscule minority, upon whom the lion's share of historical attention has been lavished – set off to Germany for scientific study in the laboratory, especially in experimental physiology.[113] But what most American physicians wanted from Germany and Austria was the same kind of ready access to practical clinical instruction (for which they expected to pay) that for so long had drawn them to the Paris hospitals. During the decades after the Civil War many American physicians continued to make their way to Paris, just as throughout the century they had included London on their itineraries, but increasingly they went to Paris only for short visits as medical tourists. 'I hope to be in Paris tomorrow evening', a young Baltimore physician who had been studying medicine in Vienna and Berlin wrote home to his father in 1877. 'How long I will stay in Paris will depend upon the collections in the Louvre which I have never seen, upon Versailles and many other things'.[114]

Story-telling and Medical Histories

Absent from the rhetoric that accompanied the shift in American migration was any indication that new ways of doing medicine played the key role in making study in Germany more appealing than study in France. In the stories about Paris and German cities that American physicians told during the years when the shift began, and in the accounts they left of their own deliberations as students, there was no sense in the 1850s and 1860s that the clinical empiricism of the Paris School had become outmoded. And certainly there was no sense that the ascendancy of laboratory medicine in Germany – the laboratory medicine that Ackerknecht said the Paris School ostracized as part of its dogged preoccupation with clinical empiricism – was what first redirected Americans to Vienna. As most Americans told the story at the time, the French model of medical science was little dimmed; what had declined, rather, was the nature of the clinical experience that they as students could acquire in Paris, compared with the opportunities to be found in Vienna.

Those who travelled to Vienna celebrated the access they found there to seeing, listening, and touching the body, just as those who remembered Paris celebrated the access to sensual experience it had given them. Over time, of course, the stories told about Paris by its American disciples changed through an ongoing process of selection, simplification, and symbolization. Increasingly they linked the broader meaning of the Paris School and of their experiences there to the clinicians they had followed in France or to the hospitals in which they had spent their days – concrete emblems that stood for the whole. Writing in 1885, for example, Edward Warren, who had studied in Paris three decades earlier, noted that the great men he had heard in Paris – Trousseau, Velpeau, Piorry, Robin, Nelaton, Jobert de Lamball, Ricord, Maisonneuve, Andral, and Dubois – were, with one exception, gone. 'But they still live in the memory of those who listened to their words of wisdom and eloquence as well as upon the proudest pages in the history of medicine'.[115] In recollections of the Paris School, the mundane realities of practical clinical experience gained through paid private instruction, a central preoccupation in the stories they told while in France, all but vanished from their narratives. Yet the essence of that experience endured, distilled into symbols – above all, the ideal of empirical truth – that stood for both the Paris of their youth and its lasting meaning.

Some Americans, though, came to tell a different story. 'There was a time when the French capital was looked upon by the medical profession throughout the world as the one and only seat of science, where alone the grand truths of our art could be discovered and taught', James Clarke White opened his commencement address at the Harvard Medical School in 1866. 'Students from every country went thither to complete their studies and to see the men whose names had been upon the lips of their teachers all through their early instruction at home as demigods in science ... . She was the acknowledged front and centre of science'. 'But', he continued, 'what position does she hold now? The earnest students of other countries no longer visit her exclusively, or even first or second, to complete their general studies, or to perfect themselves in any special branch of our art, nor is French now the universal or most important language of science, as it once was. The very names which then commanded such world-wide respect are now almost memories associated with the past, and are no more the representatives of the medicine of today'.[116]

'What is the cause of this decadence?' White went on to ask his audience. 'Why is it that the Wiener Schule holds at this moment the place then occupied by the Ecole de Médecine? The great masters in Paris have not died out and left their places to be filled by smaller men in Vienna, for with one or two exceptions the roll of French professors bears the same distinguished names that it did twenty-five years ago. Other causes have wrought the change'. As he went on to propose, 'Gradually the philosophic German mind, so sceptical and irreverent as to accept no dogmas unchallenged, and so patient and industrious in following the suggestions of nature to their very source, began to make itself heard ... ; it has made a knowledge of the German language a necessity to all who would know anything of the modern advances of science, and draws our students to Vienna and Berlin as the great schools of medicine'. White concluded by asserting that 'in the mean time Paris has been living chiefly on the reputation of her past greatness, and the slight progress she has made has seemed complete stagnation by the side of the vast advance of her indefatigable Saxon neighbors'.[117]

By the time when White spoke in 1866, his account of the decline of Paris and rise of Germany as a destination for American medical students was one that most of his compatriots would have shared. However, his explanation for that shift – rooted in the decadence of French medicine and ascendancy of the 'German mind' – was much more idiosyncratic. Through the narrative he recounted to the assembly at Harvard, White was trying to establish a new benchmark for American medicine, a new identity for his generation of physicians, and a prominent position for himself within the new order. A decade after the shift from Paris to Vienna had commenced, and at a time when Parisian experience no longer offered a very potent source of prestige to the ambitious young American doctor, White looked to Viennese experience as a new wellspring of professional distinction. He had been perhaps the first American physician of his cohort to spend a full year studying in Vienna, in 1856; was among the first of professionally respectable American physicians to declare himself a specialist, in dermatology; and was among the earliest and most vigorous American proselytizers for the Vienna School. Indeed, in 1865, the year before his address, White and five other Harvard medical graduates who had studied in Vienna during the second half of the 1850s founded the Wiener Club in Boston, a fraternity to affirm and preserve the special identity that their shared experience in Vienna conferred.[118]

The professional identity that White was crafting for himself hinged upon a representation of German medicine as special, distinct, and separate – a new departure from what had come before it. Stressing the continuities between Parisian and Viennese medicine, and between the reasons why American physicians abroad had elected to study at one or the other place, would have undercut such aims rather than have sustained them. The story that White told instead celebrated the singularity of the German mind and its ascendancy as the mark of a new era in Western medicine. His was a narrative told from the perspective of one who had cast his lot with German medicine and the special identity it promised. Elsewhere, I have explored how during the first half of the nineteenth century, the representation by American physicians of the medical empiricism they encountered in Paris as something distinctly French grew from the way they viewed and wished to portray history.[119] In particular, they depicted the Paris School as a turning point, an epistemological break with the past that inaugurated a new medical era. Both the Frenchness and newness of the Paris School helped make it an effective, distinctive banner under which the Americans could mount their campaign for reform, one that would give direction to their own lives and careers. White, in turn, was beginning the process of recasting the narrative of medical history in ways that would clarify the special mission of his generation and give meaning to its endeavours. For White, establishing the newness and Germanness of what he valued in Vienna was an essential component of a successful historical narrative. Promoting a particular version of history was a linchpin of his broader programme, for it at once explained the past, gave meaning to the present, and offered a plan for the future. Still novel in the mid-1860s, the dominant theme of White's version of history – the ascendancy of the German mind over French decadence – would become commonplace in America during the final quarter of the nineteenth century, especially as experimental laboratory science became the new hallmark of scientific medicine.

My point here has not been to refute Ackerknecht's assertion about the dead end of the Paris School: surely his case was overstated, but whether or not there was a dead end all depends on how one defines and gauges it. I have instead tried to understand what made Paris attractive to American students and why that attraction waned. More than this, I have tried to use the example of American perceptions of Paris medicine – a source of evidence Ackerknecht cited as leading testimony in support of his argument but never analyzed – to draw into question just how sharp was the discontinuity that the image of a dead end conjures up. The experiences and expectations of American physicians at the time, and the interpretations they offered for their choices, suggest patterns of change that do not mesh comfortably with the ones Ackerknecht depicted. To understand the fine structure of how and why changes in the Paris School proceeded as they did, of course, will require close study of the French medical world itself, not, as in this paper, just American perceptions of that world.

What is clear enough, though, is that the migration of American physicians to Paris during the first half of the nineteenth century cannot be taken as solid testimony to the singular intellectual vibrancy of the Paris School. Nor can the shift in American migration to Germany be interpreted as compelling evidence that the Paris School reached an intellectual dead end. Moreover, Ackerknecht's assertion that *empiricism* led to a dead end – displayed by the shift in migration – begins to appear premised upon highly stylized images not only of the Paris School but also of the Vienna School to which Americans turned, images rooted in story-telling conventions that first became established during the final third of the nineteenth century. To a significant extent, his narrative seems scripted by later images of German medicine that privileged its reliance on the experimental laboratory and the epistemological distinctiveness that came with it.

In particular, underlying the story of the Paris School Ackerknecht told is an assumed sharp distinction between the products of clinical empiricism and medical science: it was this tacit but crucial assumption that enabled him to speak of 'the superb disdain in which French medicine held medical science'.[120] Yet, at least to the American disciples of French medicine, such a statement would have made no sense at all, for one of the most powerful messages they took away from French medicine was that science meant empiricism. As much as Ackerknecht admired the sensual empiricism and concreteness of the Paris Clinical School, nowhere in his book did he explicitly make a point that was central in contemporary accounts by Americans, namely, that the clinical medicine they witnessed in Paris *was* science. It was only later polemical campaigns mounted in order to win for the laboratory a legitimate and secure place in medicine, and subsequent political programmes of discipline-building, that would begin to erode this view, leaving as one legacy a Whiggish equation of scientific medicine with medicine rooted in experimental laboratory science that remains one of the sturdiest bastions of presentism in medical historiography.[121]

It has been suggested that Ackerknecht's training as a clinician and his experience in Paris during the 1930s, and also his work as a teacher in the United States during the years when his book on the Paris School took form, may have shaped the way Paris medicine is portrayed in *Medicine at the Paris Hospital*.[122] We should ask as well about the formative influence of his training in the 1920s as a doctor in Germany, and, more than this, about the historiographic blinkers we share with him as we tell stories about medical history in a post-Flexnerian world.

Notes

This paper was supported in part by National Institutes of Health Grant LM 05013 from the National Library of Medicine. Some sections of the paper draw heavily from John Harley Warner, *Against the Spirit of System: The French Impulse in Nineteenth-Century American Medicine* (Princeton: Princeton University Press, 1998).

1. Erwin H. Ackerknecht, *Medicine at the Paris Hospital, 1794–1848* (Baltimore: Johns Hopkins Press, 1967), 123.
2. Erwin H. Ackerknecht to Henry E. Sigerist, Madison, Wisc., 13 September 1956, and Madison, Wisc., 20 July 1956, Henry Ernest Sigerist Papers, Manuscripts and Archives, Sterling Library, Yale University, New Haven, Conn.
3. Ackerknecht, *Medicine at the Paris Hospital*, xiii and dust jacket.
4. *Ibid.*, 123.
5. Richard H. Shryock, for example, took as self-evident the proposition that the American migration should be attributed to 'the scientific supremacy of the French metropolis', and assumed that the

movement of foreign students to a medical centre affirms its intellectual vibrancy. 'Their presence in large numbers had long been an excellent test of the quality of such centres. Leyden, Edinburgh, and London had been recognized in turn, before the work of Louis and Bichat brought Americans rather suddenly to Paris. Another generation would see them in Berlin, Munich and Vienna' (*The Development of Modern Medicine: An Interpretation of the Social and Scientific Factors Involved* [Madison: University of Wisconsin Press, 1979; first pub. 1936], 193 and 171). This perception has not been tempered over time; Kenneth M. Ludmerer, for example, recently described the shift in the migration of American doctors from France to Germany as 'testimony to the unchallenged superiority of nineteenth-century German medical science' (*Learning to Heal: The Development of American Medical Education* [New York: Basic Books, 1985], 32). For a more recent and immensely helpful mapping of shifting patterns in nineteenth-century medical education, see Thomas Neville Bonner, *Becoming a Physician: Medical Education in Britain, France, Germany, and the United States, 1750–1945* (New York: Oxford University Press, 1995), which has incorporated some of the argument of this paper (see esp. 189–92).

6. A. Colman to Catherine Colman, Paris, 15 April 1833, Colman (Anson) Papers, Department of Rare Books and Special Collections, Rush Rees Library, University of Rochester, Rochester, N. Y.

7. A large literature on the relationship between American physicians and the Paris School includes Henry Blumenthal, *Americans and French Culture, 1800-1900: Interchanges in Art, Science, Literature, and Society* (Baton Rouge: Louisiana State University Press, 1975), 402–67; Russell M. Jones, 'American Doctors and the Parisian Medical World, 1830–1840', *Bulletin of the History of Medicine* 47 (1973): 40–65, 177–204; idem, 'American Doctors in Paris, 1820–1861: A Statistical Profile', *Journal of the History of Medicine and Allied Sciences* 25 (1970): 142–157; idem, 'An American Medical Student in Paris, 1831–1833', *Harvard Library Bulletin* 15 (1967): 59–81; idem, 'Introduction', in *The Parisian Education of an American Surgeon: Letters of Jonathan Mason Warren (1832–1835)* (Philadelphia: American Philosophical Society, 1978), 1–69; Ronald L. Numbers and John Harley Warner, 'The Maturation of American Medical Science', in Nathan Reingold and Marc Rothenberg (eds), *Scientific Colonialism: A Cross Cultural Comparison* (Washington, D.C.: Smithsonian Institution Press, 1987), 191–214; Charles E. Rosenberg, *The Care of Strangers: The Rise of America's Hospital System* (New York: Basic Books, 1988), 82–90; Richard H. Shryock, 'The

Advent of Modern Medicine in Philadelphia, 1800–1850', in *idem*, *Medicine in America: Historical Essays* (Baltimore and London: Johns Hopkins Press, 1966), 203–32; John Harley Warner, 'The Fall and Rise of Professional Mystery: Epistemology, Authority, and the Emergence of Laboratory Medicine in Nineteenth-Century America', in Andrew Cunningham and Perry Williams (eds), *Medicine and the Laboratory in the Nineteenth Century* (Cambridge: Cambridge University Press, 1992), 310–41; *idem*, 'Remembering Paris: Memory and the American Disciples of French Medicine in the Nineteenth Century', *Bulletin of the History of Medicine* 65 (1991): 301–25; *idem*, 'Science, Healing, and the Physician's Identity: A Problem of Professional Character in Nineteenth-Century America', *Clio Medica* 22 (1991): 65–88; *idem*, 'The Selective Transport of Medical Knowledge: Antebellum American Physicians and Parisian Medical Therapeutics', *Bulletin of the History of Medicine* 59 (1985): 213–31; and *idem*, *The Therapeutic Perspective: Medical Practice, Knowledge, and Identity in America, 1820–1885* (Princeton: Princeton University Press, 1997: first published 1986).

8. See John Harley Warner, *Against the Spirit of System: The French Impulse in Nineteenth-Century American Medicine* (Princeton: Princeton University Press, 1998).

9. The phrase is from [Pierre] Louis to H[enry] I[ngersoll] Bowditch, Paris, 5 February 1840, Rare Books and Manuscripts, Francis A. Countway Library, Harvard Medical School, Boston, Mass.

10. For a fuller exploration of American attitudes toward London as a place for medical study during this period, see John Harley Warner, 'American Doctors in London during the Age of Paris Medicine', in Vivian Nutton and Roy Porter (eds), *The History of Medical Education in Britain* (Amsterdam and Atlanta: Rodopi, 1995), 341–65.

11. L. M. Lawson, 'Foreign Correspondence' (London, June 1845), *Western Lancet* 4 (1845): 145–53, p. 153.

12. Ashbel Smith to John Beard, Paris, 23 February 1832, Ashbel Smith Letters, The Center for American History, The University of Texas, Austin, Texas.

13. C. B. Chapman, 'Medical Travel in Europe' (Edinburgh, July 1851), *Boston Medical and Surgical Journal* 44 (1851): 72–5, p. 73.

14. James Jackson, Jr, to James Jackson, Sr, Bangor, Wales, 27 August 1832, James Jackson Papers, Countway Library.

15. Oliver Wendell Holmes to 'Dear Father and Mother', London, 21 June 1834, in John T. Morse, Jr, *Life and Letters of Oliver Wendell Holmes*, 2 vols (Boston and New York: Houghton, Mifflin and

Company, 1896), 1: 134.
16. James Jackson, Jr, to James Jackson, Sr, London, 12 September 1832, Jackson Papers.
17. Abel Lawrence Peirson to Harriet Peirson, Paris, 21 October 1832, Abel Lawrence Peirson Papers, Countway Library.
18. Levin S. Joynes to Thomas R. Joynes, Paris, 20 May 1841, Joynes Family Papers, Division of Archives and Manuscripts, Virginia Historical Society, Richmond, Va.
19. William Gibson, *Rambles in Europe in 1839* (Philadelphia: Lea and Blanchard, 1841), 64, 66.
20. F. Campbell Stewart, *Eminent French Surgeons, with a Historical and Statistical Sketch of the Hospitals of Paris* (Buffalo: A. Burke, 1843), xvi.
21. Joshua B. Flint, *Address Delivered to the Students of the Louisville Medical Institute, in Presence of the Citizens of the Place, at the Commencement of the Second Session of the Institute, November 13th, 1838* (Louisville: Prentice and Weissenger, 1838), 17.
22. A. Colman to Catherine K. Colman, Paris, 28 January 1833, Colman Papers.
23. Quoted in Morse, Jr, *Life and Letters of Oliver Wendell Holmes*, 1: 94.
24. Ackerknecht, *Medicine at the Paris Hospital*, 44.
25. A collection of medical theses written in Paris by Louisiana students is deposited in the Louisiana Collection, Howard-Tilton Memorial Library, Tulane University, New Orleans, La.
26. Alexander Wilcox, 'Miscellaneous' (Philadelphia, 15 November 1845), *Western Lancet* 4 (1846): 425–8, p. 426.
27. Henry Bryant to John Bryant, 21 December 1843, in letter of 11 December 1843, Bryant Collection (MS 45), New England Historic Genealogical Society, Boston, Mass.
28. F[rank] H[astings] Hamilton, 'Notes of a European Tour' (Paris), *Buffalo Medical Journal and Monthly Review* 2 (1846): 396–409, p. 398.
29. J. Y. Bassett to Marguerite Bassett, Paris, 3 July 1836, John Young Bassett Papers, Manuscripts Division, Alabama Department of Archives and History, Montgomery, Ala. Still, as one southern student described it in a letter home, 'Dissecting, for which in America we pay ten dollars for the ticket and some six or eight for subjects during the season depending on the number furnished, costs me *eight* dollars a *Month* over here. But of course the opportunities are infinitely superior' (Edward E. Jenkins to John Jenkins, Paris, 13 January 1854, John Jenkins Papers, Manuscripts Division, South Caroliniana Library, University of South Carolina, Columbia, S.C.).
30. The best study of English medical practitioners and the Paris School is

Russell C. Maulitz, *Morbid Appearances: The Anatomy of Pathology in the Early Nineteenth Century* (Cambridge: Cambridge University Press, 1987); and see John Harley Warner, 'The Idea of Science in English Medicine: The "Decline of Science" and the Rhetoric of Reform', in Roger French and Andrew Wear (eds), *British Medicine in an Age of Reform* (London and New York: Routledge, 1991), 136–64.

31. On William Wood Gerhard's 'clinique' in Philadelphia, for example, see M. H[enry] Aikins to L. S. Aikins, Philadelphia, 20 November 1856, Aikins Papers, Academy of Medicine of Toronto Collection, Thomas Fisher Rare Book Library, University of Toronto, Toronto, Canada; Elisha Bartlett to Elisabeth S. Bartlett, Philadelphia, 11 September 1841, Bartlett (Elisha) Family Papers, Department of Rare Books and Special Collections, Rush Rees Library, University of Rochester; and Levin S. Joynes to Tho[mas] R. Joynes, Philadelphia, 4 November 1839, Joynes Family Papers. And, on clinical education in America, see Rosenberg, *The Care of Strangers*, esp. 47–93, 190–211, and Dale Cary Smith, 'The Emergence of Organized Clinical Instruction in the Nineteenth Century American Cities of Boston, New York and Philadelphia' (Ph.D. diss., University of Minnesota, 1979).

32. Edward E. Jenkins to John Jenkins, Paris, 12 August 1853, Jenkins Papers.

33. Robert P. Harrison, 'Letter from Paris' (Paris, 19 November 1855), *American Medical Gazette and Journal of Health* 7 (1856): 168–71, p. 170.

34. Samuel Brown, Diary, entry for 9 July 1824, copy in Division of Special Collections, Margaret I. King Library, University of Kentucky, Lexington, Ky.

35. James Lawrence Cabell to Joseph C. Cabell, Paris, 28 January 1837, James Lawrence Cabell Papers (#1640), Special Collections Department, University of Virginia Library, Charlottesville, Va.

36. Henry Willard Williams to Abigail Osgood Williams, Paris, 6 May 1846, Henry Willard Williams Papers, Countway Library. Three weeks later he was able to tell her, 'I have the satisfaction of feeling that I am making some progress for I have the ability of *reading* French Medicine with something like facility, though I expect to wear out three Dictionaries before I am perfected in that task. Hearing and talking are yet minus, but if I continue to read a hundred pages a day I must *in time* acquire the ability to think in French and can then understand it' (Williams to Williams, Paris, 26 May 1846).

37. R. A. Kinloch, 'Medical News in Paris. Letter to the Editors' (Paris, 2 July 1854), *Charleston Medical Journal and Review* 9 (1854): 587–8, p. 587.

38. Abel Lawrence Peirson to Harriet Peirson, Paris, 26 October 1832, Peirson Papers.
39. David W. Yandell, 'Notes on Medical Matters in Paris' (Paris, February 1847), *Western Journal of Medicine and Surgery* n.s. 7 (1847): 93–113, p. 99.
40. David W. Yandell, 'Clinical Instruction in the London and Paris Hospitals', *Western Journal of Medicine and Surgery*, s. 3, 3 (1848): 392–400, p. 396.
41. Elisha Bartlett to Caroline Bartlett, Paris, 29 November 1826, Elisha Bartlett Papers, Manuscripts and Archives, Sterling Library, Yale University.
42. Austin Flint, 'Address at the Opening of the Session for 1854–55 in the Medical Department of the University of Louisville', *Western Journal of Medicine and Surgery* n.s. 2 (1854): 418.
43. Austin Flint, 'European Correspondence' (Paris, 18 May 1854), *Western Journal of Medicine and Surgery* n.s. 2 (1854): 9–17, p. 14.
44. Cabell to Cabell, Paris, 28 January 1837.
45. Austin Flint, 'Foreign Correspondence' (Paris, April 1854), *Western Journal of Medicine and Surgery* n.s. 2 (1854): 169–74, pp. 172–3.
46. Harris, 'Letter from Paris', 169.
47. Henry Bryant to John Bryant, Paris, entry of 21 December 1843 in letter of 11 December 1843, Bryant Collection.
48. Yandell, 'Clinical Instruction in the London and Paris Hospitals', 399.
49. F. P[eyre] P[orcher], 'Editorial Correspondence of the Charleston Medical Journal and Review' (Paris, 5 March 1853), *Charleston Medical Journal and Review* 8 (1853): 416–29, pp. 416–17.
50. Cabell to Cabell, Paris, 28 January 1837.
51. C. B. Chapman, 'Medical Study in Paris', *Boston Medical and Surgical Journal* 47 (1853): 286–7, p. 287.
52. Yandell, 'Clinical Instruction in the London and Paris Hospitals', 399.
53. Stewart, *Eminent French Surgeons*, 140.
54. Ashbel Smith to 'Dear Father', Paris, 26 January 1832, Smith Letters.
55. J. Y. Bassett to Marguerite Bassett, Paris, 29 April 1836, Bassett Papers.
56. J. Y. Bassett to Isaphoena Bassett, Paris, 1 June 1836, Bassett Papers.
57. P[orcher], 'Editorial Correspondence', 416.
58. L. J. Frazee, *The Medical Student in Europe* (Maysville, Ky.: Richard U. Collins, 1849), 115–16.
59. [Lundsford P. Yandell], editorial note in Austin Flint, 'Foreign Correspondence' (Paris, 18 June 1854), *Western Journal of Medicine and Surgery* s. 4, 2 (1854): 89–99, p. 97.
60. P., 'The Advantages and Disadvantages of Paris As a Place of Resort for Medical Students' (Paris, 10 July 1853), *St. Louis Medical and*

Surgical Journal 12 (1854): 79–84, p. 80.
61. Augustus Kinsley Gardner, *Old Wine in New Bottles: Or, Spare Hours of a Student in Paris* (New York: C. S. Francis & Co., 1848), 163.
62. Flint, 'Address', 417.
63. 'Correspondence' (Paris, 7 December 1853), *New Jersey Medical Reporter* 7 (1854): 66–70, p. 66. Historian Russell Jones, whose sample is eclectic and the figures no doubt low, counted 77 medical Americans who travelled to Paris in the 1820s; 222 in the 1830s; 123 in the 1840s; and 293 in the 1850s ('American Doctors and the Parisian Medical World', 42, and 'American Doctors in Paris, 1820–1861', 150).
64. 'American Physicians in Paris', *Boston Medical and Surgical Journal* 45 (1851–2): 456; and see 'American Medical Society in Paris', *Boston Medical and Surgical Journal* 47 (1853): 470; Henri Meding, *Paris médical: vade-mecum des médecins étrangers*, 2 vols (Paris: J.-B. Baillière, 1852–3), 2: 401–2.
65. Brett Randolph, 'Violation of the Natural Laws' (M.D. thesis, Transylvania University, 1848), Special Collections, Transylvania University Library, Lexington, Ky.; and see, for example, Henry J. Hawley, 'Science vs Empiricism' (M.D. thesis, Albany Medical College, 1850), and Paul Todd Taber, 'Progress of Medicine' (M.D. thesis, Albany Medical College, 1849), Archives, Albany Medical Center, Albany, N. Y.; Thomas S. Weston, 'Homeopathy' (M.D. thesis, University of Nashville, 1856), B. B. Black, 'What of Theory?' (M.D. thesis, University of Nashville, 1857), Historical Collection, Eskind Biomedical Library, Vanderbilt University, Nashville, Tenn.; and S. C. Furman, 'The Impediments to the Progress of Medical Science' (M.D. thesis, Medical College of the State of South Carolina, 1852), and W. C. Smith, 'Remarks on Empiricism' (M.D. thesis, Medical College of the State of South Carolina, 1850), Waring Medical Library, Medical University of the State of South Carolina, Charleston, S.C.
66. D. D. Slade to George Lord, Cambridge, Massachusetts, 21 November 1845, Special Collections Library, Duke University, Durham, N.C.
67. C. T. Jackson to David Henshaw, Paris, 15 June 1832, Charles T. Jackson Papers, Library of Congress, Washington, D.C.
68. James Jackson, Sr, to James Jackson, Jr, Boston, 3 April 1830, James Jackson Papers.
69. Levin S. Joynes to Thomas R. Joynes, Paris, 12 December 1841, Joynes Family Papers.
70. Henry Bryant to John Bryant, Paris, 1 July 1844, Bryant Collection.

71. 'Editorial Correspondence. Hospitals of Paris', *Boston Medical and Surgical Journal* 43 (1851): 22–4, pp. 23–4.
72. John Punnett to John W. Francis, Paris, 26 February 1836, John W. Francis Papers, Rare Book and Manuscripts Division, New York Public Library, Astor, Lenox, and Tilden Foundations, New York, N.Y.; Gabriel Manigault, Autobiography, transcript, p. 98, Manigault Family Papers, Manuscripts Division, South Caroliniana Library, University of South Carolina; Philip Claiborne Gooch, Diary, 1 January–1 September 1848, entry for Paris, 17 January 1848, Philip Claiborne Gooch Diary, Division of Archives and Manuscripts, Virginia Historical Society.
73. Gardner, *Old Wine in New Bottles*, 203.
74. George H. Doane, 'Comparative Advantages of Vienna and Paris, As Places for Medical Study, with Some Remarks on the Operation of Extraction for the Removal of Cataract', *New Jersey Medical Reporter* 7 (1854): 17–20, p. 18; and see the discussion of John Call Dalton in W. Bruce Fye, *The Development of American Physiology: Scientific Medicine in the Nineteenth Century* (Baltimore and London: Johns Hopkins University Press, 1987). And see A. C., 'Parisian Correspondence' (Paris, 15 March 1855), *American Medical Gazette and Journal of Health* 6 (1855): 203–5, p. 204; A. Peniston, Notebook on Lectures by Claude Bernard, [Paris], 1854, A. Peniston Notebook, Louisiana and Lower Mississippi Valley Collections, Louisiana State University Libraries, Baton Rouge, La.; Auguste Shurtleff, *Journal of a Trip to Europe, 1850–1852*, Ms., 2 vols, vol. 1, entry for 9 May 1851, Countway Library.
75. B., 'Letter from Paris' (Paris, 13 February 1854), *North-Western Medical and Surgical Journal* 3 (1845): 145–9, p. 146.
76. John A. Murphy, [Letter to the Editor] (Paris, March 1854), *Western Lancet* 15 (1854): 537, 538. 'No one who follows his courses can at all have any doubt in regard to the appearance of cancer cell, as differing from all others'. He went on to note that 'the difference between the older and younger part of the profession is, that the latter makes here a profound study of physiology and anatomy, while the former have received their opinions of physiology as they were studied and taught a half a century ago, oppose the present theories and facts on these subjects' (*ibid.*, 537).
77. Alfred Stillé to George Cheyne Shattuck, Vienna, 15 January 1851, Shattuck Papers, vol. 22, Massachusetts Historical Society, Boston, Mass.
78. Doane, 'Comparative Advantages of Vienna and Paris', 18. The asterisk led to a note on the preponderance of Americans in Bernard's classes.

79. Flint, 'Address', 412, 412–13, 413. On the migration of American physicians to Germany, see Thomas Neville Bonner, *American Doctors and German Universities: A Chapter in International Intellectual Relations, 1870–1914* (Lincoln: University of Nebraska Press, 1963), and, on the Vienna School, Erna Lesky, *The Vienna Medical School in the 19th Century*, translated by L. Williams and I. S. Levij (Baltimore and London: Johns Hopkins University Press, 1976).
80. David W. Yandell, 'Notes on Medical Matters and Medical Men in Paris' (Paris, July 1847), *Western Lancet* n.s. 7 (1847): 369–95, p. 374.
81. See, for example, Gooch, Journal, entry for Paris, 15 May 1848.
82. Stillé to Shattuck, Vienna, 15 January 1851.
83. Alfred Stillé to George Cheyne Shattuck, Philadelphia, 28 September 1851, Shattuck Papers, vol. 22. 'I did not succeed in finding any body who was a Republican here!' Stillé added.
84. B., 'Letter from Paris', 145, 146.
85. R. A. Kinloch, 'Medical News from Paris' (Paris, 13 January 1855), *Charleston Medical Journal and Review* 10 (1855): 159–70, p. 159.
86. *Ibid.*
87. R. A. Kinloch, 'Medical News from Paris, France', *Charleston Medical Journal and Review* 10 (1855): 58–66, p. 65. Kinloch, who clearly was referring to Nancy Talbot Clark, went on to write that 'her bearing is certainly modest, yet when at the bedside of particular patients undergoing examination, and surrounded by medical students of the other sex, you can often notice the forced action of her lips restraining a smile, prompted evidently by feeling the ludicrousness of her situation. M. Dubois, and also his excellent "Chef de Clinique", Dr. Campbell, treat her with much attention, often troubling themselves to explain to her in English, as she understands at present but little French. Mrs. C., lately applied for dissections at "Clamart" but this very properly was refused her' (p. 65).
88. Kinloch, 'Medical News from Paris', 159.
89. Henry H. Smith, *Professional Visit to London and Paris. Introductory Lecture to the Course on the Principles and Practice of Surgery. Delivered in the University of Pennsylvania, October 9, 1855* (Philadelphia: T. K. and P. G. Collins, 1855), 12.
90. Smith, *Professional Visit to London and Paris*, 11, 12, 17, 18, 19.
91. Wilcox, 'Miscellaneous', 427.
92. Yandell, 'Clinical Instruction in the London and Paris Hospitals', 398. 'A physician, who was *interne* during the existence of the law permitting it, told me, that so great was the love of money or the love of teaching, he could not say which, a short time before the law was repealed, the *internes* spent almost the entire day in the wards,

examining and reexamining the patients, very often rousing them from sleep before it was fairly light to begin the work of investigating their diseases, and, not satisfied with prosecuting it through the day, pursued it often by candle-light far into the night. Patients, at length, grew impatient and refused to submit to such torture'. Yandell further reported that 'Orfila, strict, stern and severe as he was, never succeeded in suppressing private courses on anatomy and surgery at either the Clamart or the Ecole Pratique, though he often swore he would make *cadavres* both of those who attempted to give and those who received them. They were given in spite of his watchfulness and in defiance of his threats, and would have been given had there been a score of deans all equal to Orfila. They are now given under Bouillaud's administration, and will continue to be given till there are no students willing to pay five dollars a month for a course on the former, and ten dollars for a complete course on the latter subject' (pp. 398, 399).

93. Wilcox, 'Miscellaneous', 427.
94. Edward E. Jenkins to 'Dear Sister', Paris, 27 August 1854, Jenkins Papers. Jenkins was thinking about setting up practice in St. Louis, and, in another letter, explained, 'One of the best steps preliminary to settling in St Louis would be to spend sufficient time either at Berlin or Vienna to acquire the German language' (Jenkins to Jenkins, Paris, 13 January 1854).
95. 'The Vienna Hospitals – Letter from Henry K. Oliver, Jr., M.D., of Boston' (Vienna, 1 July 1857), *Boston Medical and Surgical Journal* 57 (1857–8): 49–58, 71–7, p. 50; Warren comments on p. 49.
96. H. Z. Gill, 'Letter from Philadelphia', *Cincinnati Lancet and Observer* 11 (1868): 546–54, pp. 551, 551–2, 548, 551, 552, 553.
97. Joseph T. Webb to 'Dear Mother', Vienna, 23 June 1868, Joseph Webb Letters in Rutherford B. Hayes Papers, Rutherford B. Hayes Library, Fremont, Ohio.
98. 'Letter from S. S. Satchwell' (Paris, 2 January 1861), *Medical Journal of North Carolina* 3 (1861): 245–52, p. 251.
99. Frank J. Lutz (ed.), *The Autobiography and Reminiscences of S. Pollak, M.D., St. Louis, Mo.* (Reprinted from the *St. Louis Medical Review*, 1904), 213–14.
100. 'Medical Advantages of Vienna for American Students', *Boston Medical and Surgical Journal* 63 (1860–1): 51–3, p. 51.
101. Harris, 'Letter from Paris', 171; Robert P. Harris, 'Letter from Paris' (Paris, 25 December 1855), *Medical Examiner*, n.s. 12 (1856): 70–5, p. 74.
102. D. F. L[incoln], 'A Letter from Vienna' (Vienna, 7 June 1871), *Boston*

Medical and Surgical Journal 85 (1871): 4–7, p. 6.
103. Patrick A. O'Connell, 'A Letter from Vienna', *Boston Medical and Surgical Journal* 86 (1872): 214–17, p. 216.
104. Fred[eric]k Shattuck to George Cheyne Shattuck, Vienna, 14 March 1874, Shattuck Papers, vol. 24.
105. Lincoln, 'A Letter from Vienna', 6.
106. Joseph T. Webb to 'Dear Mother', Berlin, 1 August 1866, Hayes Papers; and Wm. P. Thornton, 'Letter to the Editors of the Lancet and Observer' (Vienna, 25 February 1859), *Cincinnati Lancet and Observer* n.s. 2 (1859): 236–8, p. 238.
107. William Williams Keen to Samuel C. and Mary Eastman, Vienna, 25 May 1865, William Williams Keen Papers, Manuscripts Division, Brown University Library, Providence, R.I.
108. Joseph T. Webb to Lu[cy] [Webb Hayes], Paris, 2 April 1867, and Joseph T. Webb to James D. Webb, Paris, 21 March 1867, Hayes Papers.
109. 'Letter from S. S. Satchwell', 245, 246.
110. Henry S. Bronson to Jeffries Wyman, Paris, 26 January 1868, Countway Library.
111. John Singleton Copley Green to James Jackson Putnam, Vienna, 5 March 1872, Countway Library; and see Abner Post to James Jackson Putnam, Berlin, 24 June 1871, Countway Library.
112. J. E., 'Foreign Correspondence' (Vienna, 26 May 1880), *Cincinnati Lancet and Clinic* 5 (1880), 13–14, p. 13.
113. A splendid study is Robert G. Frank, Jr, 'American Physiologists in German Laboratories, 1865–1914', in Gerald L. Geison (ed.), *Physiology in the American Context, 1850–1914* (Bethesda, Maryland: American Physiological Society, 1987), 11–46; and see Fye, *The Development of American Physiology*.
114. J. W. Humrichouse to C. W. Humrichouse, Lucerne, 7 September 1877, Ridgley Papers (MS 1908), Manuscripts Division, Maryland Historical Society, Baltimore, Md.
115. Edward Warren, *A Doctor's Experience in Three Continents* (Baltimore: Cushings and Bailey, 1885), 167.
116. 'The Past and Present School of Paris', *Boston Medical and Surgical Journal* 72 (1865): 389–90, p. 389.
117. *Ibid.*, 389–90.
118. 'Memorabilia des Wiener Clubs, Gegründet 1865', Countway Library. The other founding members were F. P. Sprague, Henry Kemple Oliver, B. J. Jeffries, Gustavus Hay, and H. Derby.
119. This is developed in Warner, *Against the Spirit of System*, esp. chapter 5.
120. Ackerknecht, *Medicine at the Paris Hospital*, 126.

121. I have tried to draw attention to the historical treatment of the concept of *scientific medicine* in 'Science in Medicine', *Osiris* n.s. 1 (1985): 31–58, and especially in 'The History of Science and the Sciences of Medicine', *Osiris* n.s. 10 (1995): 164–93.
122. Caroline Hannaway suggested to me the historiographic importance of Ackerknecht's training as a clinician. I hinted at the possible influence of Ackerknecht's experience teaching medical history in the United States in 'Two Tales of a City: Anglo-American Constructions of the Paris Clinical School' (presented at a conference on 'Researchers and Practitioners: Aspects of French Medical Culture in the Eighteenth and Nineteenth Centuries', Blacksburg, Va., 21 April 1990), and noted that his heavy reliance on Elisha Bartlett's *Essay on the Philosophy of Medical Science* (1844) may have informed what is in some respects a quintessentially American representation of the Paris School. Thomas Broman, after reading 'Two Tales of a City', pointed out to me the extent to which Ackerknecht's text may express a German perspective on medical history.

Selected Bibliography

This is a selected listing of the literature relating to Paris clinical medicine and to French medical institutions, medical education, and the profession, primarily for the first half of the nineteenth century. Archival and primary sources as well as additional secondary literature are referred to in notes in the essays in the volume. Limited reference only is made to sources discussing developments in the United Kingdom and other European countries.

Ackerknecht, Erwin H. 'Anticontagionism between 1821 and 1867', *Bulletin of the History of Medicine* 22 (1948): 562-93.

———. 'Aspects of the History of Therapeutics', *Bulletin of the History of Medicine* 36 (1962): 387-419.

———. 'Broussais or a Forgotten Medical Revolution', *Bulletin of the History of Medicine* 27 (1953): 320-43.

———. 'Die Pariser Spitäler als Ausgangspunkt einer Neuen Medizin', *Ciba Symposium* 7 (1959): 98-105.

———. 'Die Therapie der Pariser Kliniker zwischen 1795 und 1840', *Gesnerus* 15 (1958): 151-63.

———. 'Elisha Bartlett and the Philosophy of the Paris Clinical School', *Bulletin of the History of Medicine* 24 (1950): 34-60.

———. 'Hygiene in France, 1815-1848', *Bulletin of the History of Medicine* 22 (1948): 117-55.

———. 'Laennec et Broussais', *Revue du Palais de la Découverte* 22, spec. no. (1981): 208-12.

———. 'La médecine à Paris entre 1800 et 1850', *Les conférences du Palais de la Découverte*. Series D, no. 58. Paris: 1958.

———. 'Medical Education in 19th Century France', *Journal of Medical Education* 32 (1957): 148-52.

Selected Bibliography

———. *Medicine at the Paris Hospital, 1794-1848*. Baltimore, Maryland: Johns Hopkins Press, 1967.
———. 'Pariser Chirurgie von 1794-1850', *Gesnerus* 17 (1960): 137-44.
Albury, W. R. 'Experiment and Explanation in the Physiology of Bichat and Magendie', *Studies in the History of Biology* 1 (1977): 47-131.
———. 'French Nosologies Around 1800 and Their Relationship With Chemistry', in E. G. Forbes (ed.), *Human Implications of Scientific Advance* (Edinburgh: Edinburgh University Press, 1978) 502-17.
———. 'Heart of Darkness: J. N. Corvisart and the Medicalization of Life', in *La médicalisation de la société française, 1770-1830*. ed. Jean Pierre Goubert. Waterloo, Ontario: 1982, 17-31.
———. 'Magendie's Physiological Manifesto of 1809', *Bulletin of the History of Medicine* 48 (1974): 90-9.
———. 'The Order of Ideas: Condillac's Method of Analysis As a Political Instrument in the French Revolution', in *The Politics and Rhetoric of Scientific Method: Historical Studies*, eds. J. A. Schuster, and R. R. Yeo. Dordrecht: Reidel, 1986, 203-25.
———. 'The Productions of Truth: Body and Soul. Part 2: Displaying the Truth of the Body', in *Foucault: The Legacy*, ed. Clare O'Farrell. Kelvin Grove, Queensland: Queensland University of Technology, 1997, 356-60.
Astrow, Alan B. 'The French Revolution and the Dilemma of Medical Training', *Biology and Medicine* 33 (1990): 444-56.
Bonner, Thomas Neville. *Becoming a Physician: Medical Education in Great Britain, France, Germany, and the United States, 1750-1945*. Oxford and New York: Oxford University Press, 1995.
Bouillaud, Jean Baptiste. *Essai sur la philosophie médicale et sur les généralités de la clinique médicale*. Paris: Rouvier et le Bouvier, 1836.
Boulle, Lydie. 'La médicalisation des hôpitaux parisiens dans la première moitié du XIXème siècle', in *La médicalisation de la société française, 1770-1830*, ed. Jean Pierre Goubert. Waterloo, Ontario: Historical Reflections Press, 1982, 33-44.
Braunstein, Jean-François. *Broussais et le matérialisme: médecine et philosophie au XIXe siècle*. Paris: Meridiens Klincksieck, 1986.
Brockliss, Laurence. 'L'enseignement médical et la Révolution: essai de réevaluation', *Histoire de l'éducation* 42 (1989): 79-110.
———. 'Medical Reform, the Enlightenment, and Physician-Power in Late Eighteenth-Century France', in *Medicine in the Enlightenment*, ed. Roy Porter. Amsterdam and Atlanta: Editions Rodopi, 1995, 64-112.

Selected Bibliography

Brockliss, Laurence, and Colin Jones. *The Medical World of Early Modern France*. Oxford: The Clarendon Press, 1997.

Broman, Thomas. *The Transformation of German Academic Medicine, 1750-1820*. Cambridge and New York: Cambridge University Press, 1997.

Bynum, W. F. *Science and the Practice of Medicine in the Nineteenth Century*. Cambridge and New York: Cambridge University Press, 1994.

Canguilhem, Georges. *Etudes d'histoire et de philosophie des sciences*. Paris: Vrin, 1975.

———. *Idéologie et rationalité dans l'histoire des sciences de la vie*. Paris: Vrin, 1977.

———. *On the Normal and the Pathological*. Dordrecht: Reidel, 1978.

Caron, Jean-Claude. 'L'impossible réforme des études médicales: projets et controverses dans la France des notables (1815-1848)', in *Maladies, médecines et sociétés: approches historiques pour le présent*, ed. François-Olivier Touati, 2 vols. Actes du VIe colloque d'Histoire au Présent. Paris: L'Harmattan et Histoire au Présent, 1993, 2: 206-17.

Casey, E. S. 'The Place of Space in *The Birth of the Clinic*', *Journal of Medicine and Philosophy* 12 (1987): 351-6.

Coleman, William. 'The Cognitive Basis of a Discipline: Claude Bernard on Physiology', *Isis* 76 (1985): 49-70.

———. *Death Is a Social Disease: Public Health and Political Economy in Early Industrial France*. Madison: University of Wisconsin Press, 1982.

Coury, Charles. *L'enseignement de la médecine en France des origines à nos jours*. Paris: Expansion Scientifique Française, 1968.

———. 'La méthode anatomo-clinique et ses promoteurs en France: Corvisart, Bayle, Laennec', *Mèdecine en France* no. 224 (1971): 13-22.

Delaporte, François. *Le savoir de la maladie: essai sur le choléra de 1832 à Paris*. Paris: Presses Universitaires de France, 1990.

Delaunay, Paul. *D'une Révolution à l'autre, 1789-1848: l'évolution des théories et de la pratique médicale*. Paris: Editions Hippocrate, 1949.

Dowbiggin, Ian. *Inheriting Madness: Professionalization and Psychiatric Knowledge in Nineteenth Century France*. Berkeley: University of California Press, 1991.

Duffin, Jacalyn. 'The Cardiology of R. T. H. Laennec', *Medical History* 33 (1989): 42-71.

———. 'L'Hippocrate de Laennec repris: La fièvre à l'ombre de l'anatomie pathologique', in *La maladie et les malades dans la Collection Hippocratique*, eds. Paul Potter, Gilles Maloney, and Jacques Desautels. Actes du VIe colloque international Hippocratique ed. Quebec: Sphinx, 1990, 433-61.

———. 'The Medical Philosophy of R. T. H. Laennec (1771-1826)', *History and Philosophy of the Life Sciences* 8 (1986): 195-219.

Selected Bibliography

———. 'Private Practice and Public Research: the Patients of R. T. H. Laennec', in *French Medical Culture in the Nineteenth Century*, eds. Ann La Berge, and Mordechai Feingold. Amsterdam and Atlanta: Editions Rodopi, 1994, 118-48.

———. 'Puerile Respiration: Laennec's Stethoscope and the Physiology of Breathing', *Transactions and Studies of the College of Physicians of Philadelphia* 13 (1991): 125-45.

———. 'Sick Doctors: Bayle and Laennec on Their Own Phthisis', *Journal of the History of Medicine* 43 (1988): 165-82.

———. *To See With a Better Eye: A Life of R. T. H. Laennec.* Princeton, New Jersey: Princeton University Press, 1998.

———. 'Unity, Duality, Passion and Cure: Laennec's Conceptualization of Tuberculosis', in *Malade et maladies: histoire et conceptualisation: mélanges en honneur de Mirko Grmek*, ed. Danielle Gourevitch. Geneva: Droz, 1992. 225-71.

———. 'Vitalism and Organicism in the Philosophy of R. T. H. Laennec', *Bulletin of the History of Medicine* 62 (1988): 525-45.

Eribon, Didier. *Michel Foucault.* trans. Betsy Wing. Cambridge, Massachusetts: Harvard University Press, 1991.

Faber, Knud. *Nosography: The Evolution of Clinical Medicine in Recent Times.* New York: P. S. Hoeber, 1930.

Figlio, Karl M. 'The Metaphor of Organisation: an Historiographical Perspective on the Bio-Medical Sciences of the Early Nineteenth Century', *History of Science* 14 (1976): 17-53.

Foucault, Michel. *The Birth of the Clinic: An Archaeology of Medical Perception.* trans. A. M. Sheridan Smith. New York: Pantheon Books, 1973.

———. *Naissance de la clinique: une archéologie du régard médicale.* Paris: Presses Universitaires de France, 1963.

Foucault, Michel, B. Barret-Kriegel, A. Thalamy, F. Béguin, and B. Fortier. *Les machines à guérir: aux origines de l'hôpital moderne.* Paris: Institut de l'Environnement, 1976.

Fox, Robert, and George Weisz, eds. *The Organisation of Science and Technology in France, 1808-1914.* Cambridge and New York: Cambridge University Press, 1980.

Ganière, Paul. *L'Académie de Médecine: ses origines et son histoire.* Paris: Librairie Maloine, 1964.

———. *Corvisart, médecin de l'empereur.* Paris: Librairie Académique Perrin, 1985.

Geigenmüller, Ursula. 'Aussagen über der Französische Medizin der Jahre 1820-1847 in Reiseberichten Deutscher Arzte', Dental diss., Free University of Berlin, 1985.

Gelfand, Toby. 'A Clinical Ideal: Paris 1789', *Bulletin of the History of*

Medicine 60 (1977): 397-411.

———. 'A Confrontation Over Clinical Instruction at the Hôtel-Dieu of Paris During the French Revolution', *Journal of the History of Medicine and Allied Sciences* 28 (1973): 268-82.

———. 'Gestation of the Clinic', *Medical History* 25 (1981): 169-80.

———. *Professionalizing Modern Medicine: Paris Surgeons and Medical Sciences and Institutions in the Eighteenth Century*. Westport, Connecticut: Greenwood Press, 1980.

Goetz, Christopher, Michel Bonduelle, and Toby Gelfand. *Charcot: Constructing Neurology*. Oxford and New York: Oxford University Press, 1995.

Goldstein, Jan E. 'Foucault Among the Sociologists: the Disciplines and the History of Professions', *History and Theory* 23 (1984): 170-92.

———. *Console and Classify: The French Psychiatric Profession in the Nineteenth Century*. Cambridge and New York: Cambridge University Press, 1987.

Grmek, M. D., and Pierre Huard. 'Les élèves étrangers de Laennec', *Revue d'histoire des sciences* 26 (1973): 315-37.

Groopman, Leonard C. 'The internat des hôpitaux de Paris: The Shaping and Transformation of the French Medical Elite, 1802-1914', Ph.D. diss., Harvard University, 1986.

Gross, Michael. 'Function and Structure in Nineteenth-Century French Physiology', Ph.D. diss., Princeton University, 1974.

———. 'The Lessened Locus of Feelings: a Transformation in French Physiology in the Early Nineteenth Century', *Journal of the History of Biology* 12 (1979): 231-71.

Gutting, Gary. *Michel Foucault's Archaeology of Scientific Reason*. Cambridge and New York: Cambridge University Press, 1989.

Haigh, Elizabeth. 'The Roots of the Vitalism of Xavier Bichat', *Bulletin of the History of Medicine* 49 (1975): 72-86.

———. *Xavier Bichat and the Medical Theory of the Eighteenth Century*, London: Wellcome Institute for the History of Medicine, 1984.

Hannaway, Caroline. 'Caring for the Constitution: Medical Planning in Revolutionary France', *Transactions and Studies of the College of Physicians* 14, no. 2 (1992): 147-66.

———. 'Vicq D'Azyr, Anatomy, and a Vision of Medicine', in *French Medical Culture in the Nineteenth Century*, eds. Ann La Berge, and Mordechai Feingold. Amsterdam and Atlanta : Editions Rodopi, 1994, 280-95.

Harvey, Joy. 'La Visite: Mary Putnam Jacobi and the Paris Medical Clinics', in *French Medical Culture in the Nineteenth Century*, eds. Ann La

Berge, and Mordechai Feingold. Amsterdam and Atlanta: Editions Rodopi, 1994, 350-71.

Huard, Pierre. 'Les facettes multiples de René Théophile Hyacinthe Laennec (1781-1826)', *Bulletin de l'Académie de Médecine* 165 (1981): 249-54.

———. *Science, médecine, pharmacie de la Révolution à l'Empire (1789-1815)*. Paris: Editions Roger Dacosta, 1970.

Huard, Pierre, and Marie José Imbault-Huard. 'Concepts et réalités de l'éducation et de la profession médico-chirurgicale pendant la Révolution', *Journal des Savants* 136 (1973).

Huard, Pierre, and Marie José Imbault Huart. 'L'enseignement libre de la médecine à Paris au XIXe siècle', *Revue d'histoire des sciences* 27 (1974): 45-62.

———. 'Quelques réflexions sur les origines de la clinique Parisienne', *Bulletin de l'Académie de Médecine* 159 (1975): 583-88.

———. 'La vie et l'oeuvre de Jean Cruveilhier, anatomiste et clinicien', *Episteme* 8 (1974): 46-57.

Huguet, Françoise. *Les professeurs de la Faculté de Médecine de Paris: dictionnaire biographique, 1794-1939*. Paris: Institut National de la Recherche Pedagogique-Editions du CNRS, 1991.

Imbault-Huart, Marie José. 'L'école pratique de dissection de Paris de 1750 à 1822 ou l'influence du concept de médecine pratique et de médecine d'observation dans l'enseignement médico-chirurgical au XVIIIème siècle et au debut du XIXème Siècle', Ph.D. diss., University of Paris, 1973.

———. 'Concepts and Realities of the Beginning of Clinical Teaching in France in the Late 18th and Early 19th Centuries', *Clio Medica* 21 (1987-1988): 59-70.

Imbert, Jean. *Le droit hospitalière de la Révolution et de l'Empire*. Paris: Presses Universitaires de France, 1954.

Jacyna, L. S. 'Au lit des malades: A. F. Chomel's Clinic at the Charité', *Medical History* 33 (1989): 420-449.

———. 'Medical and Moral Science: the Cultural Relations of Physiology in Restoration France', *History of Science* 25 (1987): 111-46.

———. 'The Politics of Medicine in Restoration France', *Social History of Medicine* 40 (1987): 84-85.

———. 'Robert Carswell and William Thomson at the Hôtel Dieu of Lyons: Scottish Views of French Medicine', in *British Medicine in an Age of Reform*, eds. Roger French, and Andrew Wear. London and New York: Routledge, 1991, 110-55.

Jewson, N. 'The Disappearance of the Sick Man From Medical Cosmologies:1770-1830', *Sociology* 10 (1976): 225-44.

Selected Bibliography

Jones, Colin, and Roy Porter, eds. *Reassessing Foucault: Power, Medicine and the Body*. London and New York: Routledge, 1994.

Jones, Russell M. 'American Doctors and the Parisian Medical World, 1830-1840', *Bulletin of the History of Medicine* 47 (1973): 40-65, 177-204.

———. 'American Doctors in Paris, 1820-1861: a Statistical Profile', *Journal of the History of Medicine and Allied Sciences* 25 (1970): 143-57.

———. 'An American Medical Student in Paris, 1831-1833', *Harvard Library Bulletin* 15 (1967): 59-81.

———, ed. 'The Parisian Education of an American Surgeon: Letters of Jonathan Mason Warren (1832-1835)',. Philadelphia: American Philosophical Society, 1978.

Jordanova, Ludmilla. 'Reflections on Medical Reform: Cabanis' *Coup D'Oeil*, in *Medicine in the Enlightenment*, ed. Roy Porter. Amsterdam and Atlanta: Editions Rodopi, 1995, 166-80.

Keel, Othmar. 'Les conditions de la décomposition analytique de l'organisme: Haller, Hunter, Bichat', *Etudes Philosophiques* 1 (1982): 37-62.

———. 'La constitution de la problématique de l'anatomie des systèmes selon Laennec', *Revue du Palais de la Découverte* 22, spec. no. (1981): 189-207.

———. 'L'ecole clinique de Paris et la naissance de l'histologie', *Gesnerus* 44 (1987): 209-20.

———. *Etudes sur l'histoire de la médecine clinique et de pathologie, XVIIIe-XIXe siècle*. Montréal, Quebec: Presses de l'Université de Montréal, forthcoming 1998.

———. *La généalogie de l'histopathologie: une révision déchirante; Philippe Pinel, lecteur discret de J. C. Smyth, 1741-1821*. Paris: J. Vrin, 1979.

———. 'John Hunter et Xavier Bichat: les rapports de leurs travaux en pathologie tissulaire', in *Actes du XXVIIe Congrès International d'Histoire de la Médecine*. Barcelona: Delfos, 1981, 535-49.

———. 'Percussion et diagnostic physique en Grande Bretagne au 18e siècle', in *XXXI Congresso Internazionale di Storia della Medicina*. Bologna: Monduzzi, 1988. 869-75.

———. 'La place et la fonction des modèles étrangers dans la constitution de la problématique hôspitalière de l'Ecole de Paris', *History and Philosophy of the Life Sciences* 6 (1984): 41-73.

———. 'The Politics of Health and the Institutionalisation of Clinical Practice in the Second Half of the Eighteenth Century', in *William Hunter and the Eighteenth-Century Medical World*, eds. W. F. Bynum, and Roy Porter. Cambridge: Cambridge University Press, 1985, 207-58.

Selected Bibliography

———. 'La problématique institutionnelle de la clinique de la fin du XVIIIe siècle aux années de la Restauration', *Canadian Bulletin of Medical History* 2; 3 (1986): 183-206; 1-30.

Keel, Othmar, and Philippe Hudon. 'L'essor de la pratique clinique dans les armées européennes (1750-1800)', *Gesnerus* 54 (1997): 1-22.

La Berge, Ann. 'Alfred Donné and the Medicalization of Child Care in Nineteenth-Century France', *Journal of the History of Medicine* 48 (1991): 20-43.

———. 'The Early Nineteenth-Century French Public Health Movement: the Disciplinary Development and Institutionalization of *hygiène publique*', *Bulletin of the History of Medicine* 58 (1984): 363-79.

———. 'Medical Microscopy in Paris, 1830-1855', in *French Medical Culture in the Nineteenth Century*, eds. Ann La Berge, and Mordechai Feingold. Amsterdam and Atlanta: Editions Rodopi, 1994, 296-326.

———. *Mission and Method: The Early Nineteenth-Century French Public Health Movement*. Cambridge and New York: Cambridge University Press, 1992.

———. 'Mothers and Infants; Nurses and Nursing: Alfred Donné and the Medicalization of Child Care in Nineteenth-Century France', *Journal of the History of Medicine* 46 (1991): 20-43.

La Berge, Ann, and Mordechai Feingold, eds. *French Medical Culture in the Nineteenth Century*. Amsterdam and Atlanta: Editions Rodopi, 1994.

Lawrence, Susan C. *Charitable Knowledge: Hospital Pupils and Practitioners in Eighteenth-Century London*. Cambridge and New York: Cambridge University Press, 1996.

Léonard, Jacques. 'Les études médicales en France entre 1815 et 1848', *Revue d'histoire moderne et contemporaine* 13 (1966): 87-94.

———. *La France médicale: médecins et malades au XIXe siècle*. Paris: Gallimard, 1978.

———. *La médecine entre les pouvoirs et les savoirs: histoire intellectuelle de la médecine française au XIXe siècle*. Paris: Editions Aubier Montaigne, 1981.

———. 'La Restauration et la profession médicale', *Historical Reflections* 9 (1982): 69-84.

Lesch, John E. 'The Paris Academy of Medicine and Experimental Science, 1820-1848', in *The Investigative Enterprise in Experimental Physiology in Nineteenth-Century Medicine*, eds. William Coleman, and Frederic L. Holmes. Berkeley and Los Angeles: University of California Press, 1988, 100-38.

———. *Science and Medicine in France: The Emergence of Experimental Physiology, 1790-1855*. Cambridge, Massachusetts and

London: Harvard University Press, 1984.

Macey, David. *The Lives of Michel Foucault: A Biography*. New York: Pantheon, 1993.

Matthews, John Rosser. *Quantification and the Quest for Medical Certainty*. Princeton, New Jersey: Princeton University Press, 1995.

Maulitz, Russell C. 'Channel Crossing: the Lure of French Pathology for English Medical Students, 1816-36', *Bulletin of the History of Medicine* 55 (1981): 475-96.

——. *Morbid Appearances: The Anatomy of Pathology in the Early Nineteenth Century*. Cambridge and New York: Cambridge University Press, 1987.

Miller, James. *The Passion of Michel Foucault*. New York: Simon & Schuster, 1993.

Murphy, Terence D. 'Medical Knowledge and Statistical Methods in Early Nineteenth-Century France', *Medical History* 25 (1981): 301-19.

——. 'The French Medical Profession's Perception of Its Social Function Between 1776 and 1830', *Medical History* 23 (1979): 259-78.

Olmsted, James M. *François Magendie: Pioneer in Experimental Physiology and Scientific Medicine in Nineteenth-Century France*. New York: Schuman's, 1944.

——. 'French Medical Education As a Legacy of the Revolution', in *Essays in Biology in Honor of Herbert Evans*. Berkeley: University of California Press, 1943. 464-68.

Osborne, Thomas. 'On Anti-Medicine and Clinical Reason', in *Reassessing Foucault: Power, Medicine and the Body*, eds. Colin Jones, and Roy Porter. London and New York: Routledge, 1994, 28-47.

Outram, Dorinda. *The Body and the French Revolution: Sex, Class and Political Culture*. New Haven and London: Yale University Press, 1989.

Paul, Harry. 'The Issue of Decline in Nineteenth-Century French Science', *French Historical Studies* 7 (1972): 416-50.

Pickstone, John V. 'Bureaucracy, Liberalism and the Body in Post-Revolutionary France: Bichat's Physiology and the Paris School of Medicine', *History of Science* 19 (1981): 115-42.

Pinel, Philippe. *The Clinical Training of Doctors: An Essay of 1793*. ed. and trans. Dora B. Weiner. Henry Sigerist supplement to *Bulletin of the History of Medicine*, n.s., no. 3. Baltimore: Johns Hopkins University Press, 1980.

Piquemal, Jacques. 'Le choléra de 1832 et la pensée médicale', *Thalès* 10 (1959): 27-73.

——. 'Succès et décadence de la méthode numérique en France à l'époque de Pierre-Charles Alexandre Louis', *France Médicale* 250

(1974): 11-22.

Poirier, Jacques. 'La Faculté de Médecine face à la montée du spécialisme', *Communications* 54 (1992): 210-218.

Porter, Theodore M. *The Rise of Statistical Thinking, 1820-1900*. Princeton, New Jersey: Princeton University Press, 1986.

Ramsey, Matthew. 'The Politics of Professional Monopoly in Nineteenth-Century Medicine: the Paris Model and Its Rivals', in *Professions and the French State, 1700-1900*, ed. Gerald L. Geison. Princeton, New Jersey: Princeton University Press, 1984, 225-305.

———. *Professional and Popular Medicine in France, 1770-1830: The Social World of Medical Practice*. Cambridge and New York: Cambridge University Press, 1988.

Rey, Roselyne. 'Naissance et développement du vitalisme en France de la deuxième moitié du XVIIIe siècle à la fin du Premier Empire', Thèse de Doctorat d'Etat, Université de Paris I-Panthéon Sorbonne, 1987.

———. 'La théorie de la sécrétion chez Bordeu, modèle de la physiologie et de la physiologie vitaliste', *Dix-Huitième Siècle* 23 (1991): 45-58.

———. 'Vitalism, Disease and Society', in *Medicine in the Enlightenment*, ed. Roy Porter. Amsterdam and Atlanta: Editions Rodopi, 1995, 274-88.

Risse, Guenter B. 'The Quest for Certainty in Medicine: John Brown's System of Medicine in France', *Bulletin of the History of Medicine* 45 (1971): 1-12.

Rosen, George. 'An American Doctor in Paris in 1828: Selections From the Diary of Peter Solomon Townsend, M.D', *Journal of the History of Medicine* 6 (1951): 64-115; 209-252.

———. 'Hospitals, Medical Care, and Social Policy in the French Revolution', *Bulletin of the History of Medicine* 30 (1956): 124-49.

———. 'The Philosophy of Ideology and the Emergence of Modern Medicine in France', *Bulletin of the History of Medicine* 20 (1946): 328-39.

Rouxeau, Alfred. *Laennec après 1806*. Paris: J. B. Baillière, 1920.

Schiller, Francis. *Paul Broca: Founder of French Anthropology, Explorer of the Brain*. Berkeley and Los Angeles: University of California Press, 1979.

Shryock, Richard H. *The Development of Modern Medicine: An Interpretation of the Scientific and Social Factors Involved*. New York: Alfred A. Knopf, 1947.

Smeaton, William A. *Fourcroy: Chemist and Revolutionary*. Cambridge, England: For the author by W. Heffer & Sons, 1962.

Sournia, Jean Charles. *La médecine révolutionnaire, 1789-1799*. Paris: Payot, 1989.

Selected Bibliography

Staum, Martin S. *Cabanis: Enlightenment and Medical Philosophy in the French Revolution*. Princeton, New Jersey: Princeton University Press, 1980.
———. 'Medical Components in Cabanis's Science of Man', *Studies in the History of Biology* 2 (1978): 1-31.
Sussman, George. 'Etienne Pariset: a Medical Career in Government Under the Restoration', *Journal of the History of Medicine* 26 (1971): 52-74.
———. 'The Glut of Doctors in Nineteenth-Century France', *Comparative Studies in Society and History* 19 (1977): 293-303.
Sutton, Geoffrey. 'The Physical and Chemical Path to Vitalism: Xavier Bichat's *Physiological Researches on Life and Death*', *Bulletin of the History of Medicine* 58 (1984): 53-71.
Temkin, Owsei. 'Materialism in French and German Physiology of the Early Nineteenth Century', *Bulletin of the History of Medicine* 20 (1946): 322-27.
———. 'The Philosophical Background of Magendie's Physiology', *Bulletin of the History of Medicine* 20 (1946): 10-35.
———. 'The Role of Surgery in the Rise of Modern Medical Thought', *Bulletin of the History of Medicine* 25 (1951): 248-59.
Triaire, Paul. *Récamier et ses contemporains, 1774-1852*. Paris: Baillière, 1899.
Turner, B. S. 'The Practices of Rationality: Michel Foucault, Medical History and Sociological Theory', in *Power and Knowledge: Anthropological and Sociological Approaches*, ed. R. Fardon. Edinburgh: Athlone, 1985, 193-213.
Valentin, Michel. *François Broussais, 1732-1838, empereur de la médecine: jeunesse, correspondance, vie et oeuvre*. France: Association des Amis du Musée du Pays de Dinard, 1989.
Vess, David. *Medical Revolution in France, 1789-1796*. Gainesville: Florida State University Press, 1975.
Waddington, I. 'The Role of the Hospital in the Development of Modern Medicine: a Sociological Analysis', *Sociology* 7 (1973): 211-24.
Warner, John Harley. *Against the Spirit of System: The French Impulse in Nineteenth-Century American Medicine*, Princeton, New Jersey: Princeton University Press, 1998.
———. 'American Doctors in London During the Age of Paris Medicine', in *The History of Medical Education in Britain*, eds. Vivian Nutton, and Roy Porter. Amsterdam and Atlanta: Editions Rodopi, 1995, 341-65.
———. 'The Idea of Science in English Medicine: The 'Decline of Science' and the Rhetoric of Reform', in *British Medicine in an Age of Reform*, eds. Roger French, and Andrew Wear. London and New York: Routledge, 1991, 136-64.

Selected Bibliography

———. 'Remembering Paris: Memory and the American Disciples of French Medicine in the Nineteenth Century', *Bulletin of the History of Medicine* 65 (1991): 301-25.

———. 'The Selective Transport of Medical Knowledge: Antebellum American Physicians and Parisian Medical Therapeutics', *Bulletin of the History of Medicine* 59 (1985): 213-31.

Weiner, Dora B. *The Citizen Patient in Revolutionary and Imperial Paris*. Baltimore: Johns Hopkins University Press, 1993.

———. 'Le droit de l'homme à la santé: une belle idee devant l'Assemblée Constituante, 1790-1791', *Clio Medica* 5 (1970): 209-23.

———. *Raspail: Scientist and Reformer*. New York and London: Columbia University Press, 1968.

Weisz, George. 'Constructing the Medical Elite in France: the Creation of the Royal Academy of Medicine, 1814-20', *Medical History* 30 (1986): 419-43.

———. 'The Development of Medical Specialization in Nineteenth-Century Paris', in *French Medical Culture in the Nineteenth Century*, eds. Ann La Berge and Mordechai Feingold. Amsterdam and Atlanta: Editions Rodopi, 1994, 149-87.

———. 'The Medical Elite in France in the Early Nineteenth Century', *Minerva* 25 (1987): 150-70.

———. *The Medical Mandarins: The French Academy of Medicine in the Nineteenth and Early Twentieth Centuries*. (New York and Oxford: Oxford University Press, 1995).

———. 'The Politics of Medical Professionalization in France, 1845-1848', *Journal of Social History* 12 (1978): 3-30.

———. 'The Posthumous Laennec: Creating a Modern Medical Hero, 1826-1870', *Bulletin of the History of Medicine* 61 (1987): 541-62.

———. 'Les professeurs parisiens et l'Académie de Médecine', in *Le personnel de l'enseignement supérieur en France aux XIXe et XXe siècles*, eds. Christophe Charle, and Régine Ferré. Paris: 1985, 47-65.

———. 'The Self-Made Mandarin: The Éloges of the French Academy of Medicine, 1824-47', *History of Science* 26 (1988): 13-39.

———. 'Water Cures and Science: the French Academy of Medicine and Mineral Water in the Nineteenth Century', *Bulletin of the History of Medicine* 64 (1990): 393-416.

Wiriot, Mireille. 'L'enseignement clinique dans les hôpitaux de Paris entre 1790 et 1848', Ph.D. diss., (University of Paris, 1970).

Index

A

Abercrombie, John *142*
Abernethy, J. *141*
Academy of Medicine *15, 17, 19, 39, 52-3, 279, 289, 291-3, 296, 297*
Academy of Minute Anatomy *140, 141*
Academy of Sciences *289, 292, 293, 316*
Ackerknecht, Erwin H. *2-4, 11, 31, 34-6, 43, 45-8, 81, 119, 122, 221, 275, 276, 302-3, 313, 326-7, 337, 346, 371, 372*
aestheticization of pathology *213*
Against the Spirit of System: The French Impulse in Nineteenth-Century American Medicine *41*
Albury, W.R. *44, 51*
Alibert, Jean-Louis *44, 49, 53, 185-219*
American hospitals *347*
American medicine *338*
American physicians *337-83*
Amoreux, Pierre-Joseph *84, 86*
anatomical pathology *117-83*
anatomico-tissue pathology *150, 152*

anatomo-clinical method *266*
ancillary medical sciences *82, 85, 87*
Andral, Gabriel *4, 12, 14, 15, 22, 265, 279, 285, 327*
anthropological medicine *186*
Apothecaries Act, 1815 *146*
Arago, François *289*
Archives générales de médécine *287*
Armstrong, J. *142*
L'art de connaître les hommes par la physionomie *189, 210*
ascites *208*
auscultation *252, 258, 261, 266*
Axenfeld, Alexandre *21*

B

Badham, C. *142*
Baillie, Matthew *23, 43, 120, 122, 123, 129, 130, 133, 135, 141, 151, 154-5*
Baillière, J.B. *23*
Baron, J. *141*
Barthez, Paul-Joseph *74, 80*
Bartlett, Elisha *7, 349*
Bassett, John Young *352*
Bayle, Gaspard-Laurent *21, 126,*

Index

145, 237-8, 258, 259, 264
Beauvais de Preau, C.N. 79
Béclard, Jules 21
Bell, Charles 141
Bernardin de Saint-Pierre, Jean-
 Jacques 212
Bernard, Claude 20, 356
Berres, Joseph 284
Bibliothèque médicale 259
Bichat, Xavier 4, 12, 13, 21, 22,
 24-5, 28, 43, 120, 121, 126,
 128, 129-33, 137, 140, 152,
 153, 253
*Birth of the Clinic: An Archaeology of
 Medical Perception, The* 32, 33,
 44, 221
*Body Criticism: Imaging the Unseen
 in Enlightenment Art and
 Medicine* 187
Boerhaave, Hermann 223, 232
Boissier de Sauvages, François 74
Boissieu, Joseph de 86
Bonduelle, Michel 41
Bouchut, Eugène 21
Bouillaud, Jean-Baptiste 4, 8-15,
 18, 256, 278, 298, 302, 322,
 323, 327
Bowditch, Henry 21-2
Braunstein, Jean-François 39
Breschet, Gilbert 130
Bright, R. 142
Broca, Paul 19, 283, 294-6, 299,
 301, 302, 313, 316, 320-3
Brockliss, L.W.B. 42, 47, 50, 221
Brodie, B.C. 141
bronchitis 143
Broussais, François-Joseph-Victor
 4, 12, 14, 16, 21, 25, 29, 33, 39,
 43, 52, 122, 228-42, 251-74, 278
 agreement with Laennec 262-5
 profile 253-6
 rivalry with Laennec 257-62

Broussonet, François 80
Brown, Samuel 348
Brown-Séquard, Charles Edouard
 322
Buffon 13
Bynum, W.F. 4

C

*Cabanis: Enlightenment and Medical
 Philosophy in the French
 Revolution* 38
Cabanis, Pierre-Jean-Georges 38,
 207
Cabell, James Lawrence 350, 351
Calvet, Esprit 83, 89
cancer, diagnosis 297-302
Canguilhem, Georges 31, 124
Carpenter, William 297
Carswell, R. 135, 143
Castelnau, Henri de 318
Catholic Church 203
cell theory 26
Chambon de Montaux, Nicolas 95
Chapman, Carleton B. 343, 351
Charcot, Jean-Martin 327
Charcot: Constructing Neurology 41
Charité hospital 42, 237, 317
Chaussier, François 253
chemistry 275
Chevalier, Charles 277
Chevalier, Jean-Auguste 207
Cheyne, J. 141
Chicoyneau, J. François 74
Chomel, Auguste François 22, 317
Christianity 209
*Citizen-Patient in Revolutionary and
 Imperial Paris, The* 41
Clarke, Mrs. Nancy 360
clinical medicine 122, 280-4, 297-
 302
 1848–1872 313
 definition 313

398

Index

Clinique de l'Hôpital Saint-Louis 211, 212
Cloquet, Jules 19
Collège de France 20, 22, 264, 266
Collège de Périgord 83
Colman, Anson 339
Comptes-rendus de l'Académie des Sciences 289
Comte, Auguste 255, 265
concours system 75
Condillac, Etienne Bonnot de 43
Cooper, A. 141
Cornil, Victor 325
Corvisart, Jean-Nicolas 4, 8, 22, 27, 30, 42, 52, 87, 224-8, 232-42
Coup d'oeil général sur le XIXe siècle 23
Cours de microscopie 287
Cowan, Charles 9
Craigie, D. 142-4
Crosse, John G. 152
Cruikshank 135
Cruveilhier, Jean 4, 21, 23, 278, 280
Cusson, Pierre 84
Cuvier, Georges 238-9

D

Daguerre, Louis 288
Dahm, Susanne 186
Daremberg, Charles 7, 22-3, 293, 305, 327
d'Aumont, Arnulfe 223, 225, 233
De sedibus 123
Deidier, Antoine 76
Delafond, Onésime 282, 284
Delaitre ('La Taupe'/'The Mole') 195
Delaunay, Paul 2, 30, 31, 73
Denise, Jacques-François 78
dermatology 185
dermatose faciale 196

dermatose hétéromorphe 196
Desault, Pierre Joseph 8, 24, 30
Desbois de Rochefort, Louis 8, 30, 42, 87
Deschamps, Robert Toussaint 82
Descriptions des maladies de la peau 188, 192, 201, 210
Desgenettes, René Nicolas 16-17
Development of Modern Medicine: An Interpretation of the Social and Scientific Factors Involved, The 3
Devergie, Alphonse 290-1
Dezeimeris, J.-E. 121, 139
diatheses 200
Dictionnaire des sciences médicales (DSM) 257
Diderot, Denis 72
Donné, Alfred 278, 281-2, 286-93
Dubois d'Amiens, E.F. 124-5
Dubois, Paul 319
du Camp, Maxime 329
Duffin, Jacalyn 39, 43, 49, 51, 53
Duncan, Andrew Jr. 136
D'une Révolution à l'autre 2
Dupuytren, Guillaume 8, 9, 21, 23
Duruy, Victor 325

E

eclecticism 31, 303
Ecole de Chirurgie (Paris) 42, 94
Ecole de Médecine (Paris) 346
Ecole de Santé (Paris) 224, 234
Ecole Normale Supérieure 31
Ecole pratique de dissection 95, 145, 346, 347, 352
Ecoles de chirurgie 94
Ecoles de médecine 95
Ecoles de Santé 1, 92, 93
Elements of the theory and practice of physic designed for the use of students 137
Elliotson's Clinique 343

Index

emotional distress *194*
English hospitals *341, 343*
English tissue pathology tradition *128*
Enlightenment discourse *92*
Enlightenment positivism *10-11, 23*
Essai sur la philosophie médicale *10*
Everett, Mark Allen *185*
Examen de la doctrine médicale généralement adoptée *14*
Examen des doctrines médicales et les systèmes de nosologie *256, 258, 259, 261*
examination procedures *87*
experimental medicine *40*
experimental physiology *20, 38, 275*

F
Faber, Knud *6*
Fabre, François *315*
Faculty of Medicine of Paris *12, 17, 22, 41, 46, 145, 146, 287, 292, 303*
Ferrant, Marguerite *123, 194*
Flint, Austin *353, 358*
Follin, Eugène *19*
Ford, Brian *277*
Foucault, Michel *2, 3, 11, 31-4, 36, 43, 44, 51, 97, 98, 119, 122, 132, 221, 240, 266, 313, 327, 328*
Fourcroy, Antoine *6-7, 72, 92, 95*
Fournier, Pierre *86*
France and Great Britain *117*
French medical teaching, eighteenth century *71-115*
French medicine
 changes in *6*
 'dead-end' *275*
 Great Age of *30*
 need for reinterpretation *2-3*
 rebirth *26-7*

French Micrography School *26*
French Revolution *1, 2, 5, 24, 40, 51, 119, 200-3, 337*
French School of the Nineteenth Century *21*

G
Gardner, Augustus Kinsley *356*
gastrointestinal tract *254*
Gaudray, Élénore *199*
Gavarret, Jules *279, 322*
Gazette des Hôpitaux civils et militaires *315*
Gazette Hebdomadaire de Médecine et Chirurgie *315*
Gazette Médicale de Paris *15, 18, 315*
Gelfand, Toby *37, 41, 42, 73*
Généalogie de l'histopathologie: une révision déchirante: Philippe Pinel, lecteur discret de J.-C. Smyth (1741-1821), La *37*
gender and medicine *53-4*
Gendrin, Augustin *143*
Geoffroy, E.-F. *77*
Gibson, William *344*
Gildea, Robert *3*
Gill, H.Z. *363*
Gluge, Gottlieb *279*
Goetz, Christopher G. *41*
Gosselin, Léon *324*
Gouan, Antoine *84*
Great Age of French Medicine *30*
Great Britain and France *117*
Great Doctors, The *5*
Gregory, George *137, 138, 141*
Grmek, M.D. *123*
Gruby, David *279, 282, 284, 298*
Guerbois *123*
Guérin, Jules *18, 315*
Guy's Hospital Reports *317*

Index

H

Haigh, Elizabeth *38, 134-5*
Hamilton, Frank H. *346*
Hannaway, Caroline *98*
Harrison, Robert P. *348*
Harvey, Joy *53, 288*
Hastings, C. *142*
health and idiosyncrasy *222-4*
Hecht, Louis *313, 328, 329*
Hecquet, Philippe *76*
Hippocratic medicine *14*
Histoire de la chirurgie française au XIXe siècle 23
Histoire de la médecine 6
Histoire des sciences médicales 7, 23
Histoires des phlegmasies 257, 259
histopathological *problématique 140, 152*
Hodgkin, Thomas *128, 135, 140-1*
Hodgson, J. *130, 142*
Holmes, Oliver Wendell *343, 345*
Hôpital de la Pitié *317, 321*
Hôpital de la Ville *317*
Hôpital Saint-Louis *190-4, 197, 201, 203, 207, 214, 319, 356*
Hôpital Saint-Marcou *205*
Horeau, C.E. *236*
hospital, valorization of *236-8*
hospital-based expertise *236*
hospital gazettes *313, 314, 316, 317*
hospital journals *320*
Hospital Medicine *190, 193, 275, 337*
Hôtel-Dieu de Paris *86, 151, 200, 204, 317, 319, 348*
human individuality *221-50*
Hunter, John *23, 25, 43, 120-2, 124-6, 128-35, 137-9, 146, 151, 154*
Hunter, William *146*
Husson, Armand *319*
hypochondriasis *200*
hysteria *200*

I

iconography of disease *185-219, 209*
idéologue doctrine *207, 339*
idiosyncrasy and health *222-4*
Imbert, Jean-François *84*
individual variations *226-32*
inflammation *142, 240, 254, 258, 262*
International Exposition *1867 19*
intestinal canal *142*
irritation *258, 262, 264*

J

Jackson, Charles T. *355*
Jackson, James Jr. *343, 355*
Jacobi, Abraham *323*
Jacobi, Mary Putnam *46, 47, 313, 323-5, 327*
Jacyna, L.S. *44, 49, 53, 151*
James, J.H. *141*
Jerrold, Blanchard *320*
Jobert de Lamballe, Antoine-Joseph *317*
Journal of Morbid Anatomy 141
Joynes, Levin S. *355*
Jussieu, Antoine-Laurent de *88*
Jussieu, Bernard de *85*

K

Keel, Othmar *37, 42, 43, 74, 221*
Keen, William Williams *365*
Kinloch, Robert A. *359*
Krumbhaar, E.B. *121*

L

La Berge, Ann *45, 47, 50, 53, 322*
laboratories *275, 325, 371, 372*
Laborie, J.B. *84*
Laennec, Guillaume-François *83*
Laennec, René-Théophile-Hyacinthe *4, 12-14, 16, 21, 22,*

Index

25, 29, 39, 43, 53, 126, 140, 145, 251-74, 277, 327
  agreement with Broussais 262-5
  doctrine 263
  profile 252-3
  rivalry with Broussais 257-62
Latour, Amédée 316
Lavater, Gaspard 189, 210
Lawrence, Christopher 132
Lawrence, W. 141
Lawson, Leonidas M. 342
Le Baillif, A.C.M. 277
Le Court, Jean-François 80
Le Dran, H.F. 83
Le Roy, Alphonse 95
Le Tellier (patient) 201-2
learned societies 30
Lebert, Hermann 23, 279, 285, 286-93, 295, 296, 300
Lemoine, J.-B. 196-7
Léonard, Jacques 73
Lesch, John 38, 45, 304
life, medicalization of 240
Lincoln, David F. 364
Lister, Joseph Jackson 277
London clinicians 342
London hospitals 343
London Ophthalmic Infirmary 140, 141
Lorry, François 82
Louis, Pierre 4, 9, 22
Louisville Medical Institute 345

M

Madness and Civilization: The History of Insanity in the Age of Reason 32
Madness and Unreason: The History of Madness in the Classical Age 32
Magendie, François 13, 20, 29, 35, 38, 256, 264
Malgaigne, Joseph-François 302, 322

Mandl, Louis 279, 284, 287
Maternités 319
matière médicale 90
Maulitz, Russell 38, 125-9, 133-5, 140, 141, 145, 146, 149, 150
La Médecine: Histoire et doctrines 22
La Médecine à Paris entre 1800 et 1850 2
La Médecine et les médecins: philosophie, doctrines, intitutions 15
La Médecine Révolutionnaire 1789-1799 40
medical colleges 91
medical dominance 233-41
medical education, reform 1
medical histories 367-72
medical historiography 372
medical iconography 23, 52-3
medical journals 314-15
medical knowledge 235-6
medical management 240-1
Medical Mandarins: The French Academy of Medicine in the Nineteenth and Twentieth Centuries, The 39
medical polemics 15
medical profession, regulation 2
Medical Revolution in France, 1789-1796 36
medical scepticism 78
medical schools 96
medical statistics 275
medical theatre 52-3
medicalization of life 240
medicina practica 85
medicine
  and gender 53-4
  and religion 53-4
Medicine at the Paris Hospital, 1794-1848 2, 34, 38, 302, 337, 372
Medico-Chirurgical Society 314
Meding, Henri 50

Index

microscopy *22, 23, 25, 26, 45, 275-302, 357*
Moniteur des Hôpitaux *19, 315, 318-21*
Monographie des dermatoses *195, 196*
Monro, Alexander (secundus) *120, 137*
Monro, Alexander (tertius) *120, 135-7, 141*
Montet, Jacques *84*
Montpellier School *31, 74, 77-78, 85-86*
Morbid Anatomy of Some of the Most Important Parts of the Human Body, The *120*
Morgagni, G.B. *120-2, 128, 132, 133*
Möring, Michel *326*
Mount Sinai Hospital Reports *317*
mucous membrane *142-3*
Murphy, John A. *357*
Muséum d'Histoire Naturelle *22, 238-9*

N

Naissance de la clinique: une archéologie du regard médical, La *2, 32-4*
New York Medical Record *323, 324*
Nosographie philosophique *28*
Nosography, The Evolution of Clinical Medicine in Modern Times *6*
Nosologie naturelle *188, 203, 206, 208, 211, 214*

O

Oliver, Henry K. Jr. *362*
On Milk, and in Particular That of Nurses *288*
"On the Role of Surgery in the Rise of Modern Medical Thought" *37*

Order of Things, The *32*
Orfila, Matthew (Dean of the Faculty) *361*

P

palliative treatment *240-1*
Paris Clinical School *1, 3, 9, 19, 22, 31, 34-6, 40, 41, 43, 49, 96-8, 117-83, 275, 276, 306, 327, 346, 353*
  accomplishments *29*
  'dead end' *337, 354-67*
  definition as an entity *6*
  development *4*
  history *25*
  interchange of ideas, methods and practices *12*
  physicians *4*
  rise of *5*
  tripartite division *12*
Paris Ecole de Chirurgie *87*
Paris Médical *50*
Paris Medicine
  1794-1836 *6-18*
  1848-1872 *313*
  after Ackerknecht and Foucault *36-41*
  brilliance of *13*
  characteristics *4, 12*
  construction *27*
  continuity/discontinuity *51-2*
  demarcation *48*
  development *42*
  dynamic tension *49*
  genealogy *8*
  great era *25*
  historiography *297*
  history *2*
  indictment of *18*
  institutional changes 1794 *1*
  later nineteenth-century constructions *18-29*

Index

monolithic nature *52*
"myth" of *3-6*
new era *29*
origins *8*
perspectives past and present *1-69*
political nature *15, 50*
political tension *12*
"received view" *3-6*
received view *37*
reinterpretation *3, 42-6*
religious concerns *53*
Rise and Fall *25*
role of rhetoric *47-8*
"scientific medicine" *13*
theatrical nature *17-18, 22*
turning points *28*
twentieth century *30-7*
Parisian life *345-54*
Past in French History, The 3
Pasteurian Revolution *27, 28, 46*
pathogenesis *264*
pathological anatomy *7, 22, 25, 28, 29, 45, 152, 226, 255-6, 262, 264, 275, 278, 280-5*
Pathological and Practical Researches on Diseases of the Brain and the Spinal Chord 142
Pathological and Practical Researches on the Diseases of the Stomach, the Intestinal Canal, the Liver and other Viscera of the Abdomen 142
pathological physiology *22*
Pathological Researches on Phthisis 9
pathology *122, 139*
Peirson, Abel Lawrence *344, 348*
Peisse, Louis *15-17, 18*
Pelletan, Philippe-Joseph *17*
Petit, Antoine *84, 85, 89*
pharmaceuticals *255*
phthisis *237*
Physical and the Moral: Anthropology, Physiology and

Philosophical Medicine in France, 1750-1850, The 41
physiognomic conventions *209*
physiological medicine *28, 29, 253-6, 300*
Physiologie pathologique 279, 285, 288, 291, 296
physiology *139*
Pinel, Philippe *4, 12, 27, 28, 43, 133-5, 152, 153, 253, 258*
plica *198-200*
political transformation *5*
Porcher, E. Peyre *351*
Portal, Antoine *84*
positivism *29, 31*
Prévost, Jean-Louis *291*
private courses *49-50, 83, 84, 361*
Professionalizing Modern Medicine: Paris Surgeons and Medical Science and Institutions in the Eighteenth Century 37
Progrès Médicale 315
public courses *49-50*
Putnam (Jacobi), Mary. *See* Jacobi, Mary Putnam

Q

Quart, Thomas *197-200*

R

Ranvier, Louis Antoine *325*
Raspail, François *26, 277*
Raussin, L.-H. *79*
Rayer, Charles *12, 23, 325*
Rayer, Pierre *4, 7, 9, 278*
Récamier, Joseph *13, 29*
Récamier et ses contemporains, 1774-1852 23, 26
religion and medicine *53-4*
religious pilgrimages *204*
Restoration *203*
Revue des Deux Mondes 329

Index

Revue Médico-Chirurgicale de Paris *315*, *316*
Robin, Charles *19*, *325*, *357*
Rochard, Jules *18*, *23-6*
Rodin, A.E. *120*
Rokitansky, Karl *284*
Roussel, H.F.A. *78*
Royal College of Physicians *154*
Royal College of Surgeons *154*
Royer-Collard, A. *26*

S

Sachs, J.J. *85*
St Thomas's Hospital school *138*
Sarrau, Joseph *84*
Science and the Practice of Medicine in the Nineteenth Century *4*
scientific medicine *371*
scrofula *204*, *205*
scrophule vulgaire *188*
Shattuck, Frederick *365*
Shattuck, George Cheyne *357*, *359*
Shattuck, George Cheyne Jr. *365*
Short History of Medicine, A *3*
Shryock, Richard *3*
Sichel, Julius *356*
Sigerist, Henry *5*, *6*
Sketches of the Character and History of Eminent Living Surgeons and Physicians of Paris *15*
skin disease *187*, *194*, *201-2*
Smith, Henry *360*
Smyth, James Carmichael *128*, *133-7*, *139*, *151*
Société Anatomique *323*
Société de Biologie *292*, *323*, *325*
Société de Chirurgie *323*
Société Pathologique *323*
Société Royale de Médecine *71*, *79*, *93*
Sournia, Jean-Charles *6*, *40*
spiritual healing *203-12*

Stafford, Barbara Maria *187*
Staum, Martin S. *38*
stethoscope *252*
Stewart, F. Campbell *9*, *22*, *344*
Stillé, Alfred *357*, *359*
surgeon-apothecaries *146*

T

Tardieu, Ambroise *53*
Temkin, Owsei *37*
therapeutics *80*
Thierry, Alexandre *319*
Thomson, John *135*
tissue pathology *117-83*
   genesis *133*
   history *118*
To See With a Better Eye: A Life of R.T.H. Laennec *39*
Traité d'anatomie générale *24*
Traité des tumeurs *283*
Traité pratique du microscope *287*
Travers, B. *142*
Treatise on Auscultation *261*
Treatise on the Diseases of the Arteries and Veins *130*
Triaire, Paul *23*, *26-9*
Tribune Médicale *315*
Trichomonas vaginalis *289*
Trousseau, Armand *319-21*, *327*
tuberculosis *252*

U

L'Union Médicale *315*, *316*, *317*, *318*

V

Valentin, Michel *39*
valorization of hospital *236-8*
Valsalva, A. M. *128*
Velpeau, Alfred-Armand *19*, *283*, *296*, *298-302*, *305*, *319*, *327*
Venel, Gabriel-François *84*

Index

Verneuil, Aristide *19*
Vess, David *36*
Vidal, Auguste *124-5*
Villermé, René-Louis *138*
Vicq d'Azyr, Félix *71, 90, 96, 98*
Virchow, Rudolf *24, 295, 297*
vitalism *29, 31, 74, 77, 255, 263, 265*
Vulpian, Edmé-Félix *327*

W

Wardrop, J. *142*
Warner, John Harley *41, 45, 47, 48, 151, 327*
Warren, J. Mason *363*
Webb, Joseph *365*
Weiner, Dora *41*
Weisz, George *39*
White, James Clarke *368-70*
Willan, R. *141*
Williams, Elizabeth *41, 185*
Williams, Henry Willard *348*
Windmill Street School *138*
Wünderlich, Carl *5*
Wurtz, Adolphe *326*

X

Xavier Bichat and the Medical Theory of the Eighteenth Century 38

Y

Yelloly, J. *141*
Young Paris School *19, 327*